Thank you for your purchase of *Reconstructive Surgery of the Hand and Upper Extremity*!

Access your e-book now!

Scratch here to reveal your access code

How to redeem your code:

1. Create an account on Thieme's e-book store at **ebookstore.thieme.com/register**
2. Click the **My E-Books** link
3. Select **Redeem Access Code**
4. Enter this code to claim your e-book
5. You can now read your e-book online!

How to download your book for offline access:

On a compatible phone or tablet*:

1. Download the **Thieme Bookshelf** app from **iTunes** or **Google Play** after you've redeemed your access code
2. Validate your e-book store username and password
3. Select the e-book and tap to download it to your device
4. Your e-book is now available to read offline!

**This app is available for iPads and Android devices. The e-book cannot be downloaded to any apps or readers other than Thieme Bookshelf.*

On your PC or Mac:

1. Download **iPublishCentral Reader**** from the e-book store after you've redeemed your access code: **ebookstore.thieme.com/downloadioffline**
2. Validate your e-book store username and password
3. Select the book and click to download
4. Your e-book is now available to read offline!

***You may need to download and install Adobe Air prior to downloading iPublishCentral. Instructions are on the link provided.*

This code can only be redeemed one time. After redemption, it can be downloaded to multiple devices on your account. An internet connection is required for initial access and download. This book cannot be returned if the code has been revealed.

For any questions, please visit ebookstore.thieme.com/faqs.

Connect with us on social media

Learn the techniques with videos online at MediaCenter.Thieme.com!

Simply visit MediaCenter.Thieme.com and, when prompted during the registration process, enter the code below to get started today.

Z9P8-S648-QLW9-W8P4

	WINDOWS & MAC	TABLET
Recommended Browser(s)	Recent browser versions on all major platforms and any mobile operating system that supports HTML5 video playback. *All browsers should have JavaScript enabled.*	
Flash Player Plug-in	Flash Player 9 or higher. *For Mac users, ATI Rage 128 GPU doesn't support full-screen mode with hardware scaling.*	Tablet PCs with Android OS support Flash 10.1.
Recommended for optimal usage experience	Monitor resolutions: • Normal (4:3) 1024×768 or higher • Widescreen (16:9) 1280×720 or higher • Widescreen (16:10) 1440×900 or higher A high-speed internet connection (minimum 384 Kps) is suggested.	WiFi or cellular data connection is required.

Reconstructive Surgery of the Hand and Upper Extremity

Reconstructive Surgery of the Hand and Upper Extremity

Günter Germann, MD, PhD
Professor of Plastic and Hand Surgery,
University of Heidelberg;
Medical Director, ETHIANUM Clinic Heidelberg,
Heidelberg, Germany

Randolph Sherman, MD
Vice-Chair of the Department of Surgery,
Cedars-Sinai Medical Center;
and Professor of Clinical Surgery,
Keck School of Medicine,
University of Southern California, Los Angeles,
California, USA

L. Scott Levin, MD, FACS
Paul B. Magnuson Professor of Bone
and Joint Surgery and Chairman
of the Department of Orthopaedic Surgery;
Professor of Surgery (Plastic Surgery),
University of Pennsylvania School of Medicine, Philadelphia,
Pennsylvania, USA

ILLUSTRATOR
Amanda Tomasikiewicz

Thieme

Managing Editor: Sarah Landis
Director, Editorial Services: Mary Jo Casey
Production Editor: Sean Woznicki
International Production Director: Andreas Schabert
Editorial Director: Sue Hodgson
International Marketing Director: Fiona Henderson
International Sales Director: Louisa Turrell
Director of Institutional Sales: Adam Bernacki
Senior Vice President and Chief Operating Officer: Sarah Vanderbilt
President: Brian D. Scanlan

Cover illustrations drawn by Amanda Tomasikiewicz

Illustrators: Amanda Tomasikiewicz, Andrea Hines, Karin Arns-Germann

Library of Congress Cataloging-in-Publication Data

Names: Germann, G. (Günter), 1952- author. | Levin, L. Scott, author. | Sherman, R. (Randolph), author.
Title: Reconstructive surgery of the hand and upper extremity / Günter Germann, L. Scott Levin, Randolph Sherman.
Description: New York : Thieme, [2018]
Identifiers: LCCN 2017037097| ISBN 9781626236011 (print) | ISBN 9781626237674 (ebook)
Subjects: | MESH: Hand--surgery | Upper Extremity--surgery | Reconstructive Surgical Procedures | Atlases
Classification: LCC RD559 | NLM WE 17 | DDC 617.5/75059--dc23 LC record available at https://lccn.loc.gov/2017037097

Important note: Medicine is an ever-changing science undergoing continual development. Research and clinical experience are continually expanding our knowledge, in particular our knowledge of proper treatment and drug therapy. Insofar as this book mentions any dosage or application, readers may rest assured that the authors, editors, and publishers have made every effort to ensure that such references are in accordance with **the state of knowledge at the time of production of the book.**

Nevertheless, this does not involve, imply, or express any guarantee or responsibility on the part of the publishers in respect to any dosage instructions and forms of applications stated in the book. **Every user is requested to examine carefully** the manufacturers' leaflets accompanying each drug and to check, if necessary in consultation with a physician or specialist, whether the dosage schedules mentioned therein or the contraindications stated by the manufacturers differ from the statements made in the present book. Such examination is particularly important with drugs that are either rarely used or have been newly released on the market. Every dosage schedule or every form of application used is entirely at the user's own risk and responsibility. The authors and publishers request every user to report to the publishers any discrepancies or inaccuracies noticed. If errors in this work are found after publication, errata will be posted at www.thieme.com on the product description page.

Some of the product names, patents, and registered designs referred to in this book are in fact registered trademarks or proprietary names even though specific reference to this fact is not always made in the text. Therefore, the appearance of a name without designation as proprietary is not to be construed as a representation by the publisher that it is in the public domain.

Thieme Publishers New York
333 Seventh Avenue, New York, NY 10001 USA
+1 800 782 3488, customerservice@thieme.com

Thieme Publishers Stuttgart
Rüdigerstrasse 14, 70469 Stuttgart, Germany
+49 [0]711 8931 421, customerservice@thieme.de

Thieme Publishers Delhi
A-12, Second Floor, Sector-2, Noida-201301
Uttar Pradesh, India
+91 120 45 566 00, customerservice@thieme.in

Thieme Publishers Rio, Thieme Publicações Ltda.
Edifício Rodolpho de Paoli, 25º andar
Av. Nilo Peçanha, 50 – Sala 2508
Rio de Janeiro 20020-906, Brasil
+55 21 3172 2297 / +55 21 3172-1896

Cover design: Thieme Publishing Group
Typesetting by Debra Clark

Printed in China by Everbest Printing Ltd 5 4 3 2 1

ISBN 978-1-62623-601-1

Also available as an e-book:
eISBN 978-1-62623-767-4

MIX
Paper from responsible sources
FSC® C124385

To Karin Arns-Germann whose brilliant illustrations
enriched many presentations over the years,
my wonderful children Tina, Anna & Jonas, and to Ulli who
is a constant source of love, support and inspiration.
GG

To Martha and Max, the two irreplaceable people in my life.
RS

To my children Celia and Ben and my wife Helga—
thanks for your love, support, and sacrifice
on behalf of my patients and my profession.
LSL

Foreword

It is an honor for me to write a foreword for this text by three good friends and colleagues. The three authors are truly world experts in the field of reconstructive surgery and have close to 100 years of combined experience in reconstruction of the upper extremity. This text is the culmination of that experience and is a magnum opus on the subject. This book is particularly useful for those starting their career in reconstructive surgery as it gives a superb outline of how to manage nearly every type of problem in the upper extremity. It provides all the reasonable options for management of these problems, but it is also an excellent atlas of flaps for the hand and upper extremity. The emphasis is appropriately on primary reconstruction, but options for secondary reconstruction are covered as well. After this it covers rehabilitation protocols, which surgeons are often not familiar with. Finally, they cover various classification systems which can be overwhelming to the young surgeon. This text offers a comprehensive approach to the management of upper extremity reconstruction and should be in the library of every surgeon performing reconstruction of the upper extremity. My congratulations to the authors.

William C. Pederson, MD, FACS
Head, Hand and Microsurgery
Texas Children's Hospital
Samuel Stal Professor of Plastic Surgery
Professor of Surgery, Orthopaedic Surgery, Neurosurgery, and Pediatrics
Baylor College of Medicine
Houston, Texas, USA

Foreword

The restoration of both form and function is the ultimate goal of the hand surgeon and is possible through adherence to firmly established surgical principles, which must be constantly challenged, clarified, instituted, refined, and periodically re-evaluated. Both simple and complex clinical problems in hand trauma can present a moving target to the young surgeon, similar to specialty board examinations whose questions remain the same year after year, and only the answers change. The quantity of information can be overwhelming, possibilities for treatment unclear, newer solutions tantalizing, and both short- and long-term outcomes contradictory. Where does the uninitiated or less experienced upper extremity surgeon start?

Most traumatic and acquired hand problems simply require a thorough physical examination, knowledge of anatomy, sound judgment, and consistent care based on principles. Reflecting on their 40-plus-year careers in the trenches, Drs. Günter Germann, Randy Sherman, and L. Scott Levin have distilled their collective experience as traumatic hand surgeons into a unique, comprehensive set of algorithms, which analyze the treatment of common upper extremity injuries in a clear, succinct fashion. This approach can be used to help the young physician tailor treatment to the goals and needs of the patient, setup a strategic plan, execute the appropriate surgery, and rehabilitate the patient properly. The book is practical, clear, well organized and easy to read, especially by those who are confronted by difficult problems in the middle of the night or who are in regions where specialized care is not immediately available. The decision-making process is much easier. The summary of classification systems, illustrations of fractures, and summaries of common clinical scenarios are useful for quick reference for all surgeons.

In its revised edition, this unconventional book has become a practical guide for younger general, orthopedic, and plastic surgical hand surgeons, as well as all those in training. On our service it has been used effectively as a starting point for the young house officers on call for the hand service. It would be a mistake for even the more experienced to overlook this book, which is packed with practical pearls especially in the treatment algorithms, the precautions and pitfalls of the most commonly used flaps, and the clinical cases, all of which are clearly illustrated and anatomically accurate. There is an excellent integration of the skeletal, vascular, neural, and soft tissue aspects of reconstruction, as well as an emphasis on full-thickness coverage, early definitive reconstruction, and thoughtful rehabilitation. At the time of initial evaluation and subsequent surgical exploration, these guides will help the surgeon decide what should be discarded, prudently saved, or strategically redistributed within the injured upper limb to achieve the best functional and aesthetic outcome.

Present-day millennial medical students and surgical house officers are more comfortable with the algorithmic approach as most of their preparation starts with a Google search and subsequent scrolling down menus of possibilities. This book will clarify their options for salvage and/or reconstruction, and coupled with a comprehensive knowledge of anatomy, will help them make wiser decisions.

Rigid binary thinking and algorithms may potentially lead to oversimplification and omission of salient alternatives. Every algorithm presented in this book is debatable. However, this book can be used in a different light: to introduce different forms of treatment and to stimulate controversy and a discussion of why a particular form of treatment may be best for a given patient at a particular point in his or her life. It may stimulate the surgeon to consider both surgical and non-surgical options before making a strategic decision, which cannot be altered. No hand surgical library would be complete without this gem.

Joe Upton, MD
Hand Surgeon, Plastic and Reconstructive Surgeon
Boston Children's Hospital, Boston Shriners Hospital, Beth Israel Deaconess Hospital
Professor of Surgery, Harvard Medical School
Boston, Massachusetts

Preface

Why did three senior surgeons decide to revise a book that was published 15 years ago?

Despite changes in training paradigms and health care delivery, we believe that we can offer valuable contributions to the education of students, residents, fellows, and colleagues who are early in their practice and prepare them for the treatment of challenging clinical cases.

We began this journey almost 20 years ago with the concept of providing an algorithmic approach for clinical problem-solving in reconstructive surgery of the upper extremity. Decision-making based on “Yes” or “No” answers has dominated our own thinking and teaching for many decades. Our approach takes a complex problem and separates it into single sequential steps. The treatment plan is based on the profile of the patient, the resources that are available, and the physicians’ level of skill.

When a publisher asked us if we would be willing to update, refine, and improve the book, we didn’t hesitate to accept this request. Every aspect of the book has undergone a thorough critical analysis and revision. New techniques have been added, and others have been deleted. Illustrations have been revised to make the crucial technical points of a surgical procedure clearer to the reader.

As before, this update celebrates the privilege of combining European and North American philosophies, concepts, and approaches to create a text that we hope may be helpful for all colleagues who are treating reconstructive problems of the upper extremity.

Table of Contents

Part VI: Rehabilitation Protocols

Part VII: Classification and Zones of Injury

Introduction

The hand is one of the most extraordinary tools in nature. A combination of strength, dynamic stability, and precision movements provide the hand the ability to carry out the work of the upper extremity. Despite advances in prosthetics, targeted muscle reinnervation and vascularized composite allotransplantation, preserving and reconstructing the human hand remains the goal of the reconstructive surgeon.

Hand surgery is functional restorative surgery. The hand is one of our most important points of contact with our environment and possesses a myriad of important functions such as cognitive discrimination, tactile gnosis, and the ability to transmit and receive emotional signals. The hand serves as the eye for the blind, the ears for the deaf, and the mouthpiece for the mute. Character virtues are often attributed to size, shape, and appearance of a person's hands. Galen considered the hand an instrument of human ratio and as a mirror image of the human soul. Charles Bell reflected on the relationship of the hand to the mind. The monks of the Middle Ages used their fingers as a help in mathematic calculations ("Si tria digita scribunt, totum corpus laborat"). This tradition has now evolved to the "digital era" in which the hand is used to press buttons on a keyboard, operate a mouse, or use a cellular phone.

"Hand surgery is also aesthetic surgery": The significance of this statement by Dr. Guy Foucher, a well-recognized hand surgeon and author, becomes clear if we consider that the face and hands are usually the only points of contact in the western civilization with the exception of warmer days when, through more casual dressing, other body parts become visible. If one observes individuals with mutilated hands carefully, it becomes obvious that the majority of these patients attempt to conceal their injured and disfigured hands.

In such cases this may lead to psychological disturbances in some patients whose professions require frequent contact with the public. The goal of reconstruction of this complicated biomechanical tool, with restoration of appearance, function, and tactile gnosis, is to achieve general well-being and professional and social reintegration.

Specific tactics and overall strategy depend on many variables that evolve as the surgeon's experience increases. They have to be integrated into a complex decision-making process which involves comparing and evaluating all factors that affect outcome.

Reconstructive procedures should be tailored to the individual needs of the patient. For example, application of only one coverage technique to different wounds and injuries may result in solutions that may not match the patient's needs. The principle of "one technique fits all" has little place in hand and upper extremity reconstruction. The main goal of reconstructive surgeons should be to achieve functional reconstruction using the most similar tissue possible, thus preserving or restoring hand aesthetics so that patients may resume their daily activities as soon as possible.

This book will help to explain decision-making processes developed by the authors throughout many years of clinical practice. The method of using algorithms has been selected to achieve the greatest possible clarity. This book is not all encompassing; there will always be exceptions and clinical situations for which the described categories do not apply.

The Key to the Map—How to Use the Book

As the cover implies, this text is designed to be a guide to decision-making through the labyrinth of problems we face in treating patients with hand and upper extremity problems. Using algorithms, specific injuries and clinical situations can be managed in a logical, deductive fashion. These algorithms constitute the centerpiece of the book. They serve as a map to guide reconstructive surgeons from point of origin to intended destination.

The other information in the book are designed to support your use of the algorithms.

The utility of the algorithms will be maximized by understanding how we have highlighted certain parts of each diagram. A summary of the key below will appear as necessary throughout the book.

Light blue boxes contain different parameters used for decision-making, either anatomical discriminators or supplemental information used as a navigational aid.

Dark blue boxes provide additional explanations, treatment options, or guidelines.

Dark red boxes contain warnings, precautions, or pitfalls.

Orange outlines emphasize particular waypoints. *Waypoints* are select parameters in decision-making, guidelines, warnings, and options.

Glossary

ABD: abduction
ADD: adduction
ADL: activity of daily living
ADM: abductor digiti minimi
AIN: anterior interosseous nerve
ALT: anterolateral thigh
AMT: anteromedial thigh
AO/ASIF: Association for Osteosynthesis/Association for Stable Internal Fixation
APB: abductor pollicis brevis
APL: abductor pollicis longus
AR: axial radial
AROM: active range of motion
AU: axial ulna
AxRI: axial radial instability
AxUI: axial ulnar instability
BR: brachioradialis
CIC: carpal instability complex
CID: carpal instability dissociative
CIND: carpal instability nondissociative
CMC: carpometacarpal
CPM: continuous passive motion
CRP: C-reactive protein
CT: computed tomography
DBS: dorsal blocking splint
DD: differential diagnosis
DIEP: deep inferior epigastric perforators
DIP: distal interphalangeal
DISI: dorsal intercalated segment instability
DMCA: dorsal metacarpal artery
DMSO: dimethyl sulfoxide
DT: dorsal translation
ECRB: extensor carpi radialis brevis
ECRL: extensor carpi radialis longus
ECU: extensor carpi ulnaris
EDC: extensor digitorum communis
EDM: extensor digiti minimi
EDQ: extensor digiti quinti
EI: extensor indicis
EIP: extensor indicis proprius
EMG: electromyogram
EPB: extensor pollicis brevis
EPL: extensor pollicis longus
FCR: flexor carpi radialis
FCU: flexor carpi ulnaris
FDP: flexor digitorum profundus
FDS: flexor digitorum superficialis
FPB: flexor pollicis brevis
FPL: flexor pollicis longus
FTSG: full-thickness skin graft
FMC: fine motor coordination
ICAM: Immediate controlled active motion
ICG: indocyanine green
IP: interphalangeal
IV: intravenous
K-wire: Kirschner wire
LT: lunotriquetral
MCI: midcarpal instability
MP: metacarpophalangeal
MRI: magnetic resonance imaging
MVA: motor vehicle accident
OR: operating room
ORIF: open reduction internal fixation
PA: posterioanterior
PET: positron emission tomography
PGA: polyglycolic acid
PIN: posterior interosseous nerve
PIP: proximal interphalangeal
PL: palmaris longus
PROM: passive range of motion
PT: palmar translation (carpal instability)
PT: physical therapy
PT: pronator teres
RMCI: radiomidcarpal instability
RMO: relative motion orthosis
ROM: range of motion
RT: radial translation
SL: scapholunate
SLAC: scapholunate advanced collapse
SNAC: scaphoid nonunion advanced collapse
STSG: split-thickness skin graft
STT: scaphotrapeziotrapezoidal
TBSA: total body surface area
TFCC: triangular fibrocartilage complex
TFL: tensor fascia lata
TGE: tendon gliding exercise
TH: triquetrohamate
TPF: temporoparietal fascia
UMCI: ulnar midcarpal instability
UT: ulnar translation
VISI: volar intercalated segment instability
WBC: white blood cell [count]
WHO: wrist-hand orthosis

Part I

General Principles

Chapter 1

General Principles of Upper Extremity Reconstruction

Reconstructive surgery of the upper extremity as it relates to trauma, tumor, and sepsis has progressed significantly over the past 50 years. The introduction of microsurgical techniques—including a wide variety of new flaps, functional free muscle transfer, nerve conduits, motor nerve transfers and allografts, and even hand transplantation—complements the vast array of sophisticated treatment concepts, which now include vascularized composite allotransplantation. These additions have greatly expanded the number of options available to the reconstructive surgeon.

The current philosophy of treatment in combination with early functional rehabilitation represents a significant evolution; historically, treatment was much more limited and sequential. It involved multiple-stage interventions that simply covered defects, with functional restoration not being considered until later in the process. More recently, surgeons have demonstrated the ability to perform "one-stage" multiphase reconstructions with the use of precisely tailored composite flaps of skin, tendons, nerves, vessels, and, often, vascularized bone for the earliest possible definitive and appropriate repair.

Today, the reconstructive surgery plan may be fully executed during the initial operative exploration (i.e., replantation) or after a "second-look" procedure and definitive wound closure. Definitive reconstruction during the primary injury period saves time, shortens the postinjury morbidity interval, and allows for earlier rehabilitation intervention, thereby maximizing functional outcomes.

This combined treatment strategy reduces overall professional and hospital expenditures and speeds the patient along a path toward faster recovery and reintegration with family, work, and community. A growing body of literature supports primary reconstruction as highly cost effective. This approach decreases the time and cost of disability resulting from injury.

Secondary reconstruction, when necessary, is often performed in scarred tissue planes in extremities that may be contracted and dysfunctional. Despite the surgeon's best efforts, it is not always possible to keep a patient's joints and soft tissues mobile with the use of passive motion exercise while awaiting secondary reconstruction. Such delays inevitably lead to compromised outcomes and further morbidity.

Our ultimate treatment goal must be to quickly and definitively restore the best possible form and function of the injured upper extremity. By implementing the latest techniques for immediate bony stabilization, restoring joint congruency, repairing motor tendon units—and mobilizing these repairs rapidly, with aesthetically oriented soft tissue coverage—our patients will achieve personal, social, and professional reintegration.

Treatment Goals

The goals of patient care and treatment throughout the process of restoring an upper extremity include the following:

- Extremity salvage
- Preservation and restoration of function
- Correction of acquired defects (i.e., after trauma or tumor)
- Optimization of aesthetic appearance
- Social and professional reintegration
- Cost-effective therapy

After an injury, the selection of specific treatment concepts and preferred reconstructive procedures is based on a thorough analysis that includes the following considerations:

- Clinical evaluation of the patient
- Pertinent medical and demographic profiles
- Wound assessment, including tissue loss and functional impairment
- Injury classification as an adjunct to guide management

Compliance with these guidelines will lead to the use of standardized treatment protocols with sufficient flexibility to select the best operative procedure for each patient and each injury. The upper extremity should be thought of as a highly integrated and multidimensional functional organ. The hands and arms are the primary mechanisms by which we, as humans, physically interact with the world and with each other. The skin, tendons, muscles, nerves, joints, and bones of these extremities should not be thought of as isolated structures; rather, they must be recognized as meticulously calibrated interacting parts of a highly complex machine. Subsequently, reconstructive procedures to address complex defects should not be thought of as repairing isolated structures; they represent an orchestrated process that is performed in the service of the integral restoration of the function of the hand and the upper extremity.

The following chapters present a comprehensive and detailed roadmap for upper extremity reconstruction. They will provide definitions, classifications, guidelines, algorithms, and procedures. These chapters were developed with the intent of offering both the surgical student and the master upper extremity surgeon a framework for achieving the best outcomes possible for their patients.

Chapter 2

Assessment and Management Strategy

Traumatic wounds should be evaluated as soon as possible after the patient has been admitted to the emergency department. When the patient's condition permits, an operative exploration should be performed. After adequate debridement, primary structure repair should occur if at all possible.

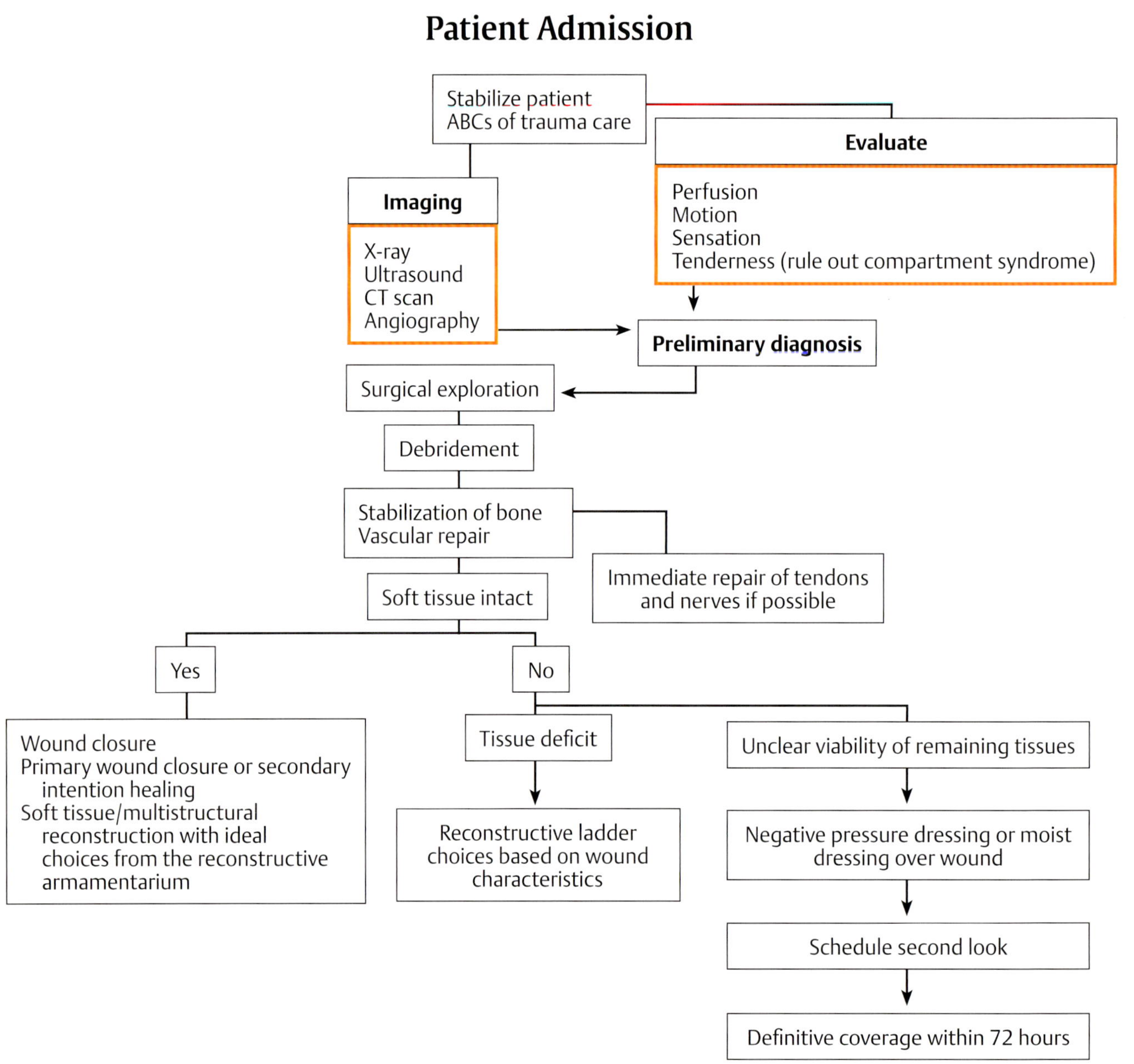

Algorithm 2.1

Parameters in decision-making	Additional options or guidelines	Warnings, precautions, or pitfalls	Emphasis on a particular waypoint

During the first surgical exploration, all nonviable tissue is debrided. The skeleton must be stabilized first, and blood flow must be re-established if the limb is avascular. A shunt should be considered if prolonged ischemia has occurred or is anticipated. If possible, vital structures such as vessels, nerves, tendons, and bones should be repaired primarily. Depending on the mechanisms of injury, the condition of the patient, and the options available, primary wound closure is preferred. If there is any doubt about the viability of the tissues that remain in the wound, the wound should be managed temporarily with the use of topical saline dressings or a negative pressure device, which can maintain a moist wound environment for 48 to 72 hours. A second-look procedure should be scheduled within 24 to 48 hours.

During the second procedure, definitive coverage should be performed. In rare cases (i.e., after crush, avulsion, burn, or electrical injuries), this "second look" may not allow for the adequate determination of the viability of the tissues. When this occurs, delayed closure is preferred so that sufficient debridement can be assured.

Patient Evaluation Algorithm

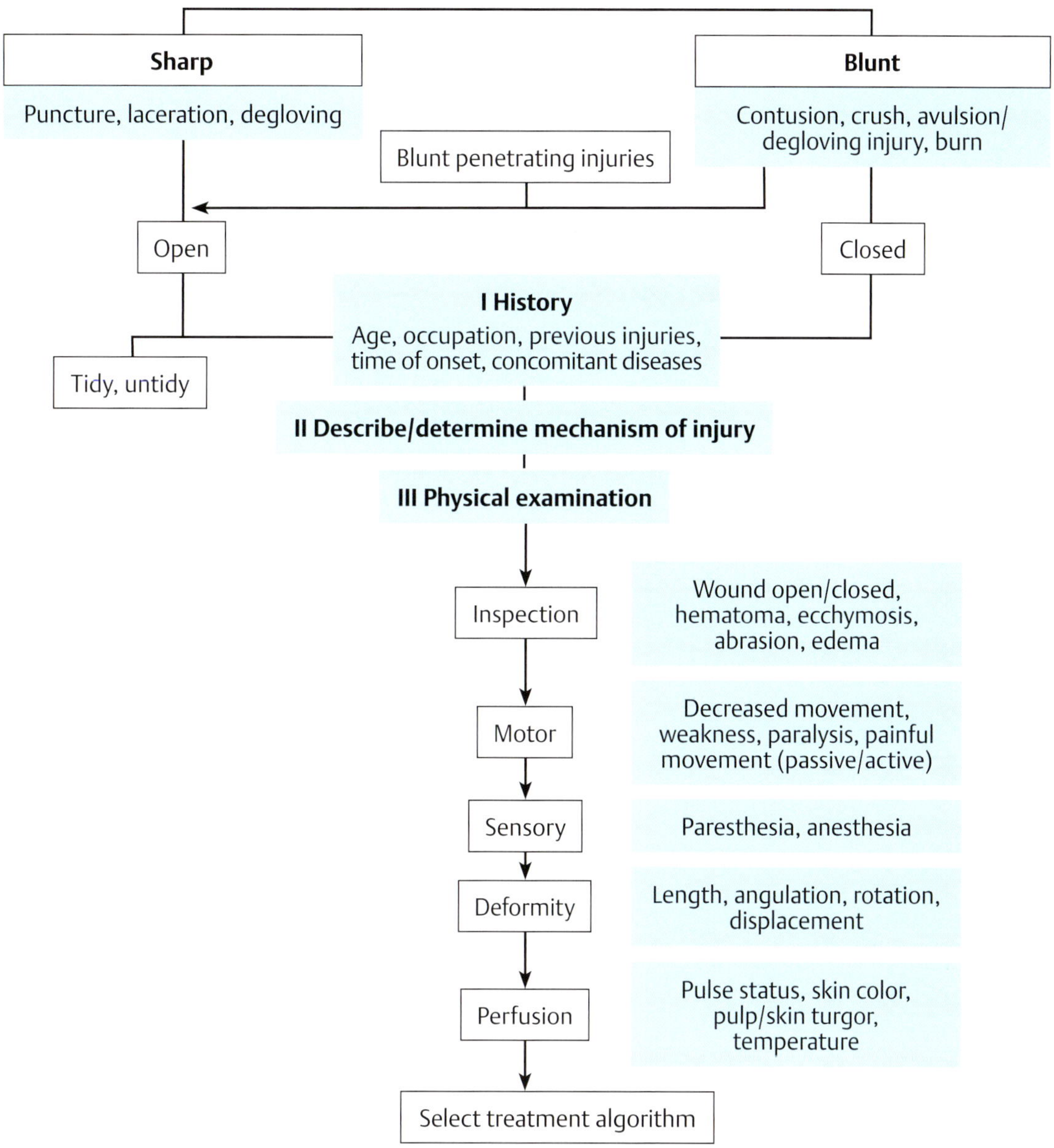

Algorithm 2.2

Parameters in decision-making	Additional options or guidelines	Warnings, precautions, or pitfalls	Emphasis on a particular waypoint

Workup of Hand Edema

Location
(anatomical description)

Individual digit
Hand
Forearm
Arm

Duration

Constant
Intermittent
Chronic
Acute

Aggravating and alleviating factors

Rest
Position
Dependency
Compression
Medication
Immobilization
Activity
Temperature

Severity

Slightly noticeable
Obscures anatomical landmarks
Decreases AROM

Algorithm 2.3

Parameters in decision-making	Additional options or guidelines	Warnings, precautions, or pitfalls	Emphasis on a particular waypoint

Pain

Type

Sharp
Dull
Electric
Radiating
Burning

Location

Digits, palm, forearm, brachium
Volar, dorsal
Pinpoint, diffuse
Superficial, deep

Duration

Constant
Intermittent
Chronic
Acute

Onset

Injury, activity, at rest
Spontaneous

Aggravating and alleviating factors

Movement
Position
Dependency
Compression
Medication
Cold (i.e., Raynaud's phenomenon or glomus tumor)

Severity

Visual analog scale
0 = no pain
10 = most severe pain

Algorithm 2.4

Parameters in decision-making	Additional options or guidelines	Warnings, precautions, or pitfalls	Emphasis on a particular waypoint

Chapter 3

Clinical Examination

After a detailed patient history is obtained, a careful physical examination of the upper extremity is essential in order to make a diagnosis and formulate a treatment plan. Despite the ever-expanding technology available for patient imaging, the physical examination is key to the appropriate assessment and treatment of these patients.

In this video chapter (**Video 3.1**), the techniques of physical examination are highlighted; these include manual muscle testing, sensory testing, and provocative maneuvers that can help to define upper extremity pathology. A complete examination should be performed on each patient to optimize clinical decision-making.

The following points should be included in the examination of the hand.

- Skin
- Vascularity, color, pulp, and refill
- Nerves: two-point, sharp, and dull
- Tendon movement: isolate (extrinsic and intrinsic)
- Bone and joint: palpation, motion, and pain
- Ligaments
- Nails
- Finkelstein test: de Quervain's disease
- Tinel test: nerve irritation and regeneration
- Phalen test: median nerve compression
- Froment test: ulnar nerve palsy
- "OK" sign: anterior interosseous palsy
- Hitchhiker sign: posterior interosseous nerve palsy
- Allen test: vascular integrity
- "Grind" test: basilar joint and arthritis
- Watson test: scapholunate instability
- Lumbrical plus test: intrinsic muscles
- Flexor tendons
- Bunnell test: intrinsic tightness

Chapter 4

Principles of Treatment and Management

General Strategy

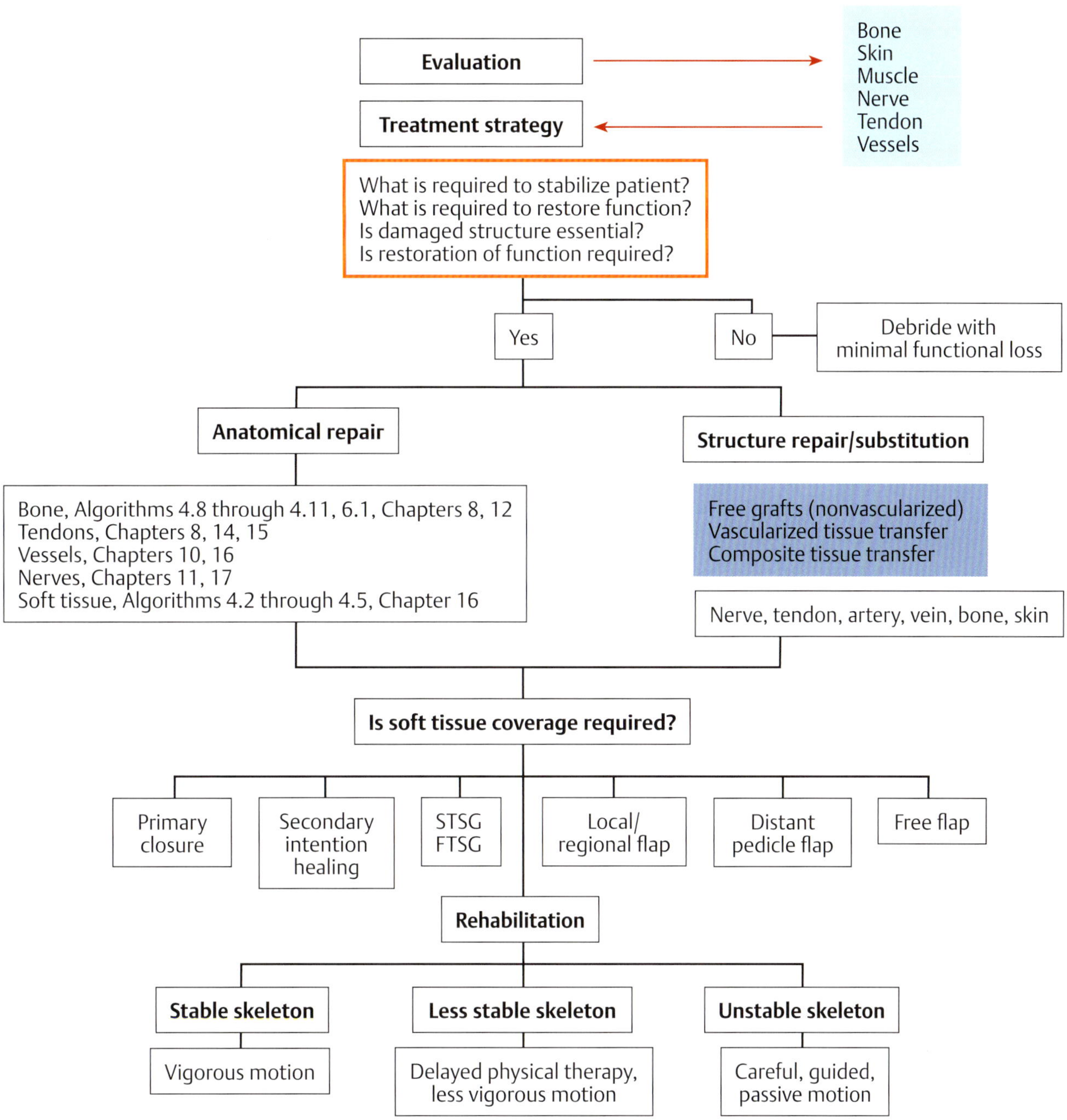

Algorithm 4.1

Parameters in decision-making	Additional options or guidelines	Warnings, precautions, or pitfalls	Emphasis on a particular waypoint

Skin and Soft Tissue Loss

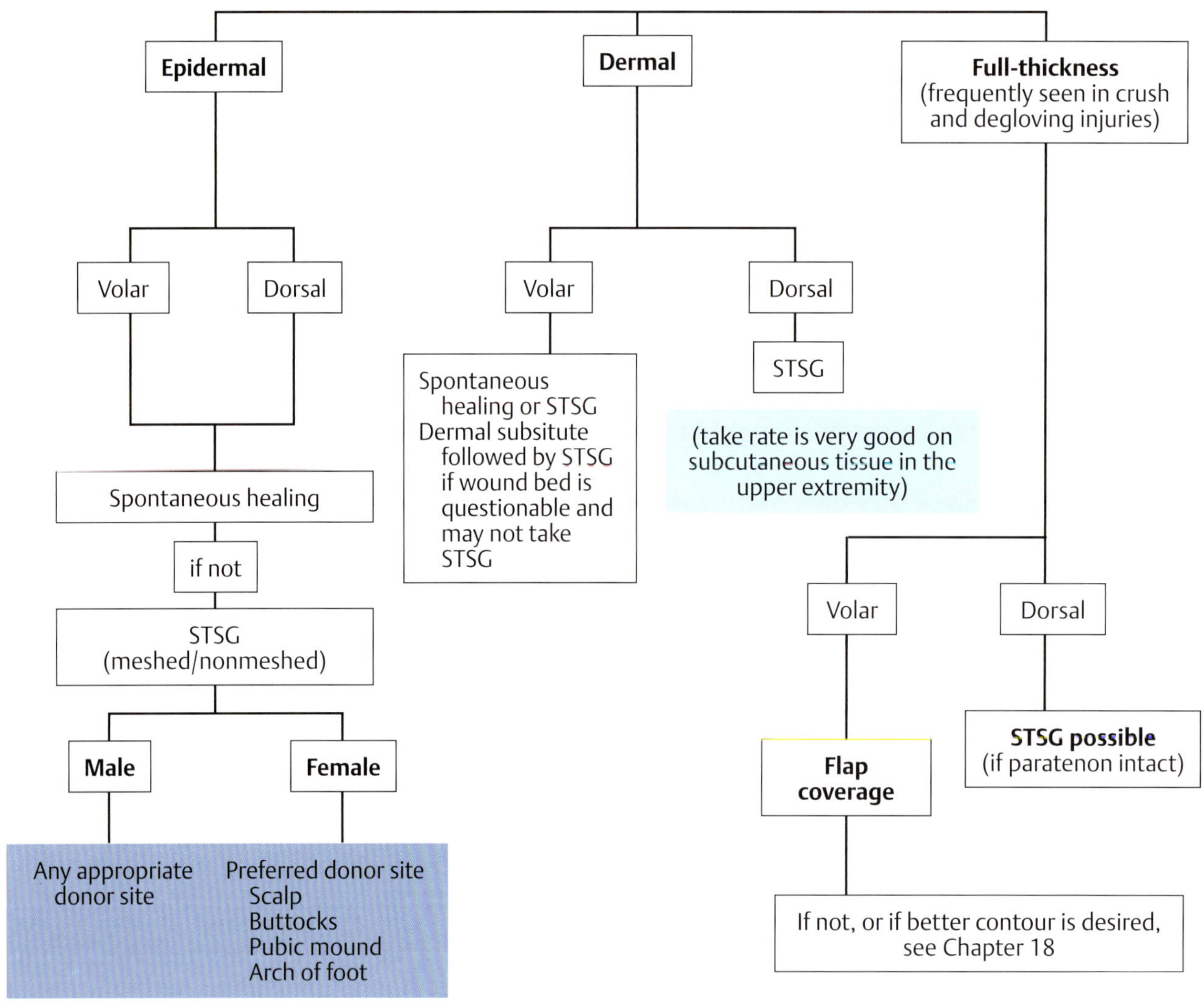

Algorithm 4.2

Parameters in decision-making	Additional options or guidelines	Warnings, precautions, or pitfalls	Emphasis on a particular waypoint

Skin and Soft Tissue–Closed Injury

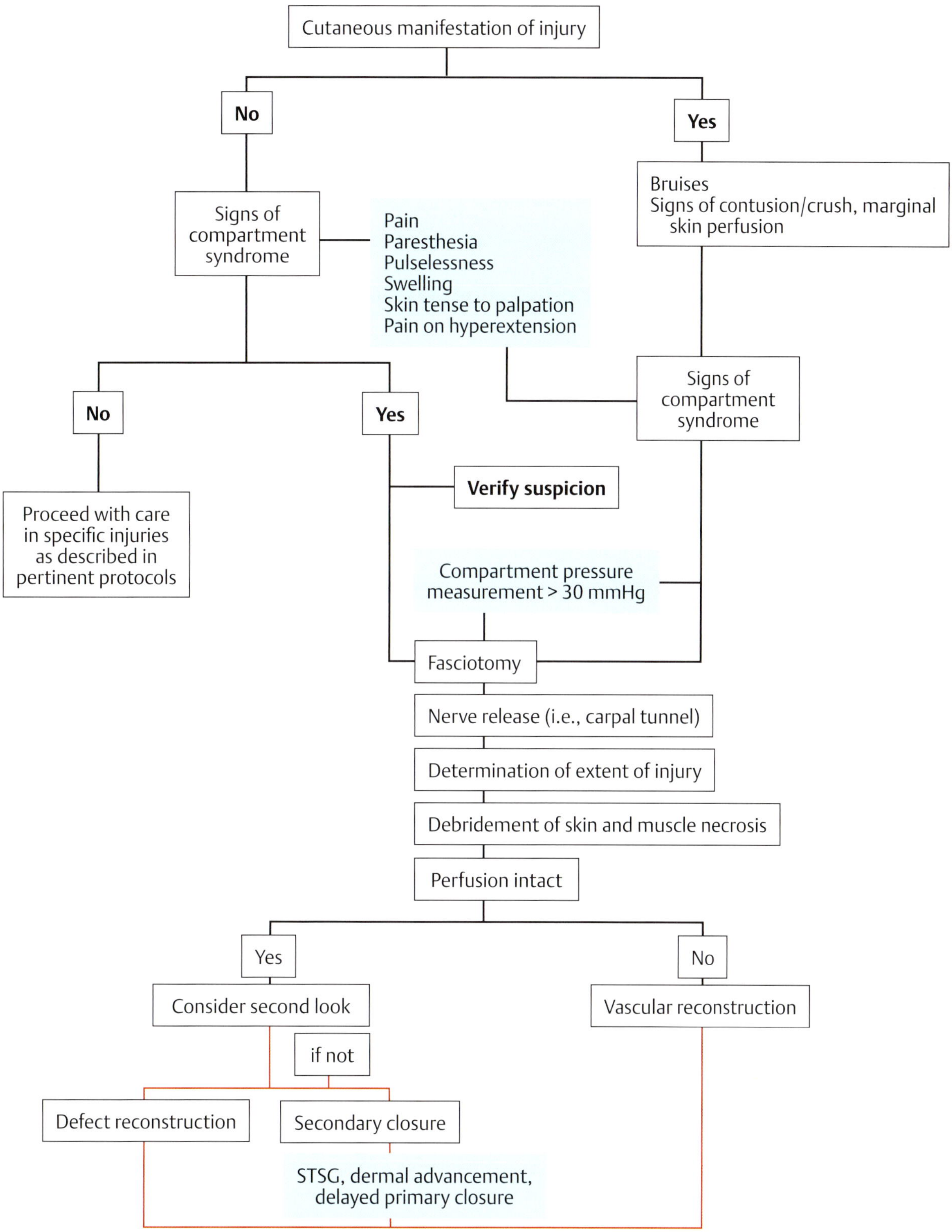

Algorithm 4.3

Parameters in decision-making	Additional options or guidelines	Warnings, precautions, or pitfalls	Emphasis on a particular waypoint

Skin and Soft Tissue–Open Injury

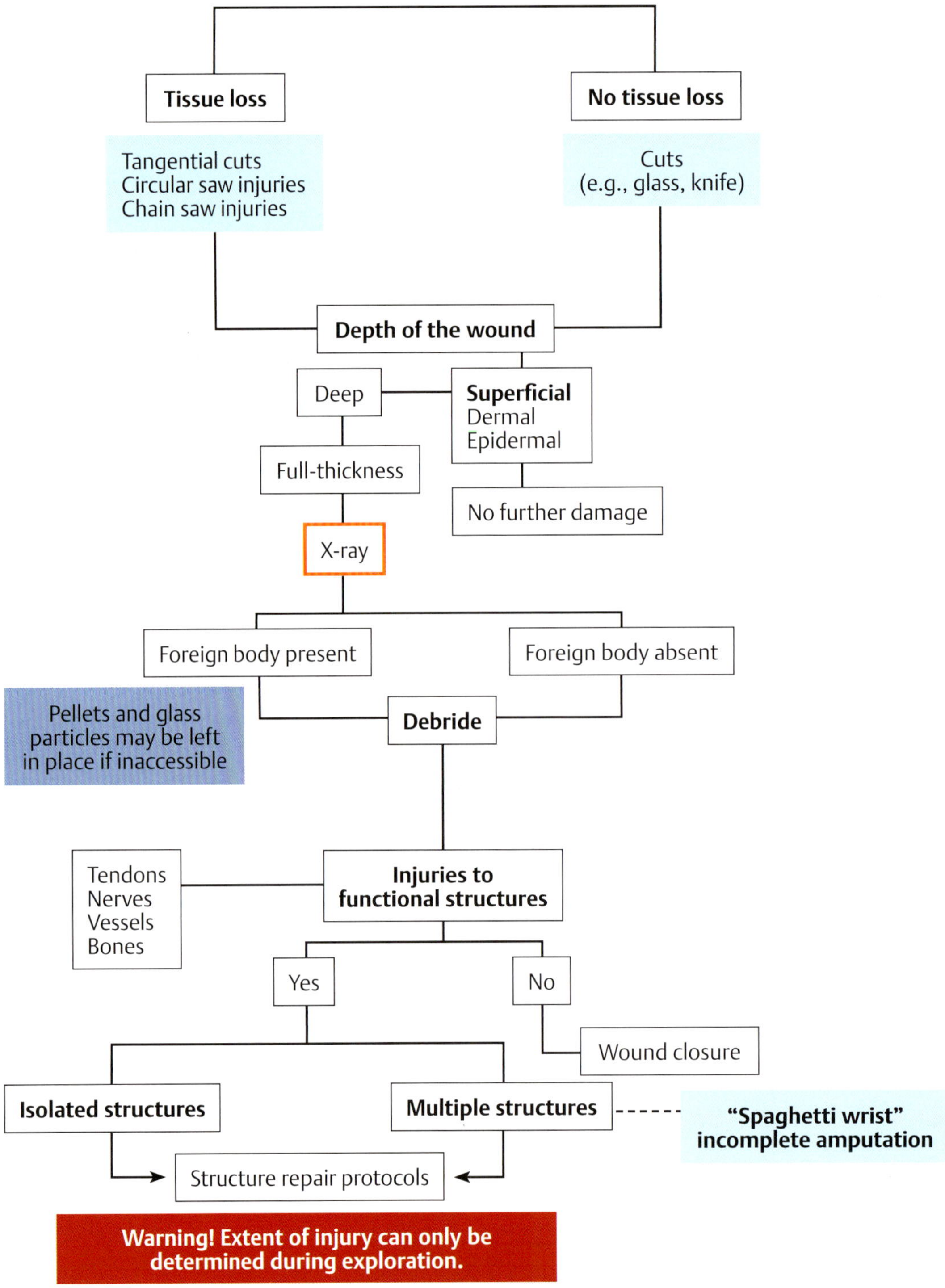

Algorithm 4.4

Parameters in decision-making	Additional options or guidelines	Warnings, precautions, or pitfalls	Emphasis on a particular waypoint

Blunt Injuries

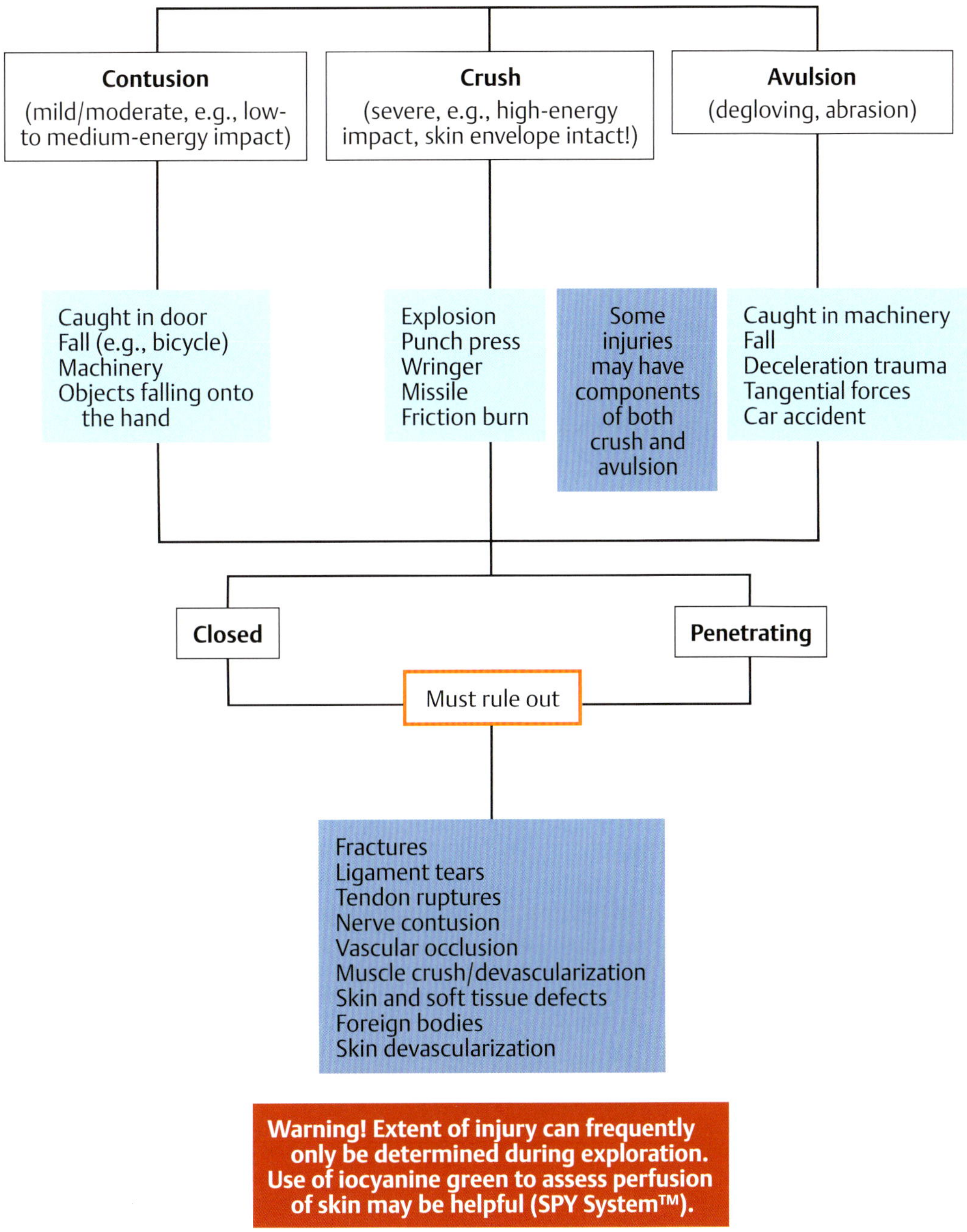

Algorithm 4.5

Parameters in decision-making	Additional options or guidelines	Warnings, precautions, or pitfalls	Emphasis on a particular waypoint

Thermal Burns

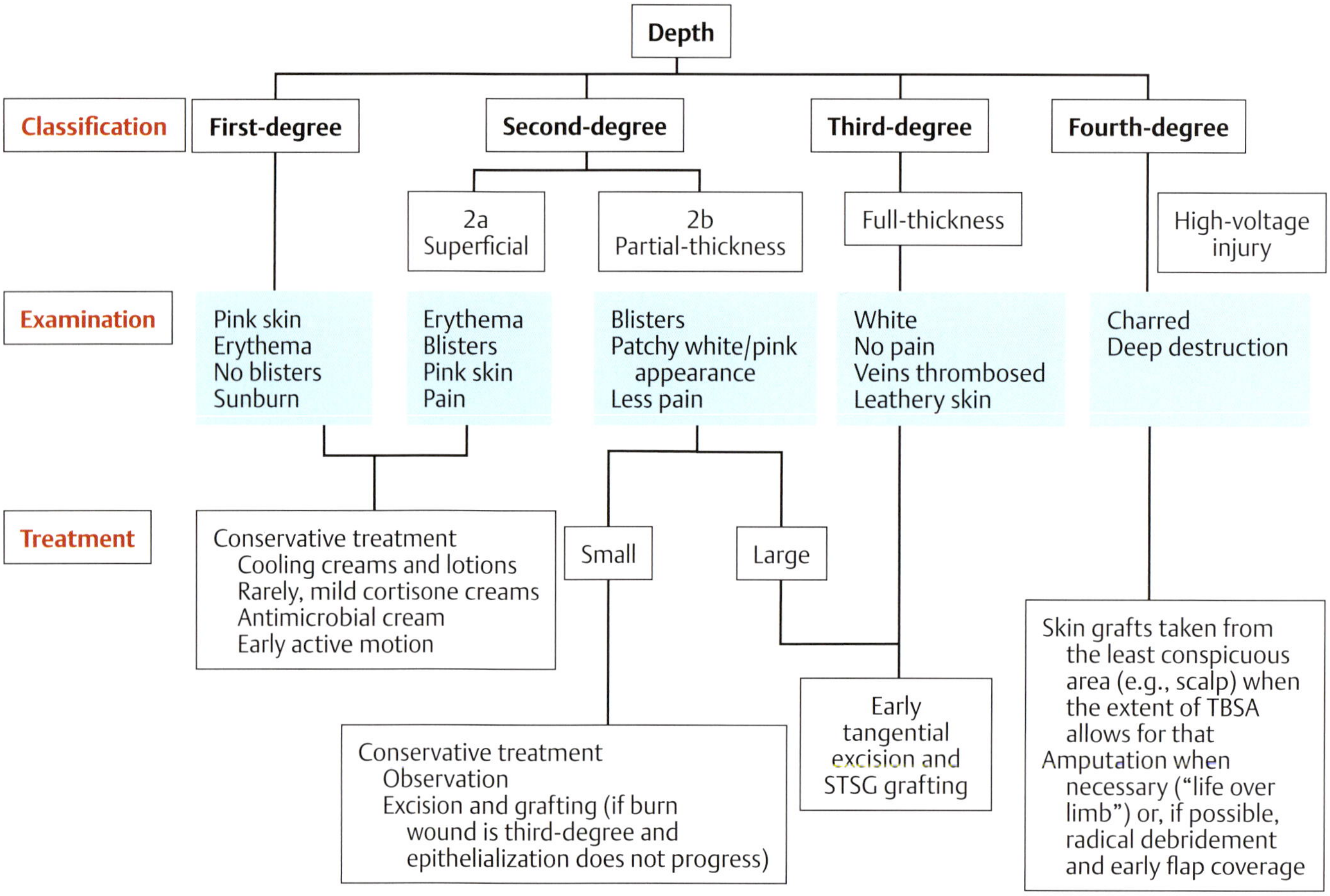

Note: In volar hand burns, conservative treatment is encouraged due to the tremendous capacity for re-epithelialization and the difficulty of adequate reconstruction.
Indications for volar excision only are nonhealing second- to fourth-degree burns.
Criteria for referral to Burn Center are > 15% TBSA; face, genital area, hands involved; inhalation trauma; full-thickness burns.

Algorithm 4.6

Parameters in decision-making	Additional options or guidelines	Warnings, precautions, or pitfalls	Emphasis on a particular waypoint

Chemical Lesions

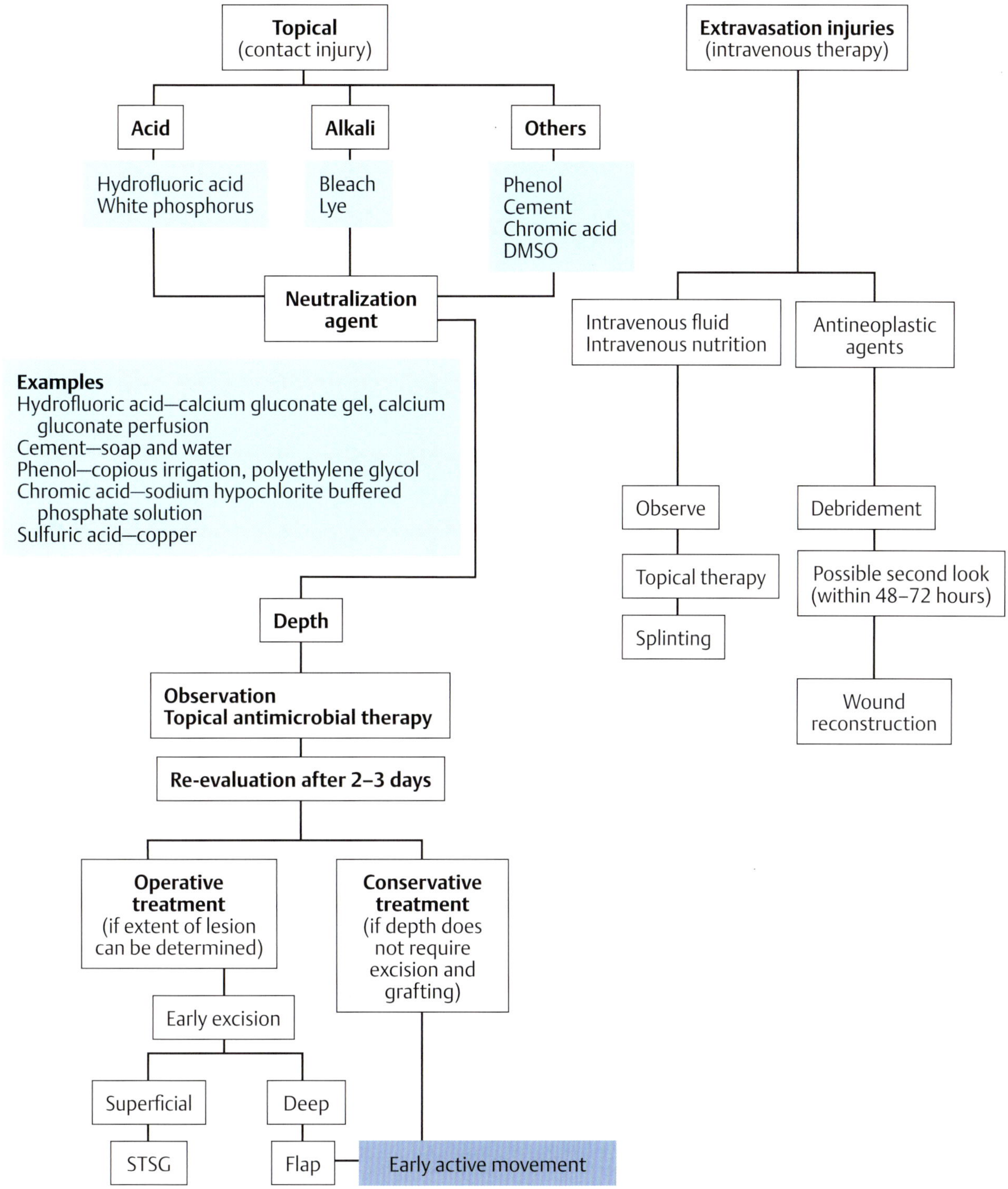

Algorithm 4.7

Parameters in decision-making	Additional options or guidelines	Warnings, precautions, or pitfalls	Emphasis on a particular waypoint

Management of Open Fractures

Assessment

Patient profile
Medical risk factors
Classification (e.g., AO/ASIF)
Mechanism of injury
Delay between injury and hospital admission

↓

Bone

X-ray (simple, complex, degree of comminution)
CT
Joints above and below
Bone loss (yes, no) (see Algorithms 4.9, 4.10)
Associated injuries (abdomen, spine, pelvis)

↓

Soft tissue

Skin (laceration—simple, complex; defect of skin, skin and muscle; amputation—complete, incomplete)
Contamination (dirt, grease, organic material, e.g., grass and twigs; metal, e.g., gunshot pellets and wadding)
Neurovascular injury (artery–vein–nerve combination)
Motor system (tendon laceration, defect)

↓

Treatment

1. Debridement (see Algorithms 4.12, 4.13)
2. Fracture fixation (see Algorithm 4.11)
3. Wound care after 1 + 2 above

- Definitive (see Algorithms 4.9, 4.10)
- Provisional (bead pouch, porcine allograft topical, wound vacuum)

Algorithm 4.8

Parameters in decision-making	Additional options or guidelines	Warnings, precautions, or pitfalls	Emphasis on a particular waypoint

Fractures

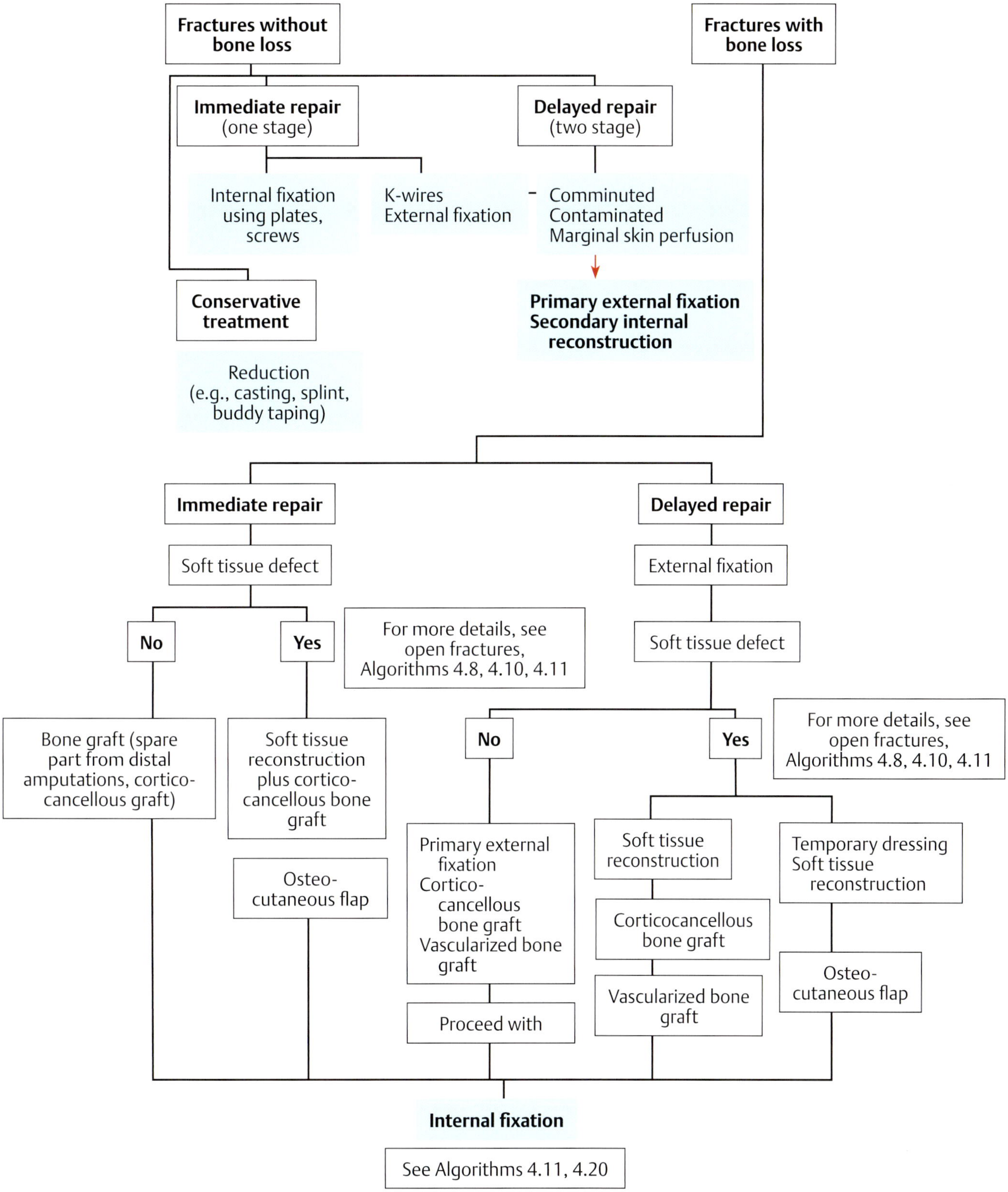

Algorithm 4.9

Parameters in decision-making	Additional options or guidelines	Warnings, precautions, or pitfalls	Emphasis on a particular waypoint

Management of Fractures with Associated Soft Tissue Involvement

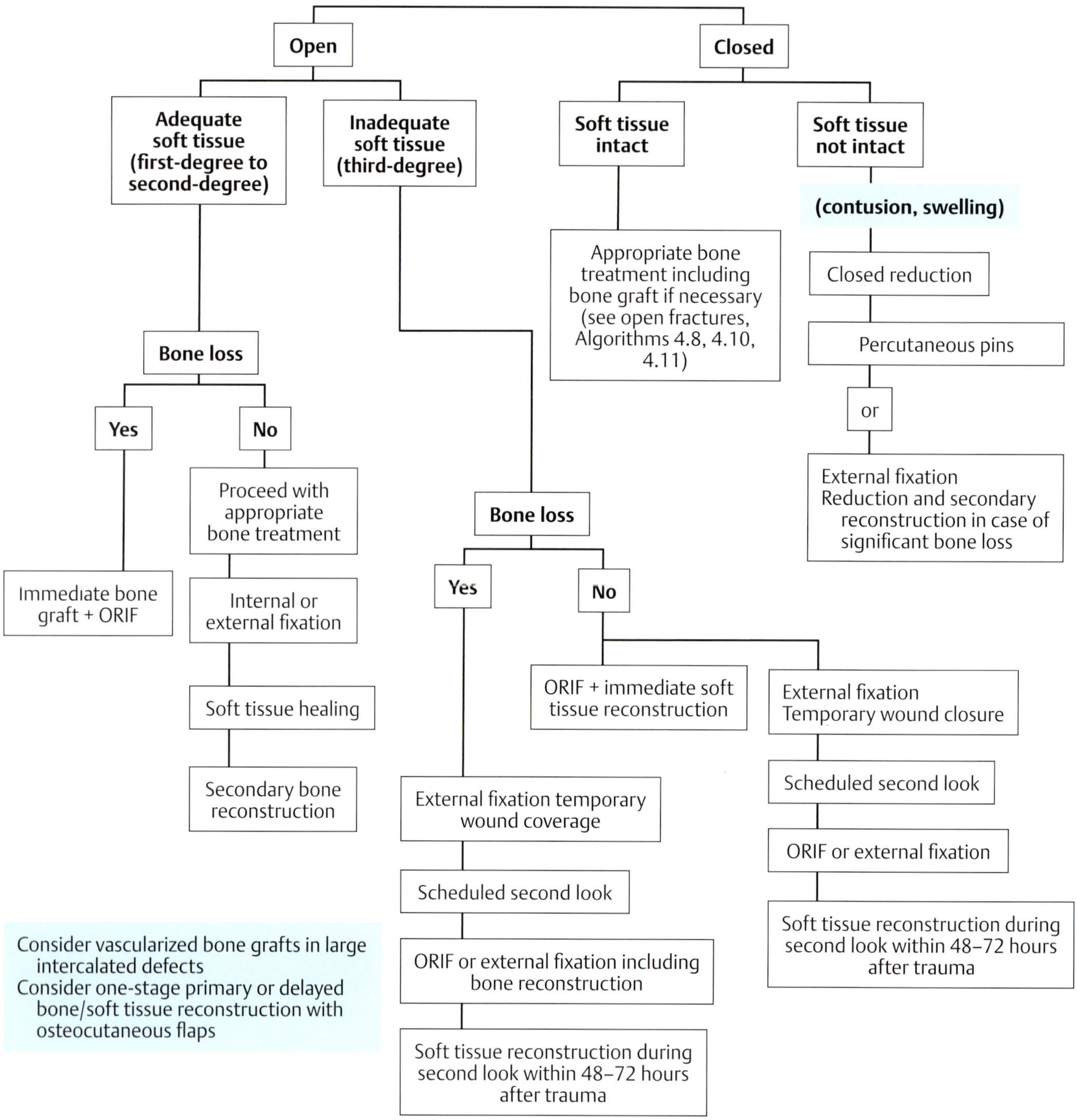

Algorithm 4.10

Parameters in decision-making	Additional options or guidelines	Warnings, precautions, or pitfalls	Emphasis on a particular waypoint

Choice of Fracture Fixation

External fixation

- Bone comminuted
- Severe contamination
- Long delay from injury to OR
- If unable to achieve wound closure in a timely fashion
- If second look and debridement are required
- If bone or soft tissue is devascularized
- Major soft tissue defects

Internal fixation

- Intact soft tissue
- Fracture accessible with minimal stripping (in open injuries)
- Clean wounds
- Internal fixation possible
- Bridge or span locking plate can be used with bone graft after wound closure (i.e., flap)
- Intra-articular injuries–absolute indications even in open injuries

Algorithm 4.11

Debridement

All wounds in the upper extremity will require debridement to optimize wound conditions that will allow for wound closure. In cases of open fractures, debridement and stabilization are the most important prophylaxis against sepsis.

Sequence

I. Timing

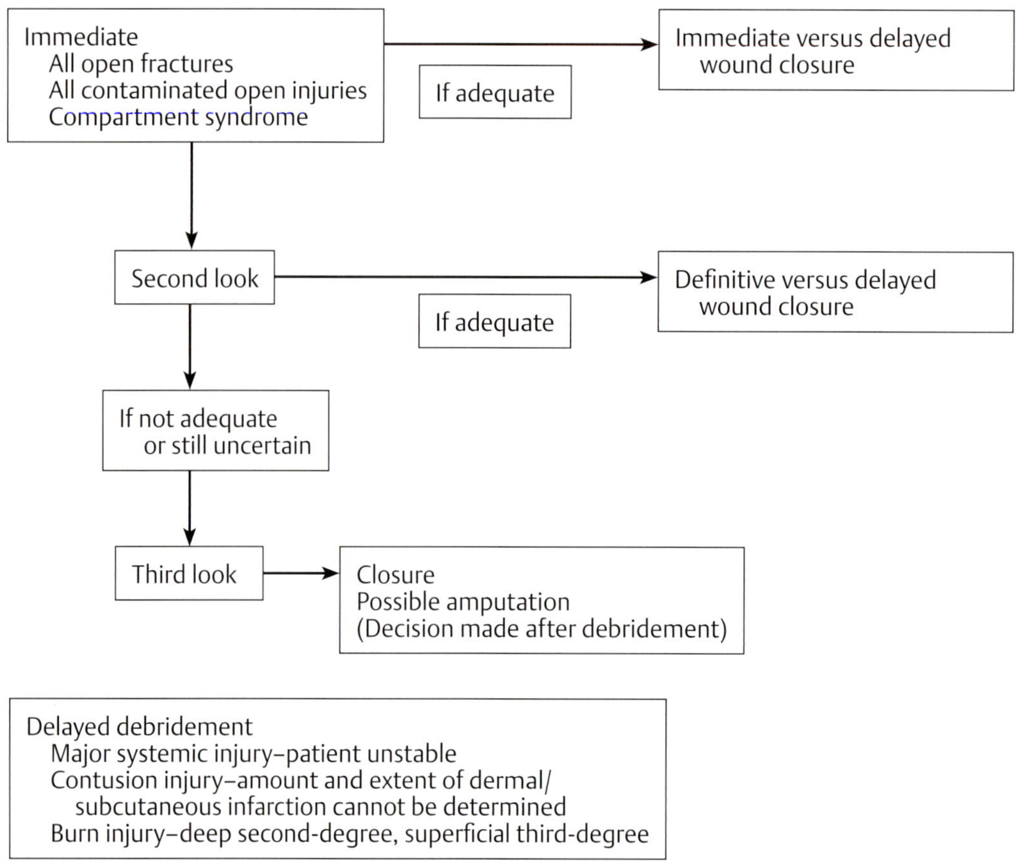

II. Tourniquet inflation

III. Wound inspection

IV. Centripetal debridement by structure

Algorithm 4.12

Parameters in decision-making	Additional options or guidelines	Warnings, precautions, or pitfalls	Emphasis on a particular waypoint

Debridement–Structures

Skin, Subcutaneous tissue Dissect to bleeding dermis using a scalpel. Trim edges 1–2 mm to create clean wound edge. Cut skin back to healthy fat (punctate bleeding, with minimal hemosiderin staining).

Fascia May be debrided sharply and should always be removed if not vascularized. Liberal opening/extensive exploration of compartments.

Muscle Debride to contractile muscle (color is pink, bleeding from cut muscle tissue).

Bone Remove all fragments devoid of significant soft tissue attachments.

Nerve Be aware of cutaneous nerves—they may cause painful neuromas. Epineurium can be removed if contaminated (median, radial, and ulnar nerve) with fascicles remaining. If nerve is not vascularized it can remain, provided it does not desiccate, and wound closure is achieved early.

Vessels Remove any perforated, thrombosed segments. Identify main vascular trunks. If not intact and if there is no flow, perform segmental vascular debridement; ligate major vessels, clip minor. Identify, mark, and protect major viable vessels that can be used for vascular access during immediate/delayed free tissue transfer.

V. Pulsatile irrigation

Caveat: avoid implosion of foreign material, hydrodissection of tissue planes, and insufflation of tissues.

VI. Deflate tourniquet
Evaluate structures for bleeding.

VII. Decision-making on wound closure

Algorithm 4.13

Parameters in decision-making	Additional options or guidelines	Warnings, precautions, or pitfalls	Emphasis on a particular waypoint

Infections–Overview

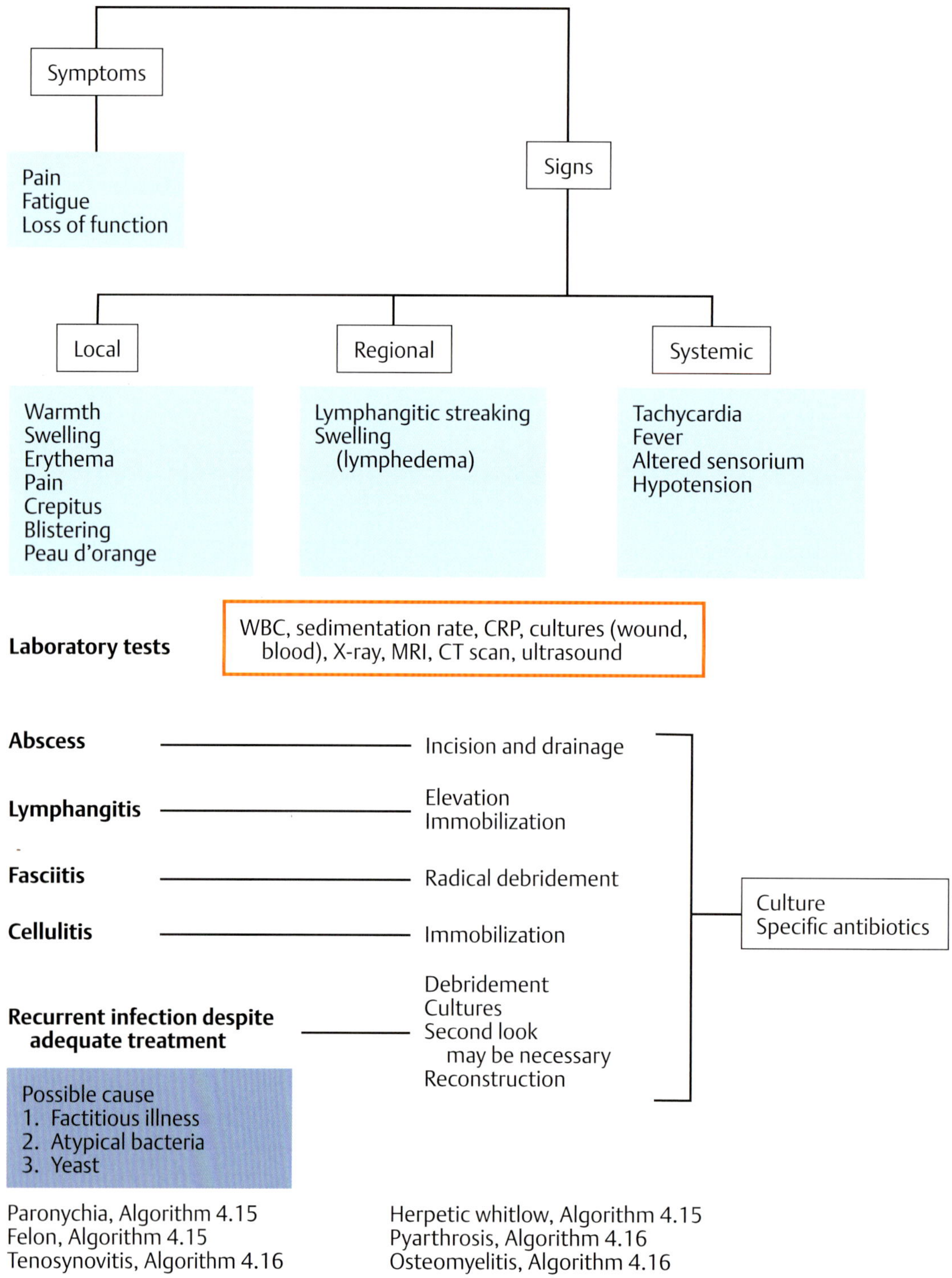

Algorithm 4.14

Parameters in decision-making	Additional options or guidelines	Warnings, precautions, or pitfalls	Emphasis on a particular waypoint

Infections

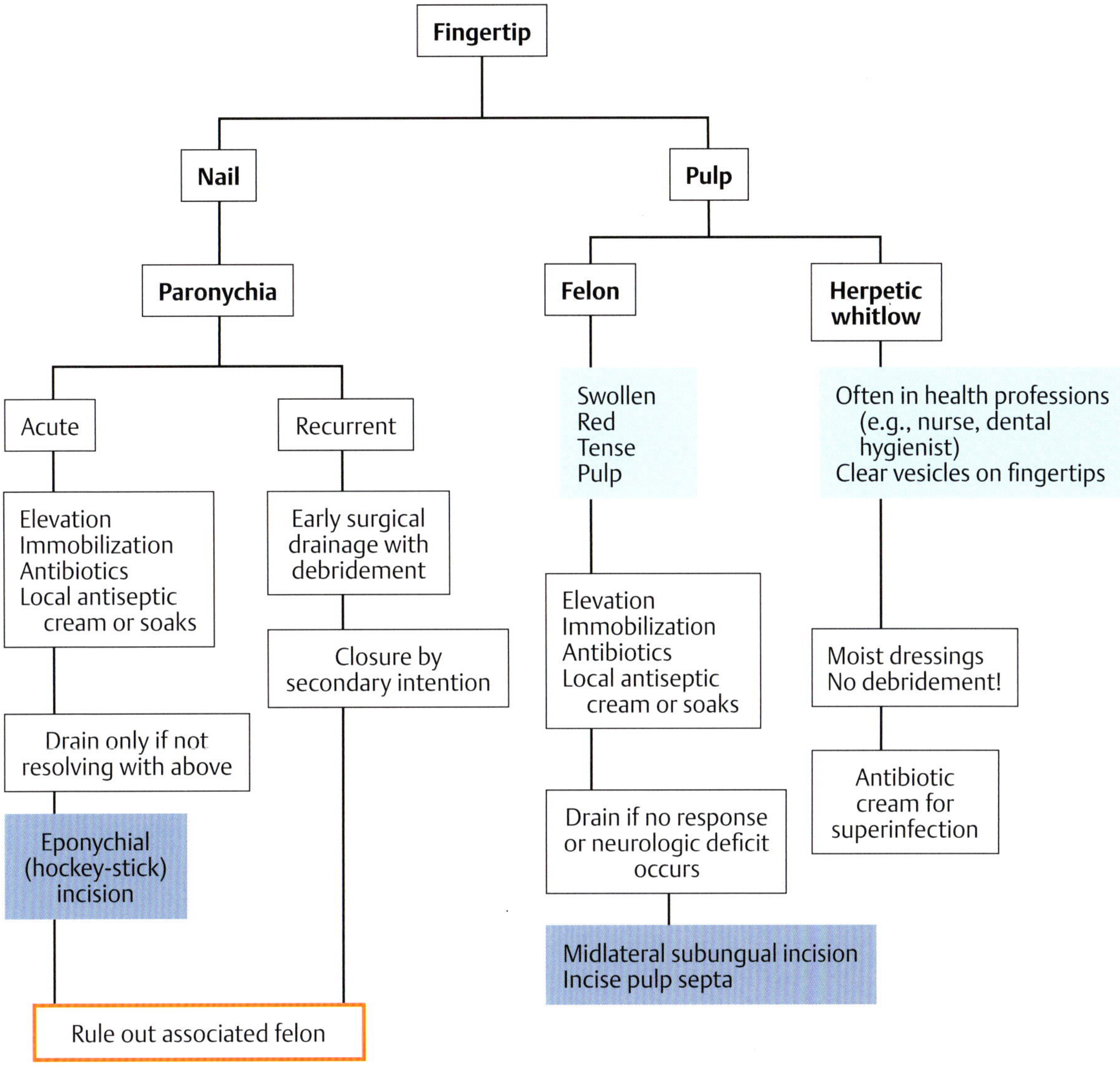

Algorithm 4.15

Parameters in decision-making	Additional options or guidelines	Warnings, precautions, or pitfalls	Emphasis on a particular waypoint

Infections

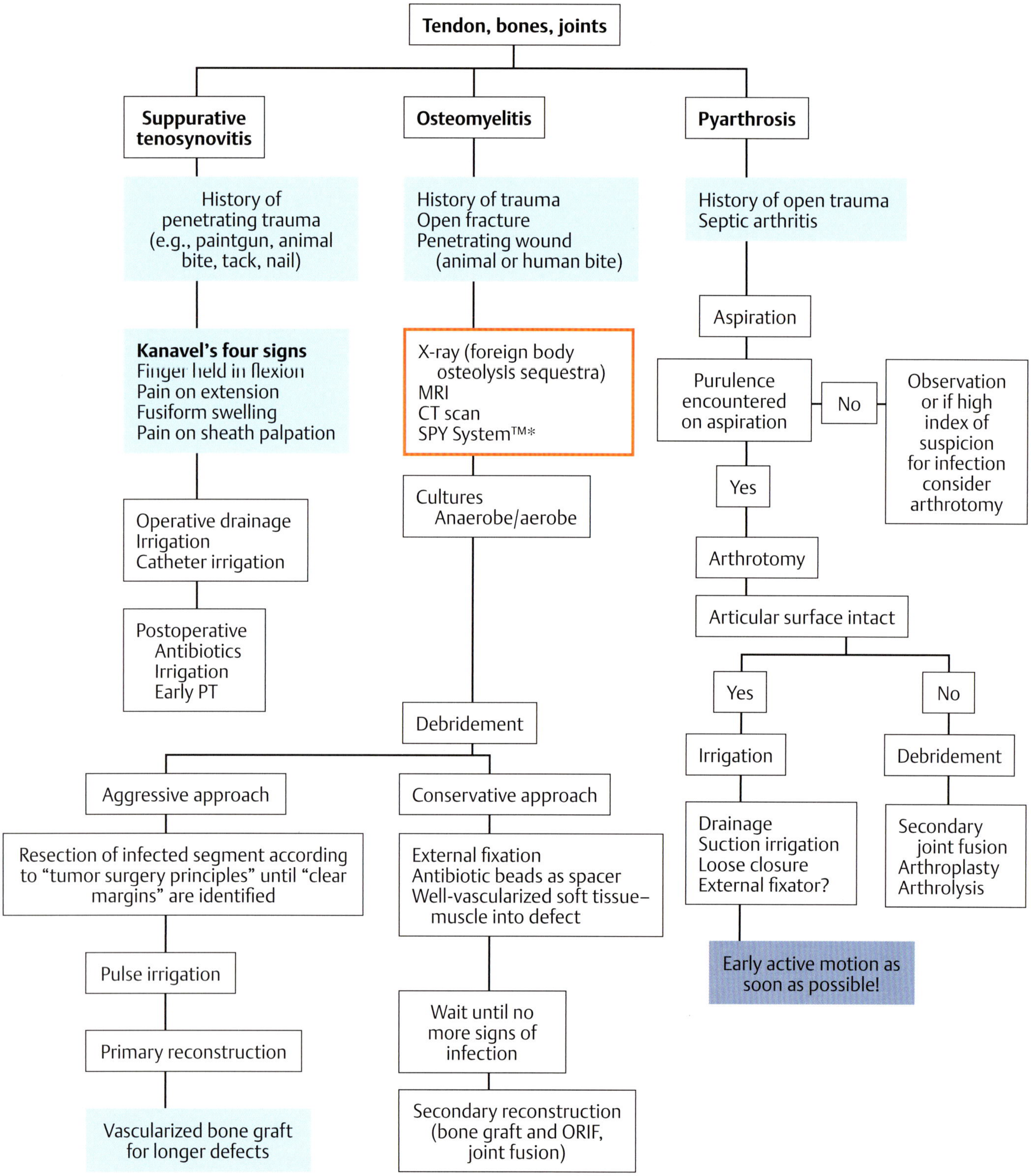

Algorithm 4.16

*ICG tissue perfusion monitoring system.

Parameters in decision-making	Additional options or guidelines	Warnings, precautions, or pitfalls	Emphasis on a particular waypoint

Contractures I

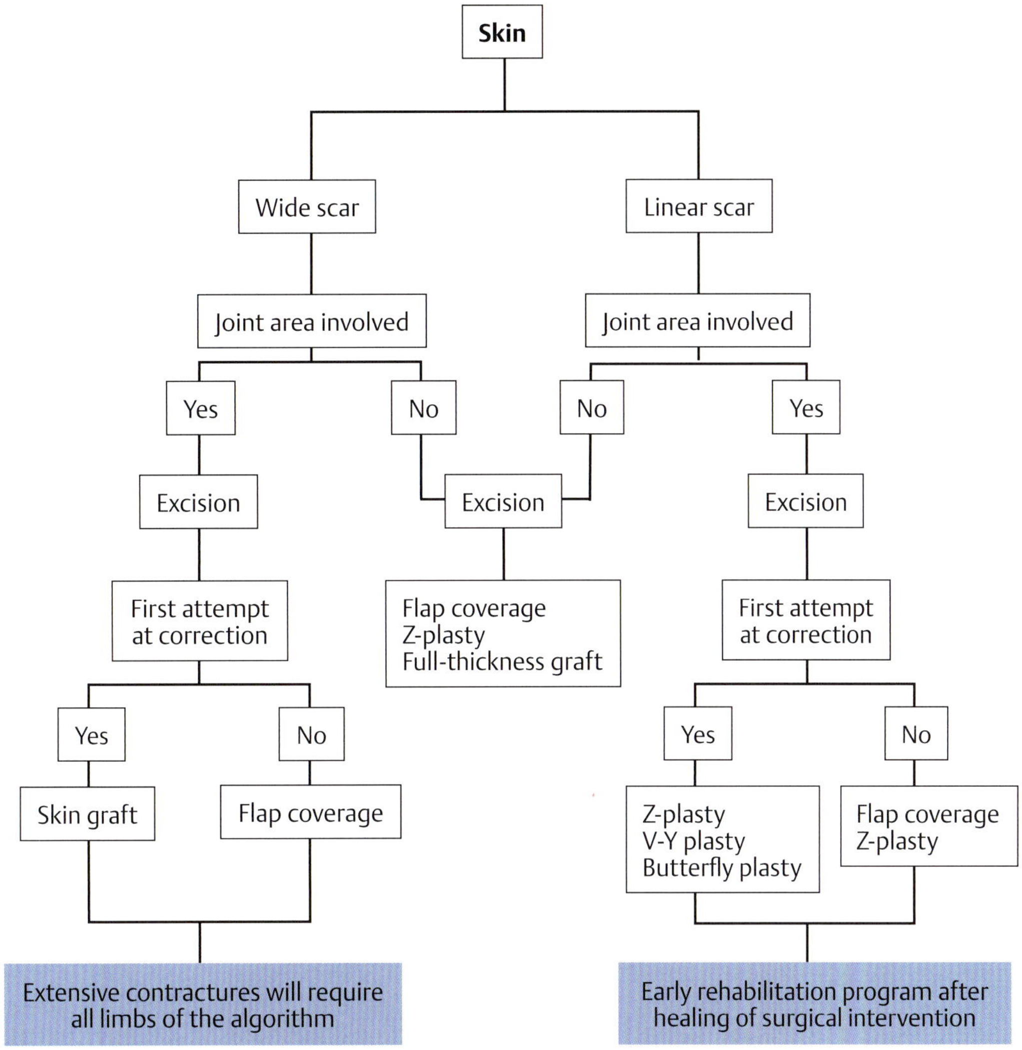

Algorithm 4.17

Parameters in decision-making	Additional options or guidelines	Warnings, precautions, or pitfalls	Emphasis on a particular waypoint

Contractures II

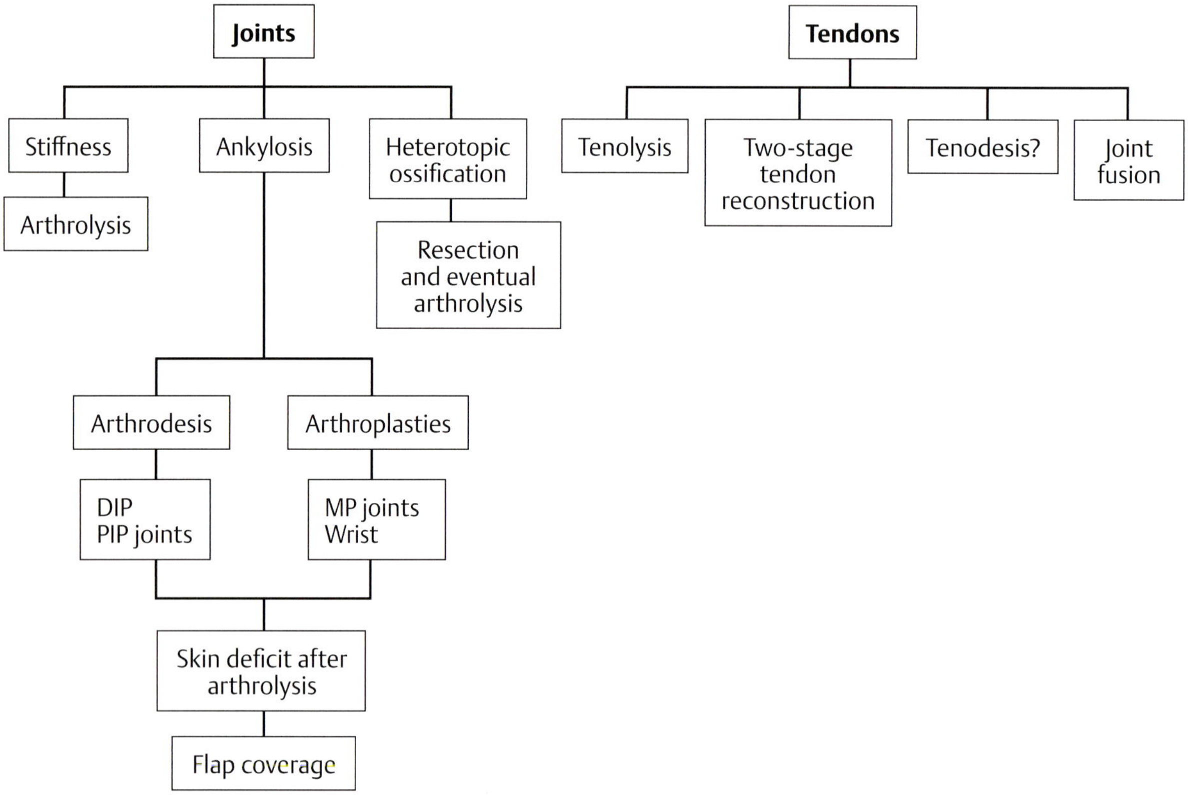

Extensive contractures will require all limbs of the algorithm
Early rehabilitation program after healing of surgical intervention

Algorithm 4.18

Parameters in decision-making	Additional options or guidelines	Warnings, precautions, or pitfalls	Emphasis on a particular waypoint

Tumors

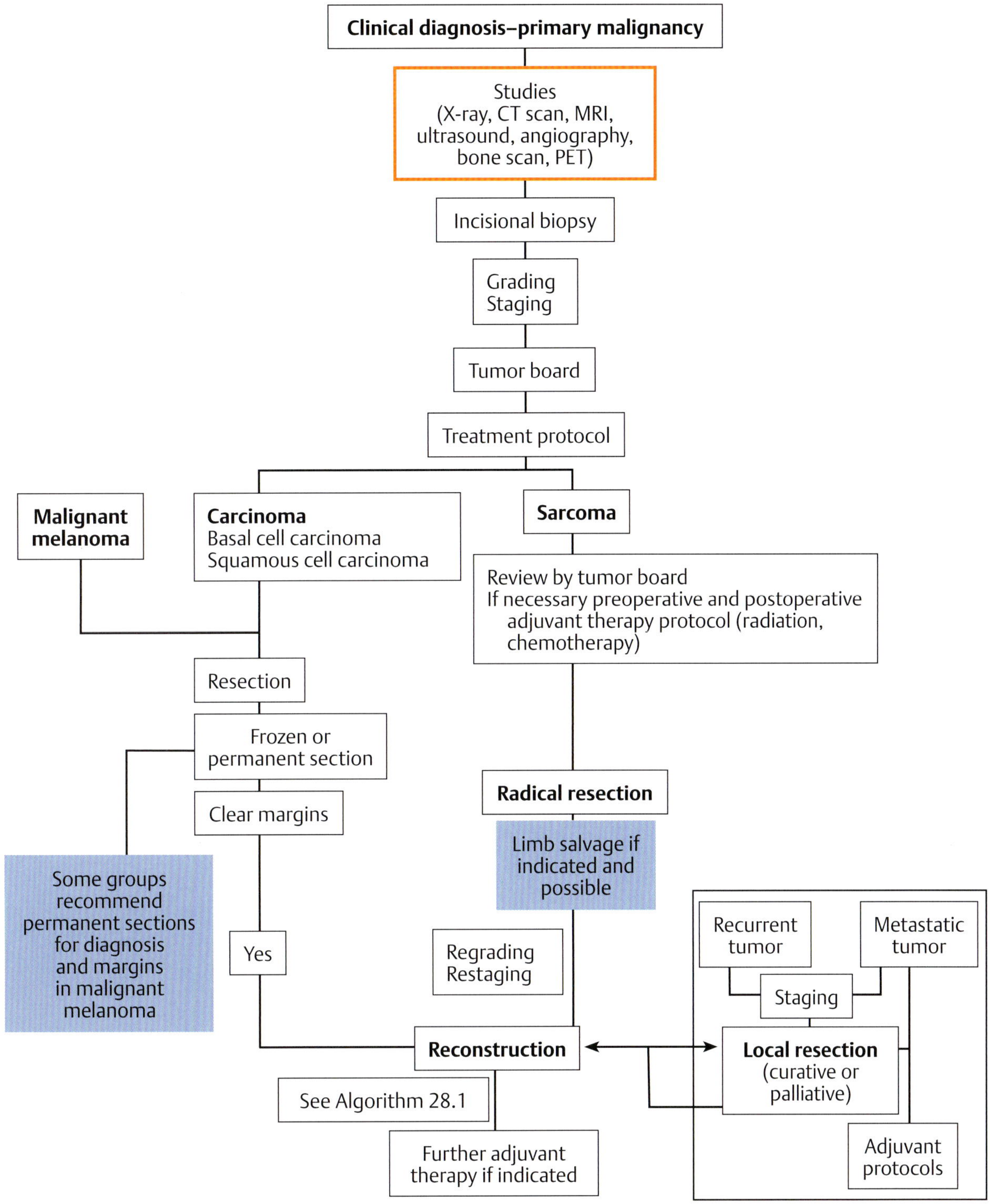

Algorithm 4.19

Parameters in decision-making	Additional options or guidelines	Warnings, precautions, or pitfalls	Emphasis on a particular waypoint

Monitoring of Flaps and Impending Flap Failure

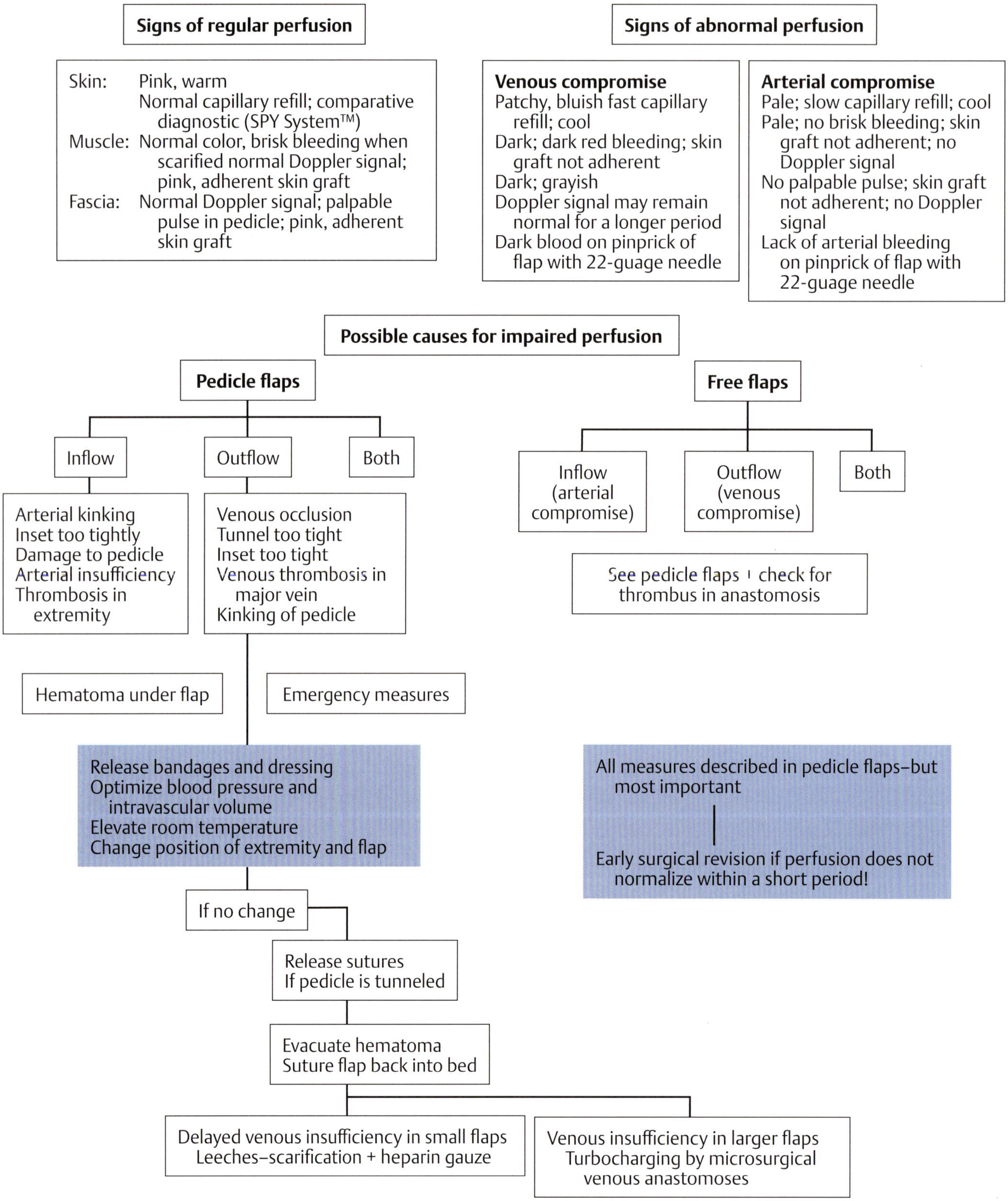

Algorithm 4.20

Parameters in decision-making	Additional options or guidelines	Warnings, precautions, or pitfalls	Emphasis on a particular waypoint

Splinting

Splints play a critical role in the acute care and rehabilitation of hand and upper extremity injuries. The appropriate understanding, selection, and use of these devices will maximize the potential for positive outcomes after relatively insignificant injuries to the most devastating traumatic events. Casts should be considered as more durable and resilient. Both casts and splints fulfill several fundamental needs for an injured extremity: rest, comfort, protection, hygiene, mechanically advantageous, static positioning, dynamic assist potential in selected instances, and aesthetic and psychological support. Common materials for their fabrication include plaster, fiberglass, and thermoplastic sheeting. Casts are best suited for fracture management and should be prudently applied when significant soft tissue swelling is present during the acute injury phase. Most importantly, the maintenance of an optimal hand position is the key to successful splint application and use. The terms *position of function, intrinsic plus,* and *neutral position* have been used to describe the most elemental position for a hand that is to be placed in a cast or splint (**Fig. 4.1**).

Four key components apply when positioning a patient's hand for splinting or casting:

1. The wrist should be positioned between 0 and 10 degrees of extension.
2. The metacarpophalangeal joints should be placed at 70 degrees of flexion.
3. The interphalangeal joints should be slightly flexed.
4. The thumb should be abducted, either volarly (most common) or dorsally.

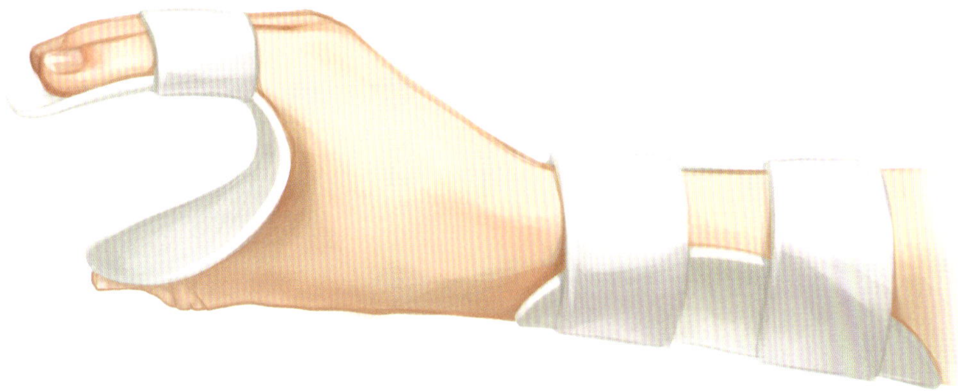

Fig. 4.1 Splinted arm showing position of function.

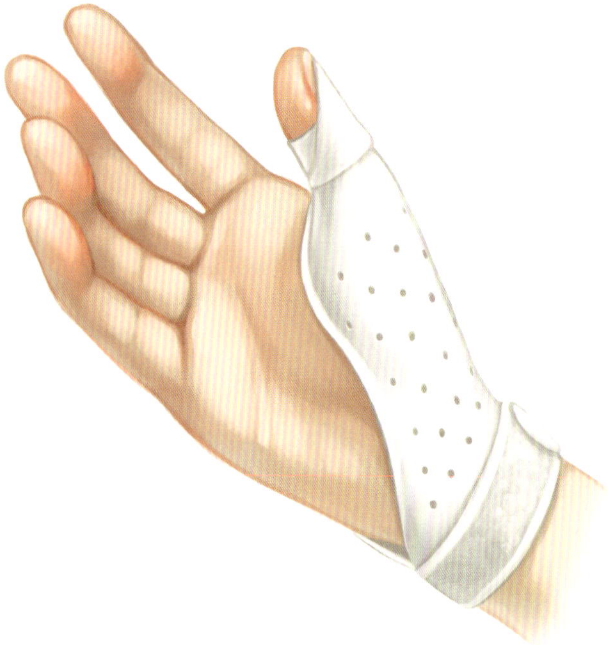

Fig. 4.2 Thumb spica splint.

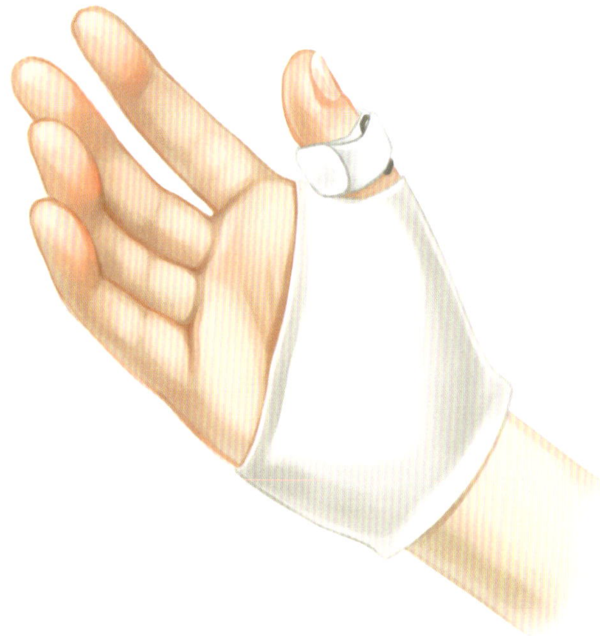

Fig. 4.3 First web space splint.

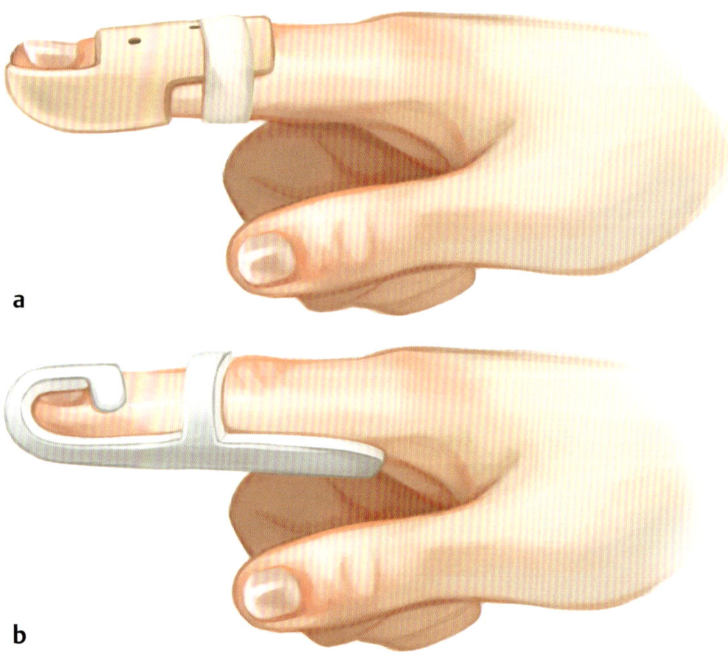

Fig. 4.4 Dorsal digital splints for fingertips.

Either rolled cotton padding or tubular cotton stockinette must be applied to the arm first to protect the skin. The radiographic verification of the hand position after splint placement is recommended.

Spica splints may be used to isolate injured digits or joints while maintaining as much hand mobility as possible (**Fig. 4.2**).

Simple first web space splints are effective for maintaining abduction during the healing phase of penetrating soft tissue injuries or burns in this area (**Fig. 4.3**).

Prefabricated dorsal digital splints are easily placed for fingertip injury, mallet finger, or other isolated phalangeal fractures (**Fig. 4.4**).

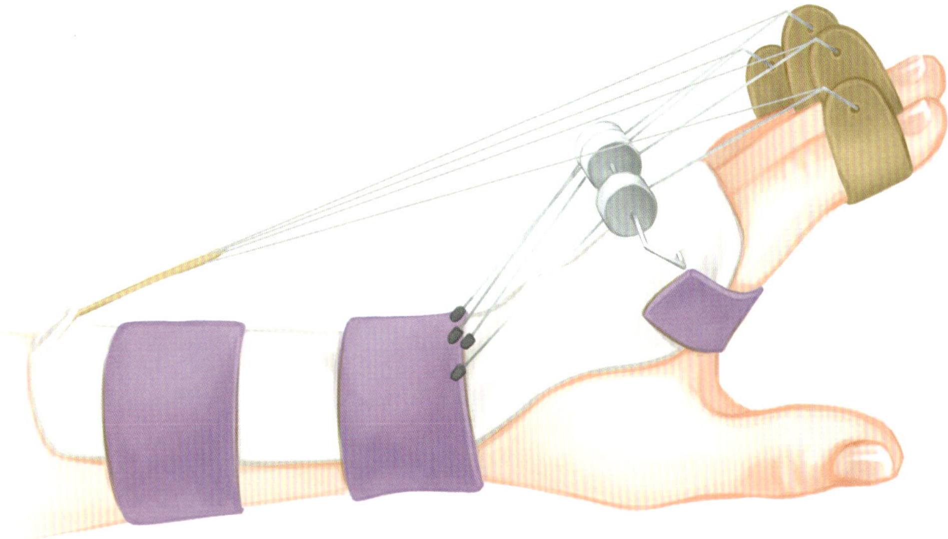

Fig. 4.5 Dynamic splinting for extensor repair.

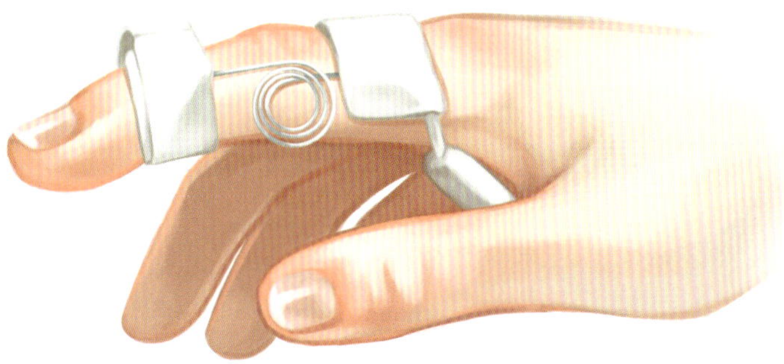

Fig. 4.6 Dynamic splinting for flexor repair.

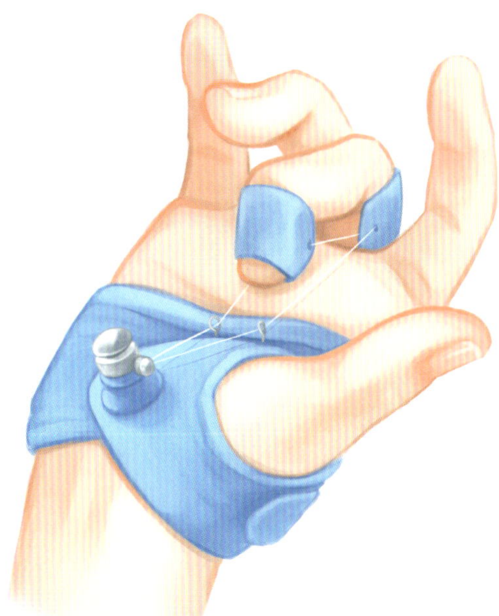

Fig. 4.7 Dynamic splinting for flexor repair.

After extensor lacerations are repaired, the joints are splinted in extension to offload tension on the tenorrhaphy (**Fig. 4.5**).

Dynamic splinting for flexor tendon rehabilitation using either the Duran protocol, the Kleinert protocol, or another protocol provides protected early movement at the repair site without loading the suture repair site (**Fig. 4.6**). Correctly constructed dynamic splints should be well monitored (preferably by a hand therapist) and should optimize the patient's long-term range of motion while minimizing tendon rupture and adhesion as early postoperative complications (**Fig. 4.7**).

Part II

Techniques of Structure Repair

Chapter 5

The Reconstructive Ladder

Based on a careful analysis of the injury and the defect, missing structures and missing functions are identified. Options for reconstruction are then considered and selected from the entire armamentarium of tools available.

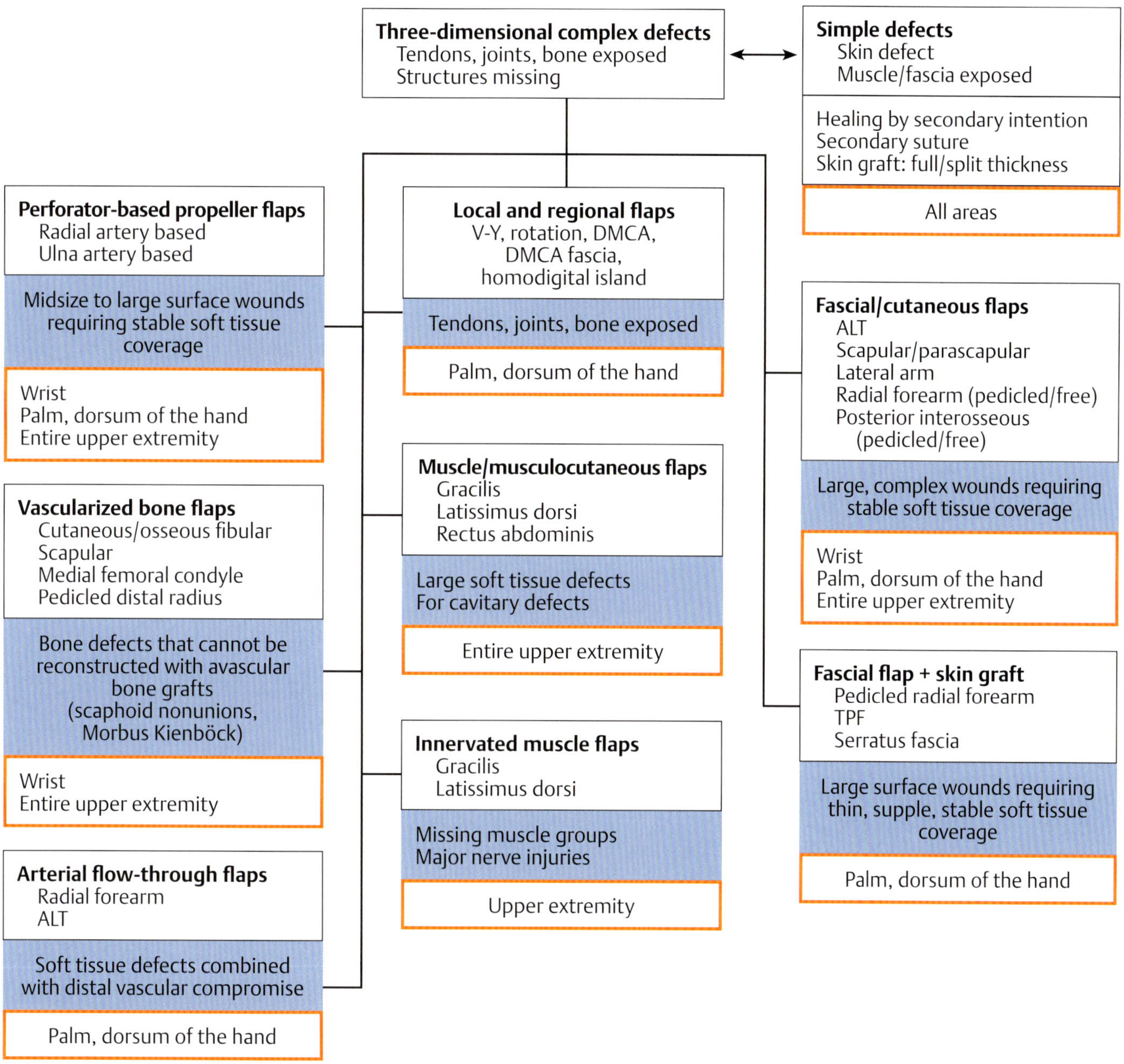

Fig. 5.1 Reconstructive ladder.

Parameters in decision-making	Additional options or guidelines	Warnings, precautions, or pitfalls	Emphasis on a particular waypoint

Chapter 6

Skin Grafts

Skin Grafts

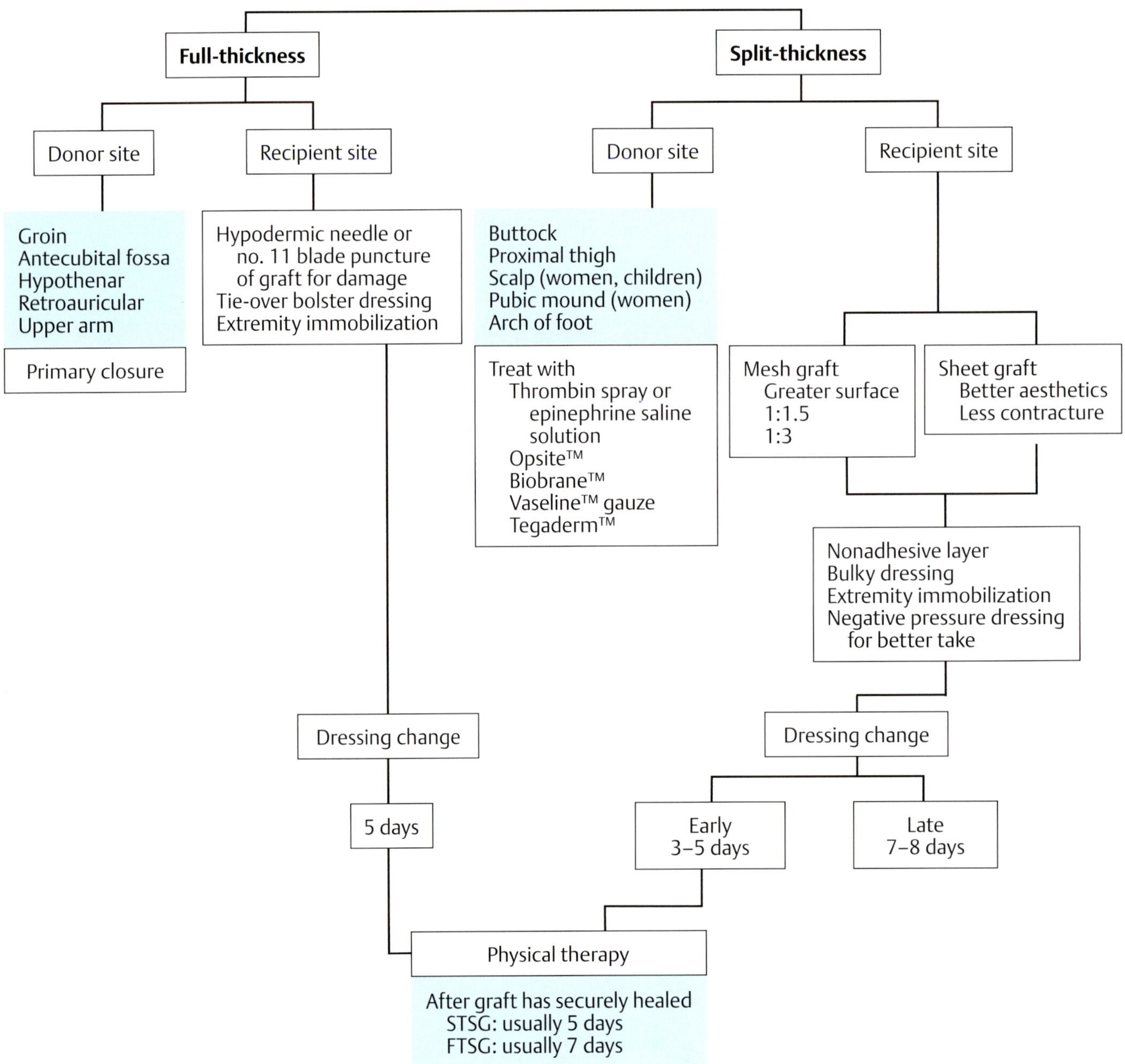

Algorithm 6.1

Parameters in decision-making	Additional options or guidelines	Warnings, precautions, or pitfalls	Emphasis on a particular waypoint

Chapter 7

Techniques of Osteosynthesis

Options–Osteosynthesis

Internal
- K-wire
- Plate/screws
- Rod
- Biodegradable pins
- Suture (ligaments)

External
- Traction
- Casting
- External fixation
  - Unilateral
  - Delta

Combination
- External fixation + plate
- External fixation + screws
- K-wire + external fixation

Implant characteristics

K-wire
- Simple
- Percutaneous
- Less rigid
- Tension possible (in tension band wiring)
- Rapid
- Easily removed
- Inexpensive
- Buried

Screws
- Neutralization device
- Compression device (lag screw)
- Alone or with plate
- For interfragmental compression, a 3:1 ratio is recommended in terms of fracture length and bone width

Intramedullary rod
- Limited approach
- Minimum soft tissue stripping
- Good for gross alignment
- Compression limited

Plate
- Rigid if combined with screw
- Requires soft tissue stripping
- Hazardous if used in inadequate soft tissue
- Compression
- Neutralization
- Spanning
- Bridging
- Buttress
- Locking

External fixation
- Helpful in open fractures
- Stabilizes comminuted fractures
- Less rigid
- Helpful in skin contusion
- Pins can cause infection
- Can be combined with ORIF if soft tissue is stable

Biodegradable implants (pins)
- Not rigid
- Good for small osteochondral fragments
- Early mobilization may be delayed

Algorithm 7.1

Chapter 8

Techniques of Bone Repair

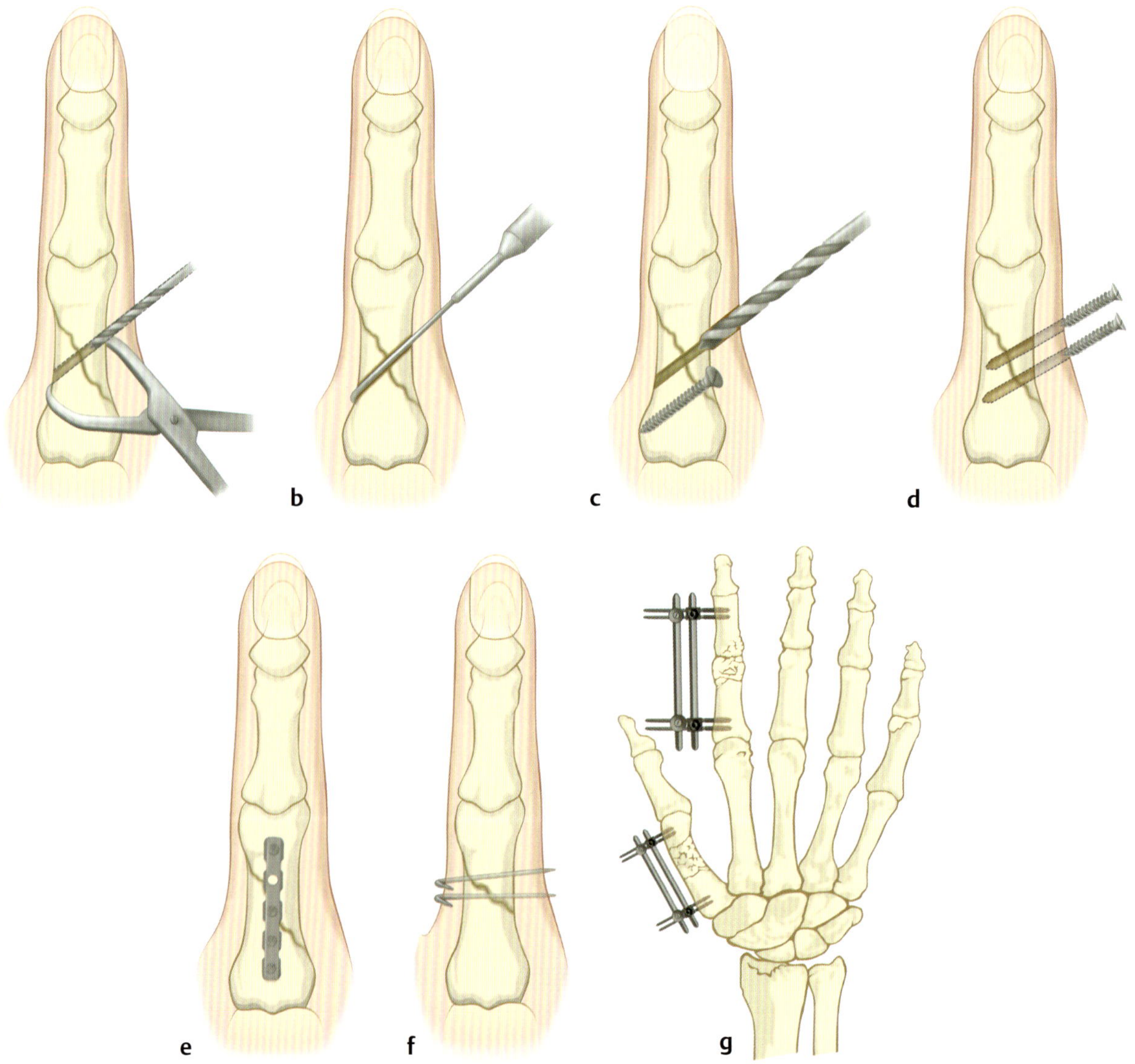

Fig. 8.1 (a) Bicortical drilling after fracture reduction. **(b)** Measurement of screw length with a depth gauge. **(c)** Fixation with interfragmentary compression screws. For this fixation, the proximal hole—where the screw enters the bone—is drilled so that it is slightly larger. **(d)** Correct screw placement. **(e)** Plate fixation for horizontal or comminuted fractures. **(f)** For a horizontal fracture that is stabilized with pins, crossing of the pins in the fracture line must be avoided. **(g)** External fixation of intra-articular and/or comminuted diaphyseal fractures.

Chapter 9

Techniques of Tendon Repair

Basic technique is a rectangular suture which has undergone numerous modifications after Kirchmayer's first description in 1917.

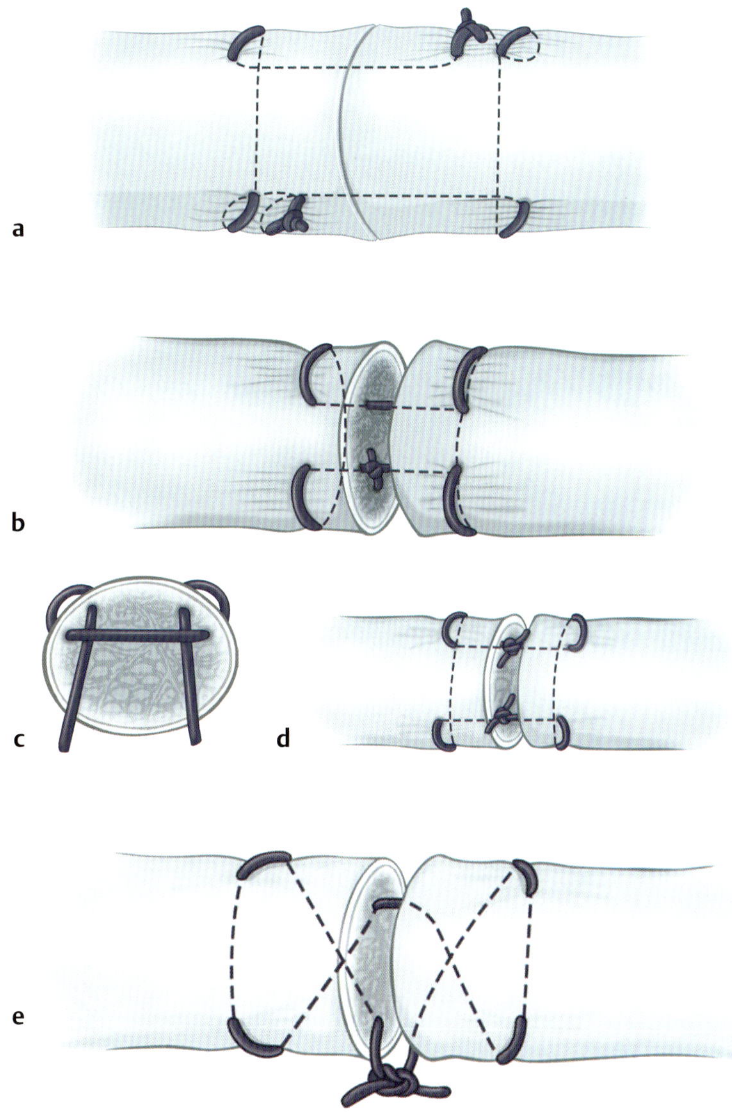

Fig. 9.1 (a) Original Kirchmayer/Kessler: Two sutures (two-strand) with knots buried in the tendon outside the suture line. A two-strand core suture with knots. In the suture line or burled in the tendon outside the suture line. Intratendinous knots may have better gliding properties, but have more suture material in the tendon gap. Theoretically, sutures should be placed insofar as possible at the volar aspect of the tendon to avoid disturbance of the dorsally situated vessels. Too much compression at the suture line should be avoided to prevent bulging of the tendon repair with subsequent impairment of gliding. **(b–e)** Modified Kessler: One or two sutures (two-strand) with intratendinous knots. Cross section demonstrates optimal position of core sutures (*continued*).

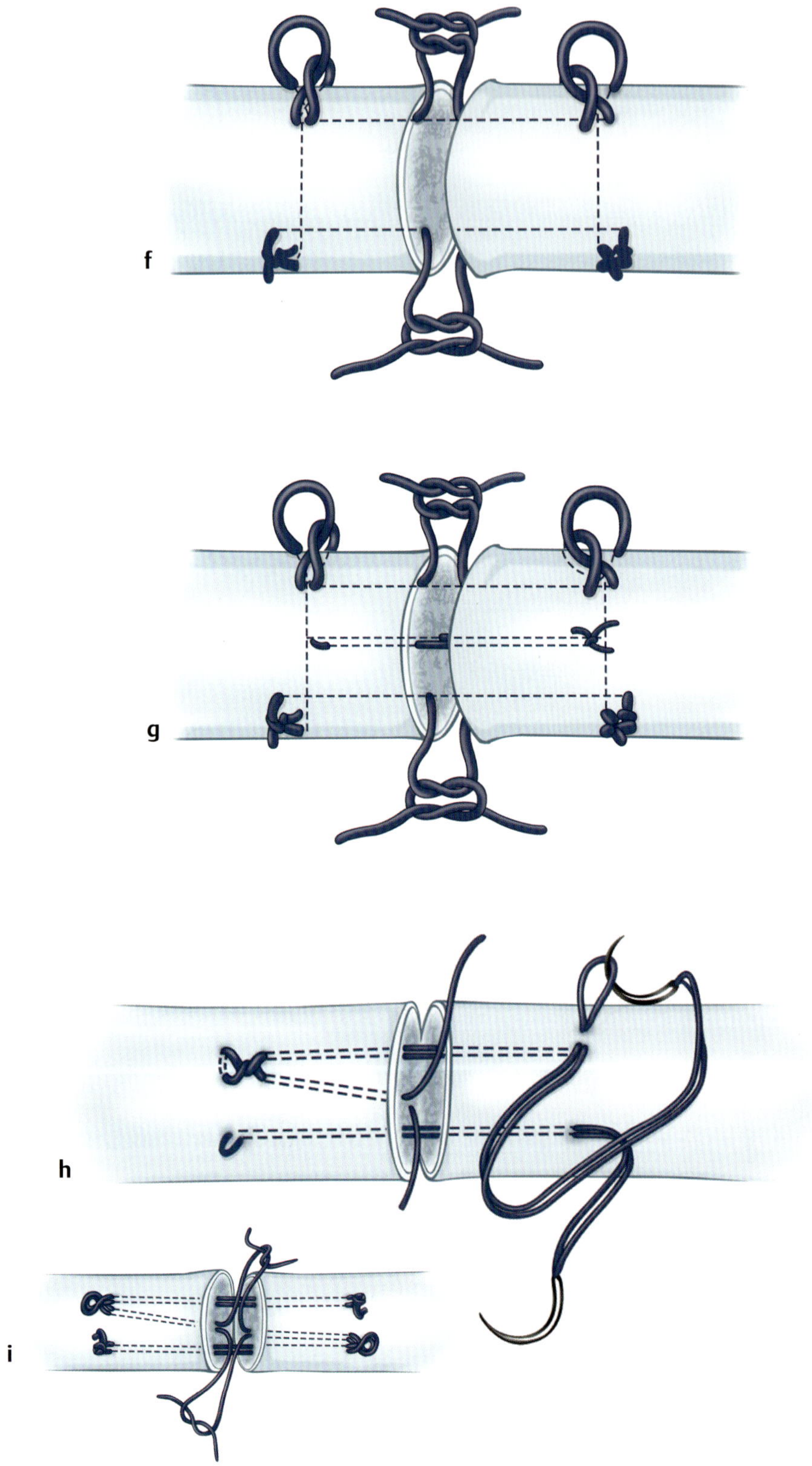

Fig. 9.1 (*continued*) **(f)** Strickland's "double grasp" modification of the Kirchmayer-Kessler technique (two-strand). **(g)** "Double grasp" technique with an additional rectangular mattress suture (four-strand). **(h,i)** Tsuge's loop technique: Double loop (six-strand)(*continued*).

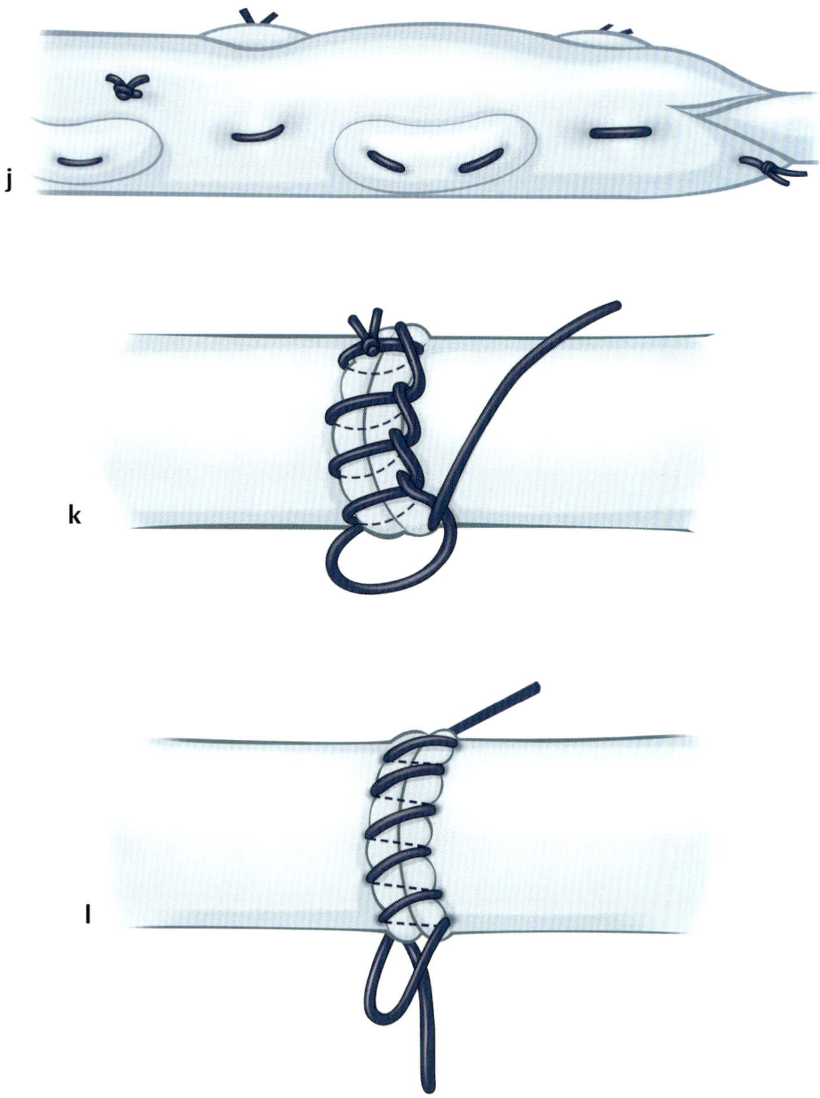

Fig. 9.1 (*continued*) **(j)** Pulvertaft technique: The tendon stumps are connected in a braided pattern—excellent tensile strength, allows early active mobilization. **(k,l)** Epitenon sutures: Epitenon sutures add considerable tensile strength to the tendon repair. They also smooth the contour of the tendon repair, thereby improving gliding properties. The two most commonly used patterns are running stitches (5–0) or interlocking sutures (5–0). A modification is a crisscross pattern that may increase tensile strength.

Chapter 10

Techniques of Vascular Repair

Several techniques are used for vascular repair. Best results are usually achieved with familiar techniques. Four techniques are described below:

- End-to-end anastomosis, 180-degree technique
- End-to-side anastomosis
- End-to-end anastomosis, 120-degree technique
- End-to-end anastomosis, “back-wall-first” technique

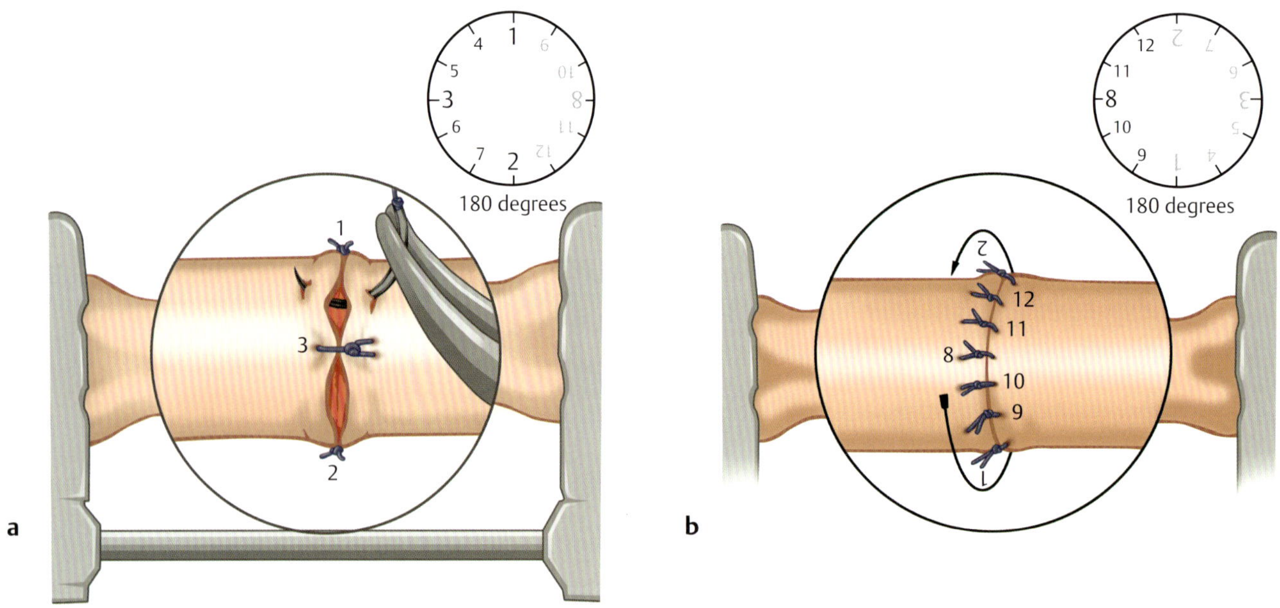

Fig. 10.1 End-to-end anastomosis, 180-degree technique. **(a)** Two corner sutures are placed 180 degrees apart (*1,2*). A third stitch (*3*) is placed equidistant from stitches 1 and 2. Stitches 4 through 7 complete the front wall sutures. **(b)** The vessel is then flipped over, and a stitch is placed in position 8. Sutures 9 through 12 complete the procedure.

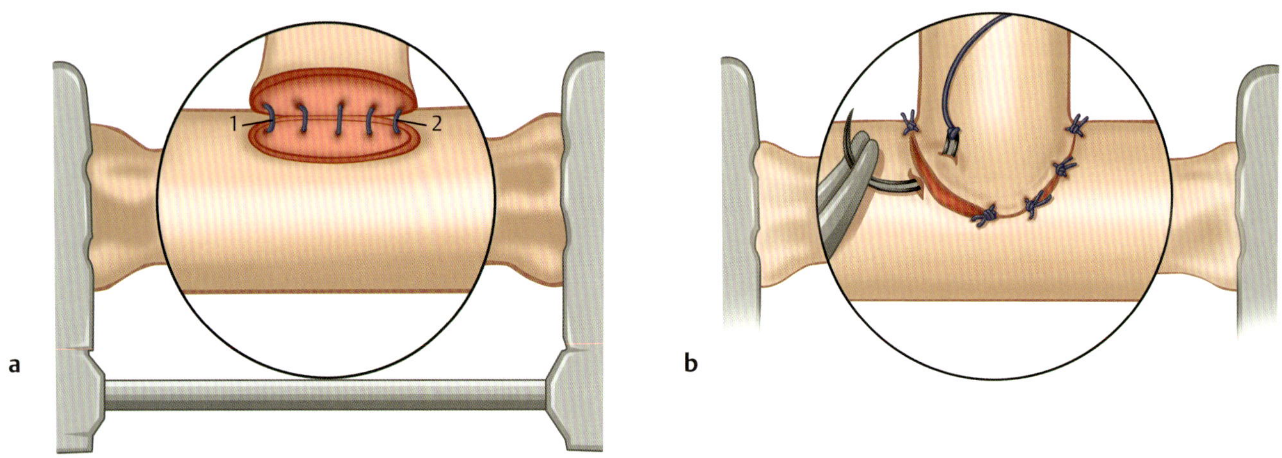

Fig. 10.2 End-to-side anastomosis. **(a)** Two corner sutures are placed 180 degrees apart (*1,2*). **(b)** Interrupted stitches (in larger vessels, running suture) are used for the vessel wall, with the more difficult access to complete the most difficult part first. Rinsing of the vessel lumen with heparinized saline solution ensures proper visualization of intima. Inspection of the correct placement of stitches is critical upon completion of the anterior wall. Trick: place two sutures close together at either side of the corner sutures to prevent leakage from the angles. Take great care not to grasp the intima of the recipient vessel.

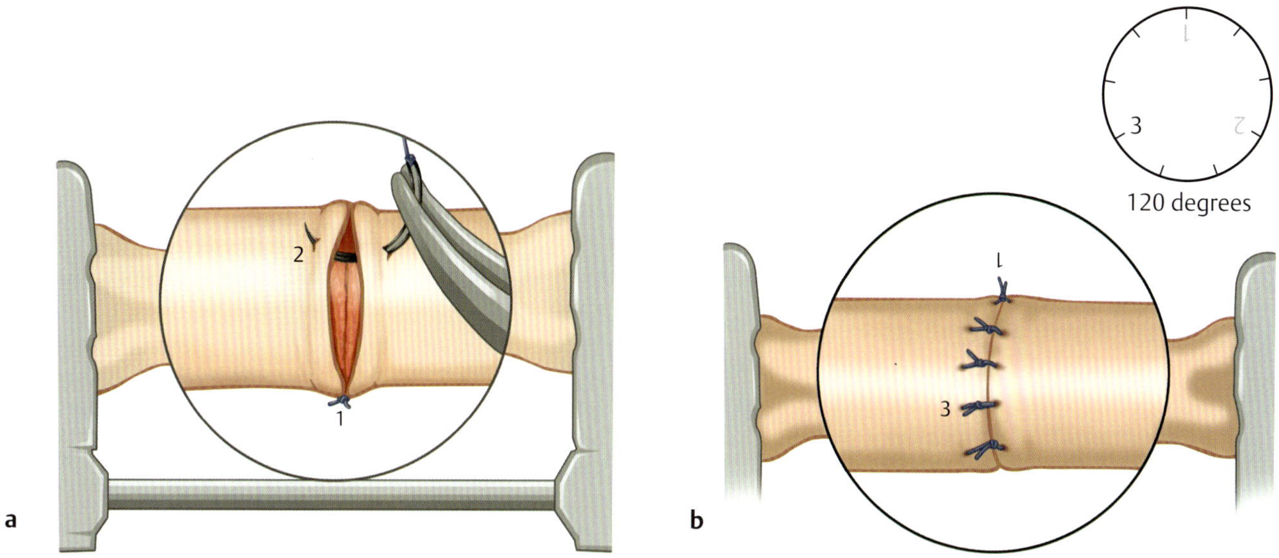

Fig. 10.3 End-to-end anastomosis, 120-degree technique. **(a)** Two corner sutures are placed at a 120-degree position on the front wall. The vessel is flipped over. A third stitch is added 120 degrees from the first, for the segmental completion of the back wall. **(b)** The vessel is flipped again to complete the front wall.

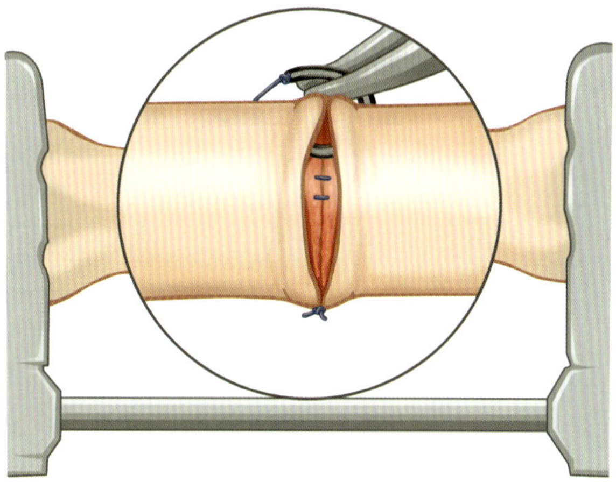

Fig. 10.4 End-to-end anastomosis, back-wall-first technique. One everting suture is placed in the center of the back of the back wall. The back wall is subsequently completed under vision. Completion of the anastomosis is achieved by working from both sides toward the center of the vessel. The vessel is not flipped over during the anastomosis.

Chapter 11

Techniques of Nerve Repair

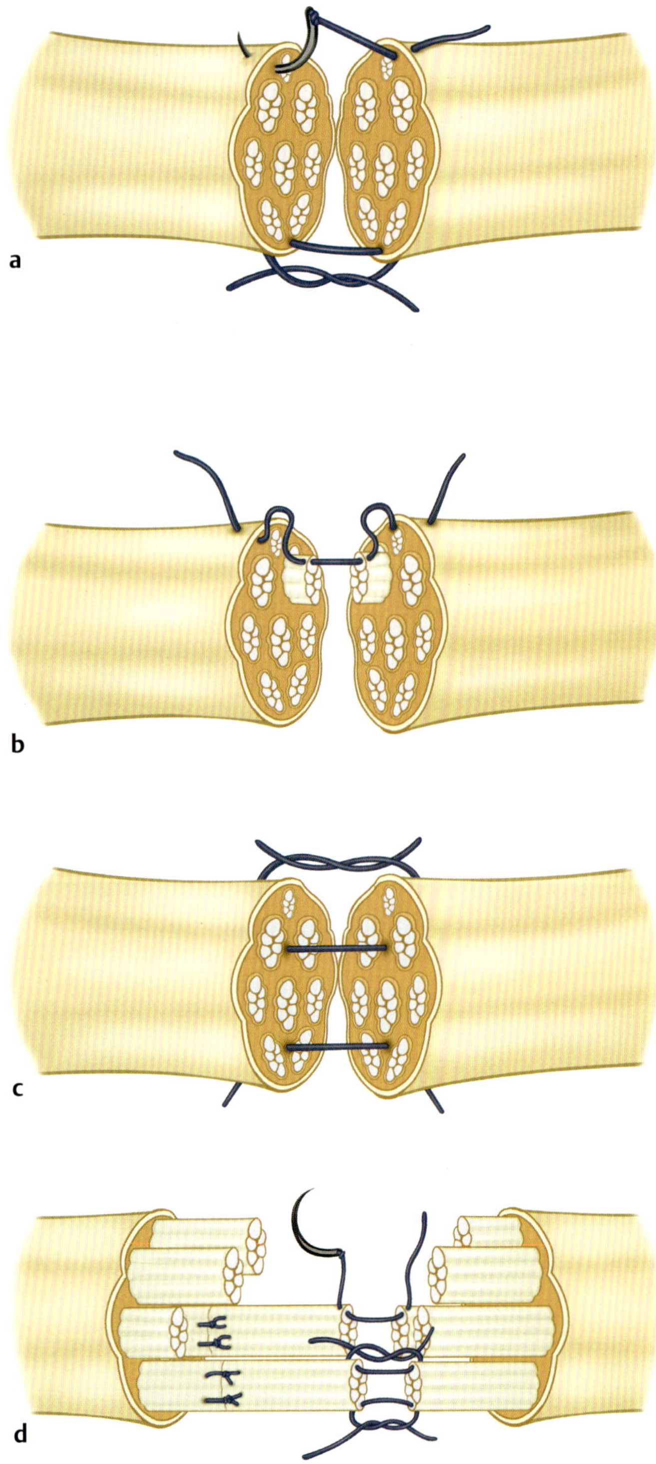

Fig. 11.1 Techniques of nerve repair.

(a) Epineural suture

- By far the most common repair in smaller peripheral nerves
- Trim edges perpendicular to long axis of the nerve
- Mobilize proximal and distal nerve segments
- Use microscope to visually enhance precision
- Use 180-degree technique to guarantee maximal coaptation
- Avoid tension at the neurorrhaphy site at all costs
- Use the smallest suture possible to achieve tension-free, stable coaptation
- Avoid focal increase of pressure on the suture line to prevent bulging and poor alignment of the fascicle

(b) Epi-perineural suture

- Indicated in nerves with few fascicular bundles
- Allows fascicle matching techniques (visual/staining)
- Stronger suture in the epineurium of the back wall may reduce the tension on the suture line. The same goal can be achieved by using a strip of fascia/tendon that is anchored to the back wall of both nerve stumps
- Maximize alignment of nerve stumps and simultaneous sealing of the epineurial envelope
- Avoid focal increase of pressure on the suture line to prevent bulging and/or poor alignment of the fascicles

(c) Nerve graft donor sites

- Sural nerve
- Medial antebrachial cutaneous nerve
- Lateral antebrachial cutaneous nerve
- Avoid tension on grafts
- Venous conduit—short peripheral defects (less than 2 cm)
- Nerve allograft (i.e., Axogen™)
- Fibrin glue may be used in place of sutures in selected cases

(d) Individual fascicular suture

- Indicated only in nerve grafting and in most distal targets where differentiation can be assured (i.e., motor branch of median nerve just before entry into the muscle; otherwise, too much suture material is brought into the nerve)
- Secure well-perfused soft tissue envelope in case of nerve grafting
- Use 10–0 or maximum 9–0 for exact neurorrhaphy

Part III

Treatment Algorithms

Chapter 12

Bones

Distal Phalanx

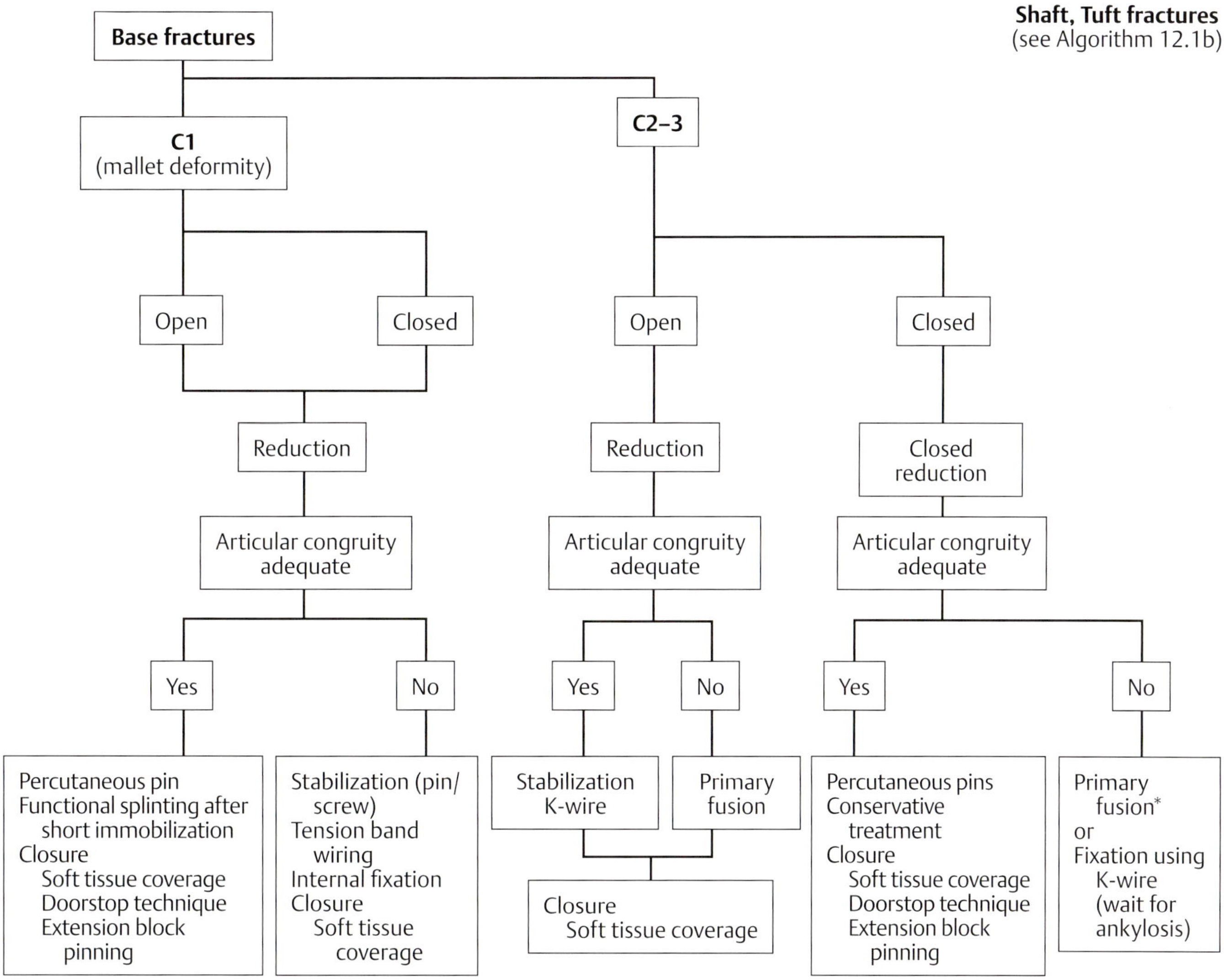

*Primary fusion if attempt at joint reconstruction is not likely to restore pain-free motion or if patient desires definitive solution

Algorithm 12.1a

Parameters in decision-making	Additional options or guidelines	Warnings, precautions, or pitfalls	Emphasis on a particular waypoint

Distal Phalanx

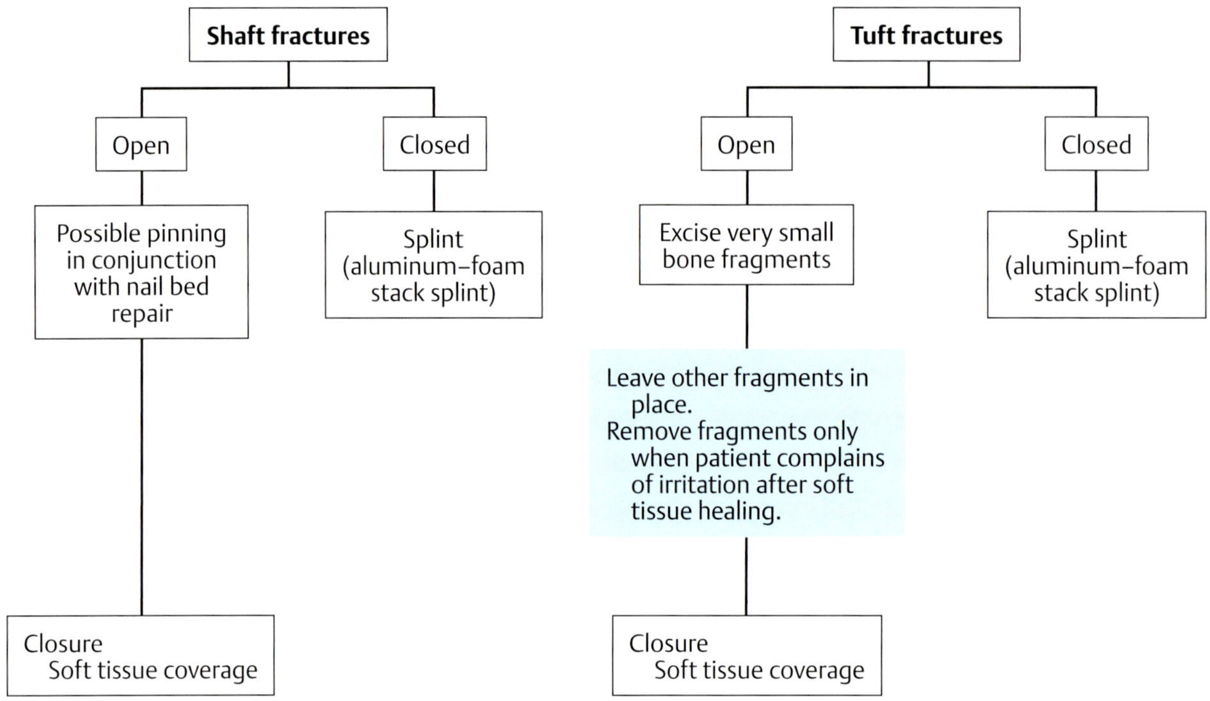

Algorithm 12.1b

Parameters in decision-making	Additional options or guidelines	Warnings, precautions, or pitfalls	Emphasis on a particular waypoint

Metacarpals, Proximal and Middle Phalanges

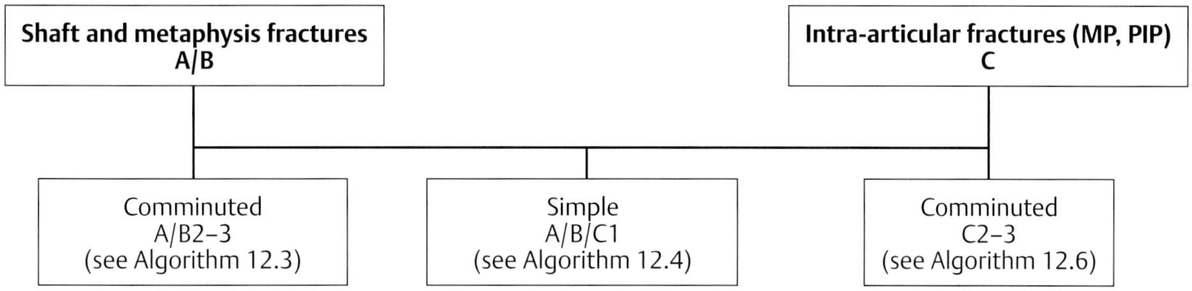

Algorithm 12.2

Metacarpals, Proximal and Middle Phalanges

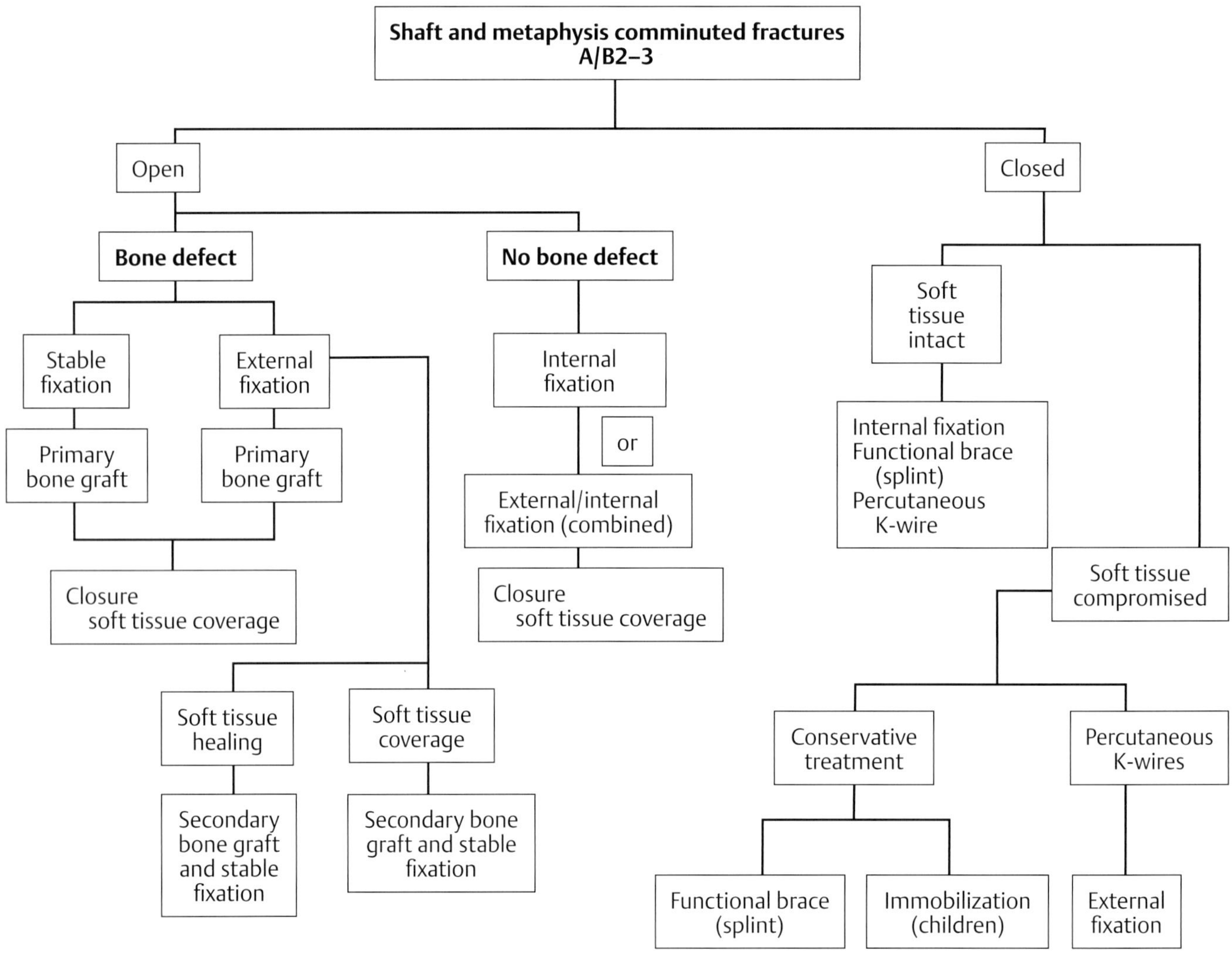

Algorithm 12.3

Metacarpals, Proximal and Middle Phalanges

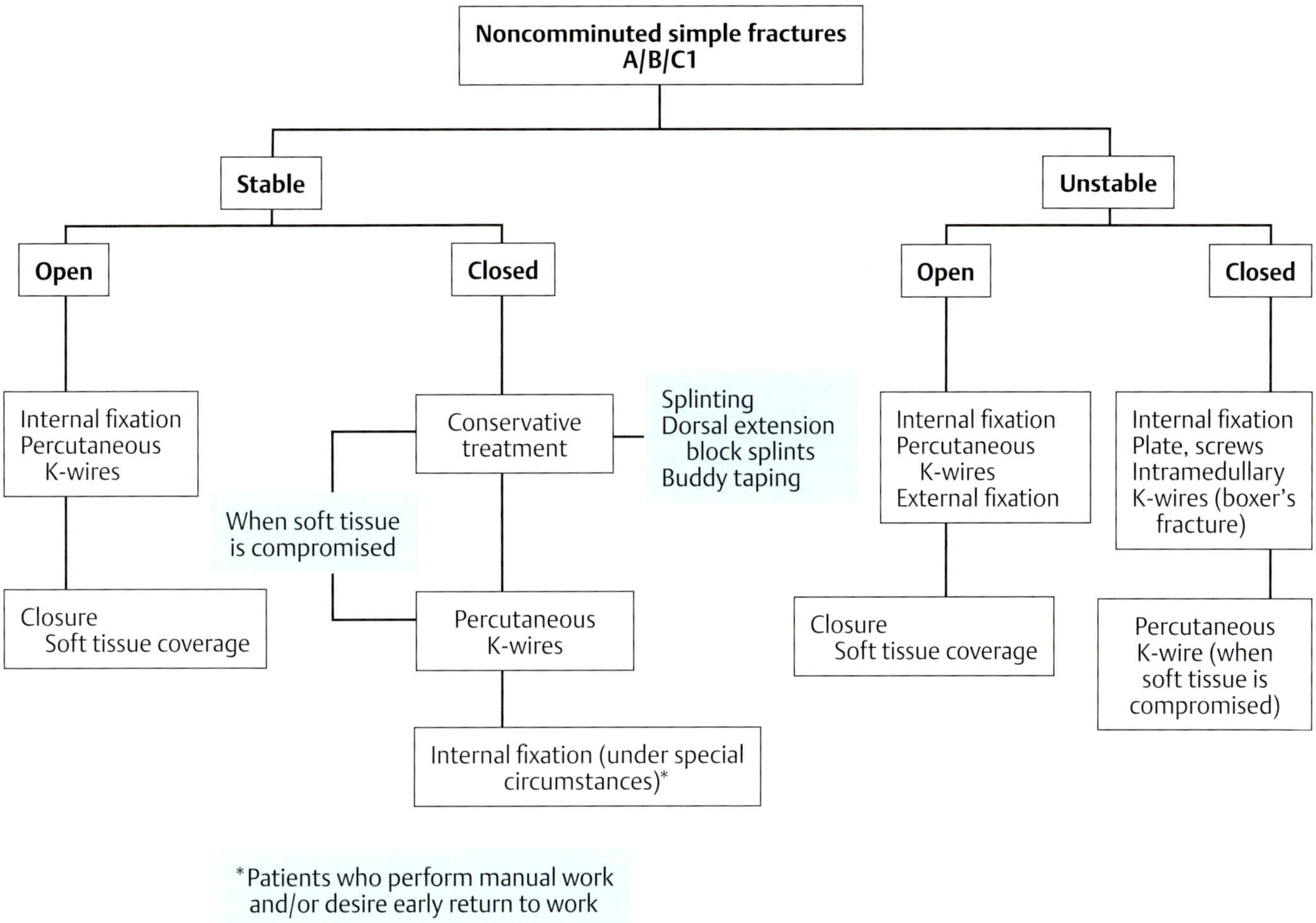

Algorithm 12.4

Parameters in decision-making	Additional options or guidelines	Warnings, precautions, or pitfalls	Emphasis on a particular waypoint

Metacarpals, Proximal and Middle Phalanges

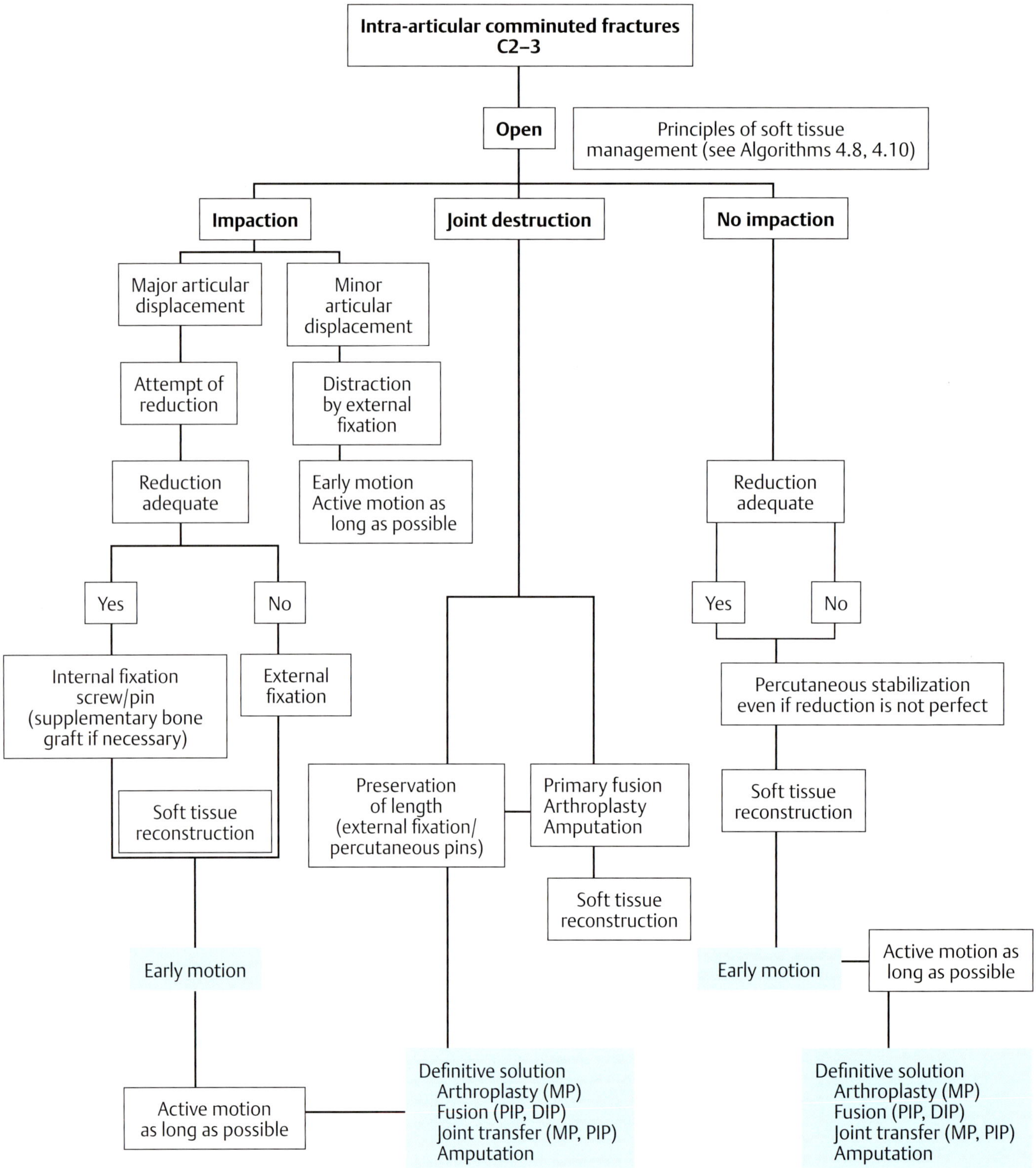

Algorithm 12.5

Parameters in decision-making	Additional options or guidelines	Warnings, precautions, or pitfalls	Emphasis on a particular waypoint

Metacarpals, Proximal and Middle Phalanges

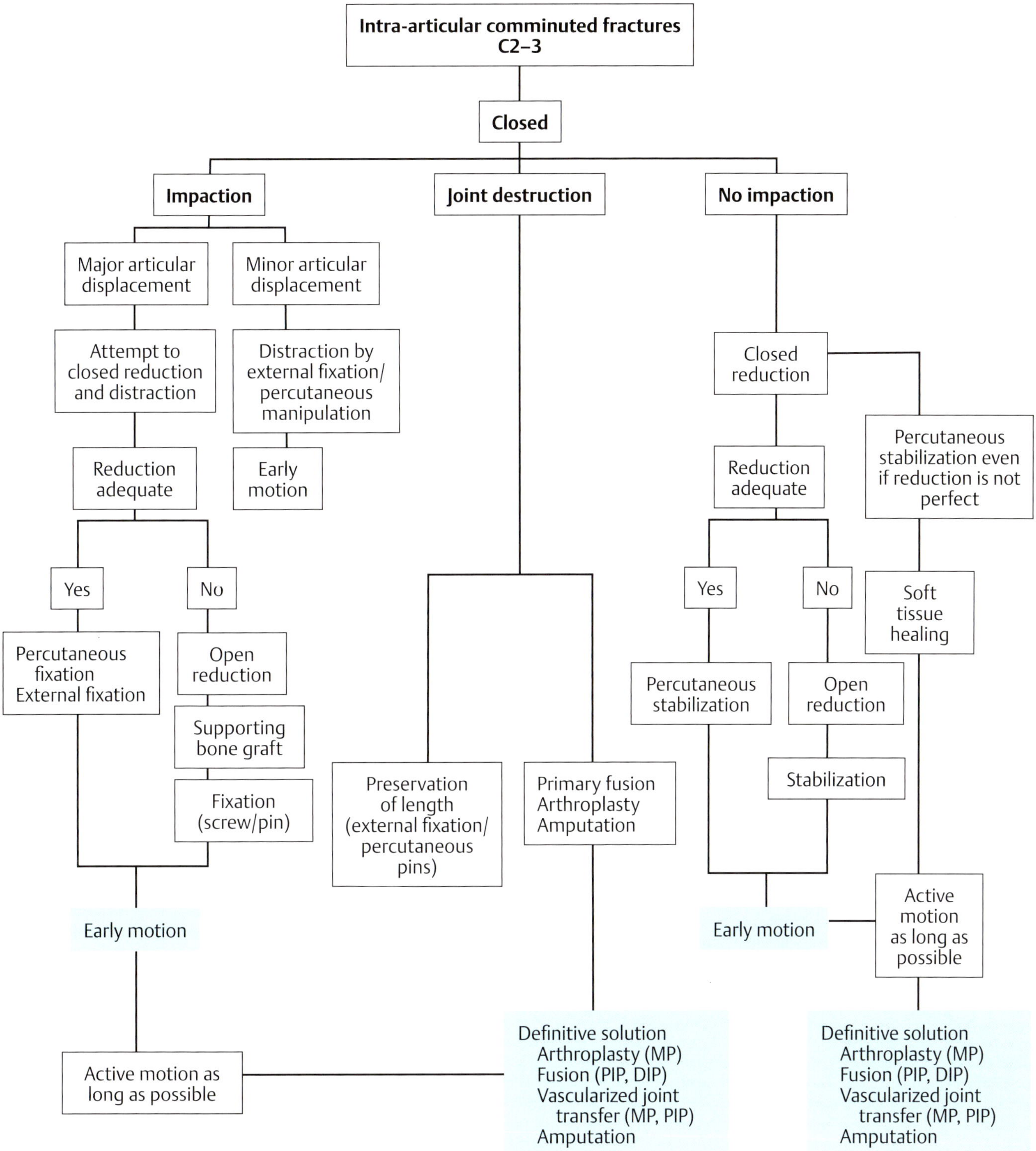

Algorithm 12.6

Parameters in decision-making	Additional options or guidelines	Warnings, precautions, or pitfalls	Emphasis on a particular waypoint

Carpus

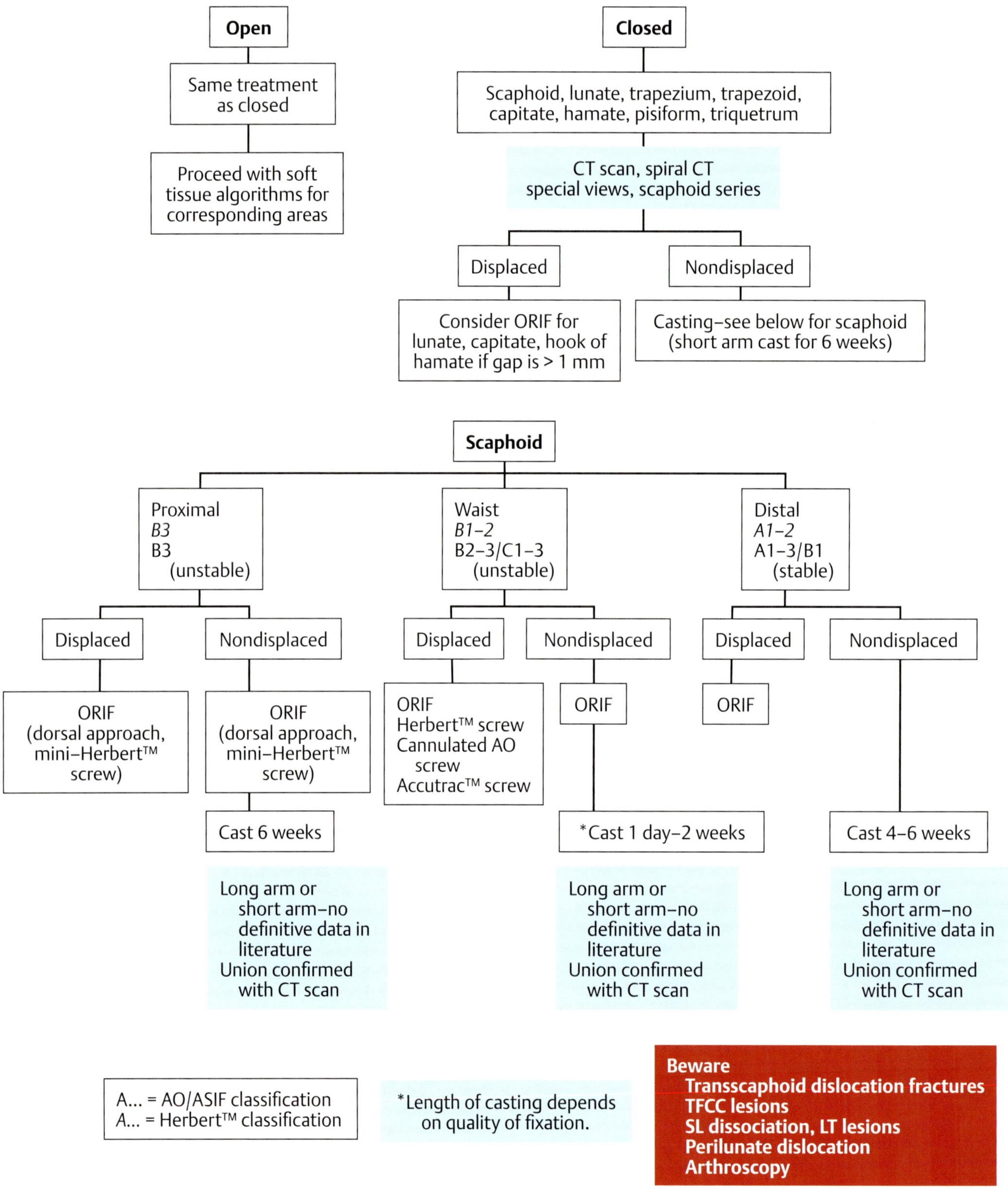

Algorithm 12.7

Parameters in decision-making	Additional options or guidelines	Warnings, precautions, or pitfalls	Emphasis on a particular waypoint

Radius

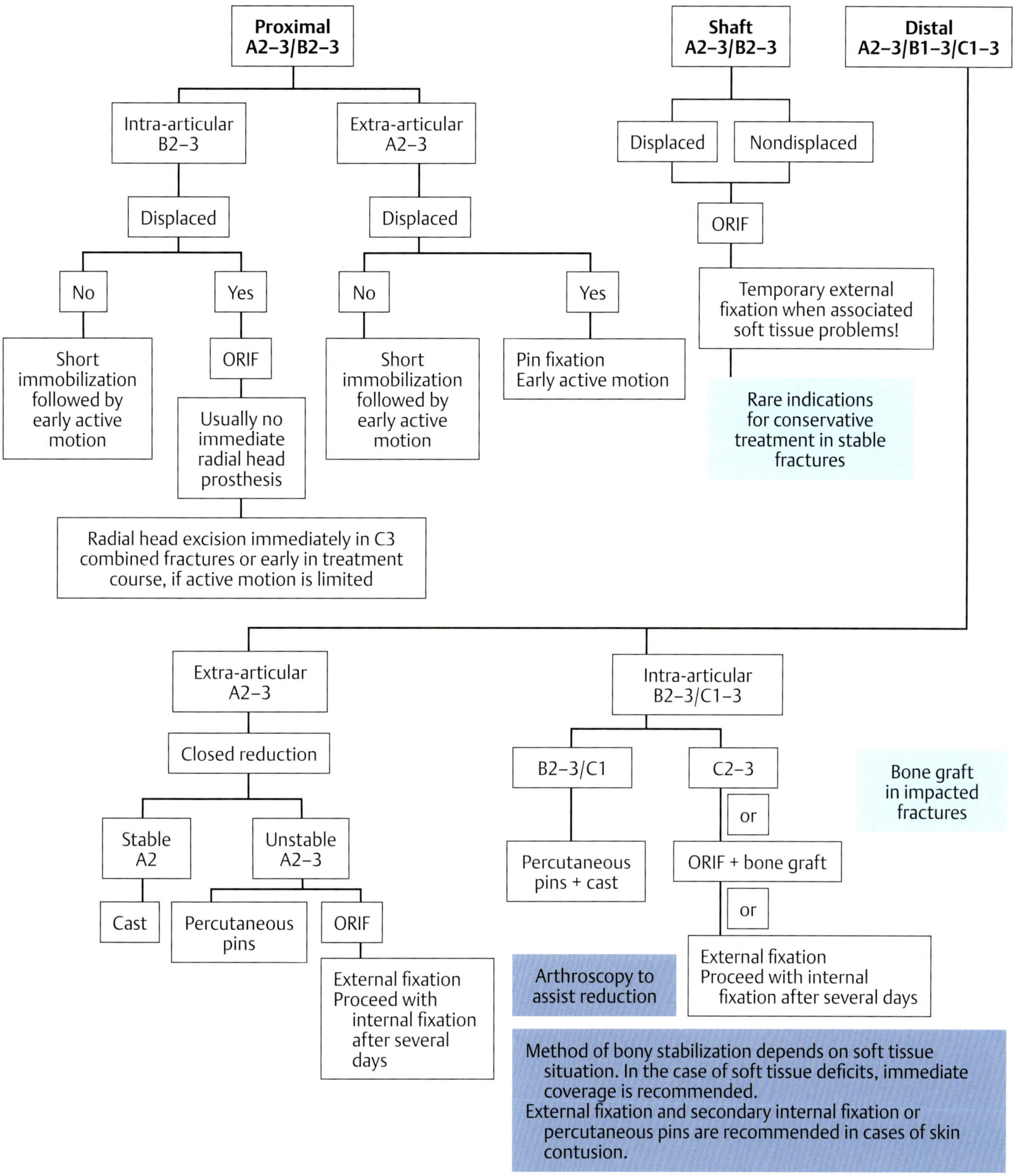

Algorithm 12.8

Parameters in decision-making	Additional options or guidelines	Warnings, precautions, or pitfalls	Emphasis on a particular waypoint

Ulna

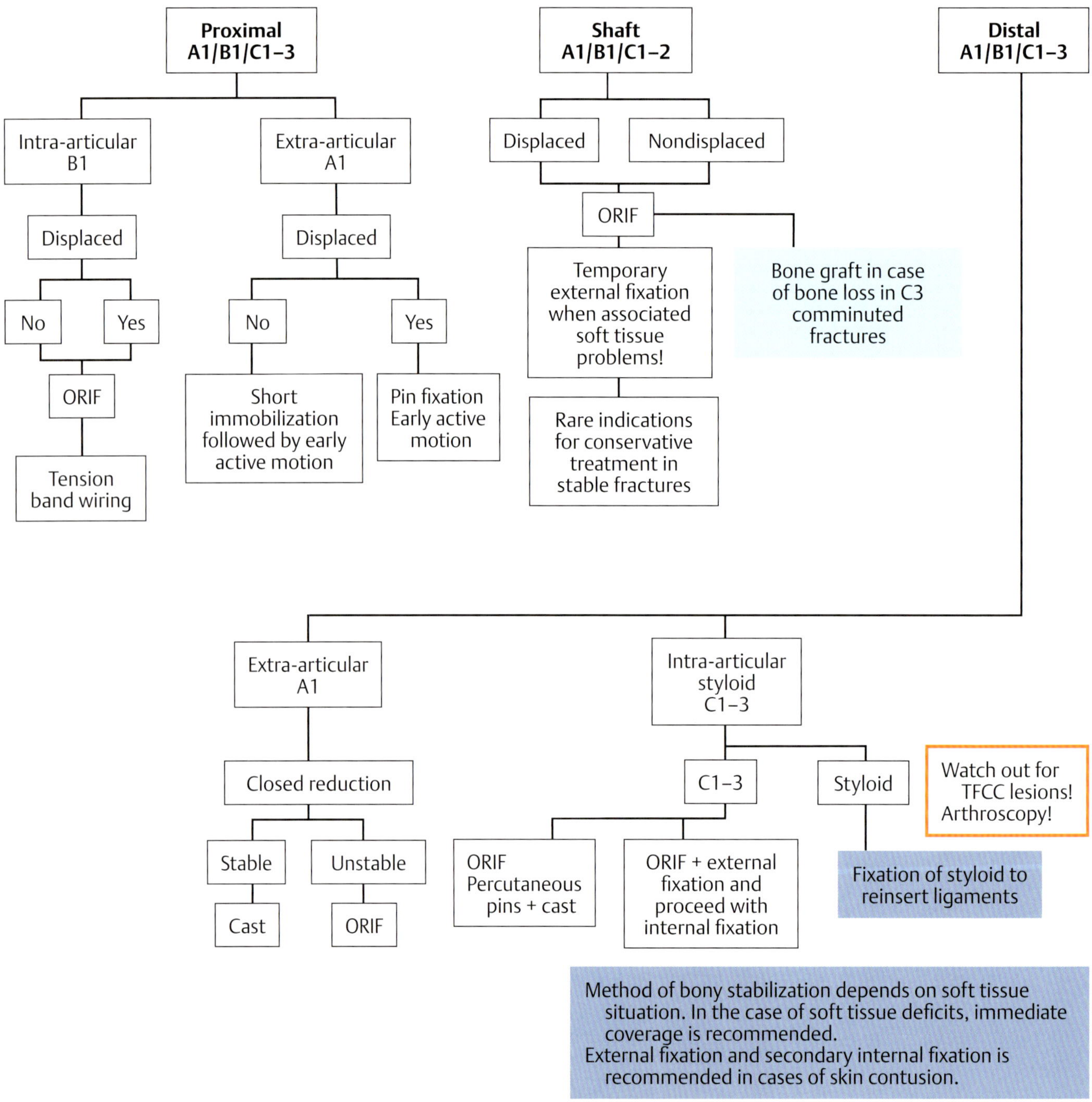

Algorithm 12.9

Parameters in decision-making	Additional options or guidelines	Warnings, precautions, or pitfalls	Emphasis on a particular waypoint

Both-Forearm Fractures

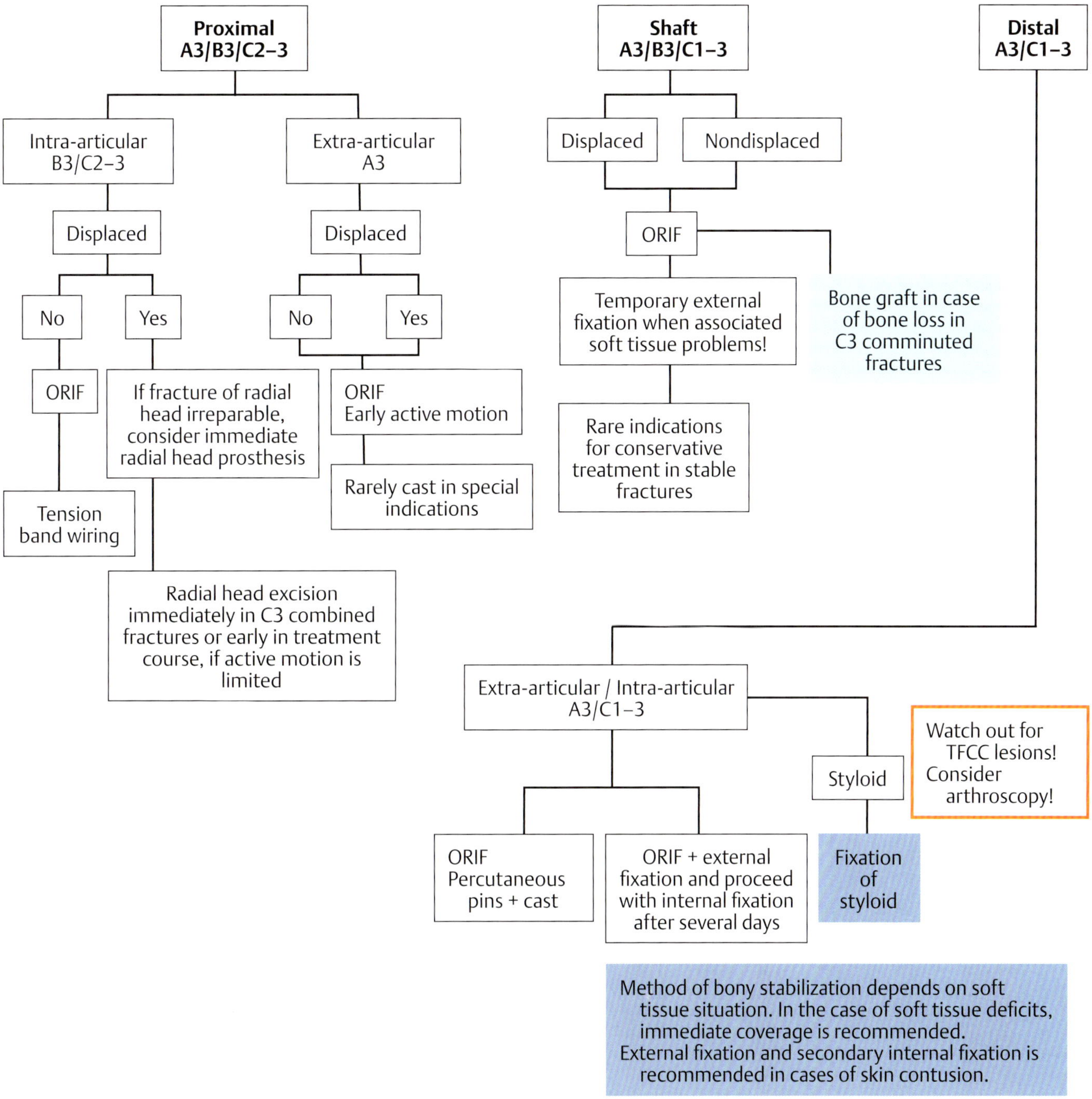

Algorithm 12.10

Parameters in decision-making	Additional options or guidelines	Warnings, precautions, or pitfalls	Emphasis on a particular waypoint

Humerus

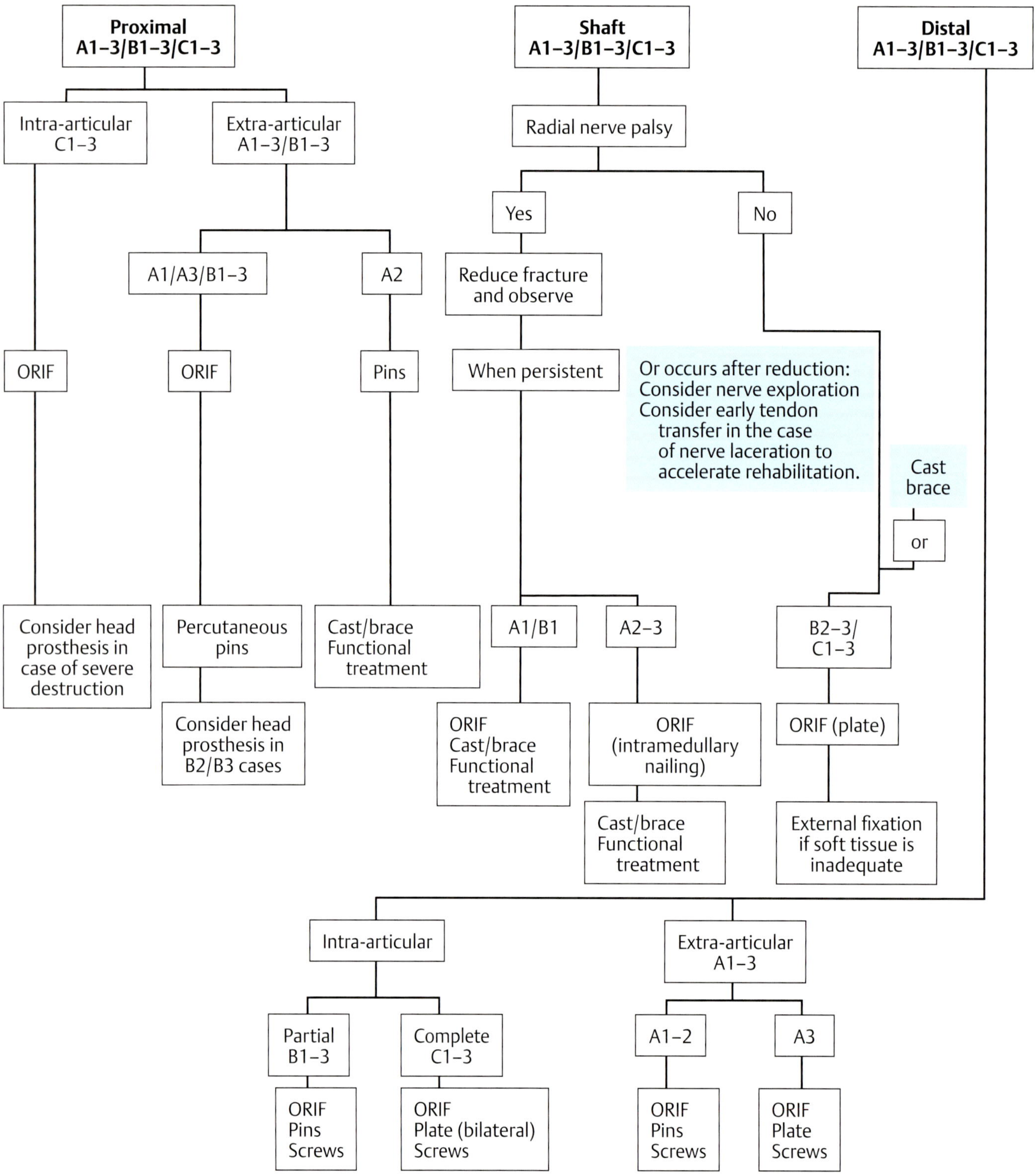

Algorithm 12.11

Parameters in decision-making	Additional options or guidelines	Warnings, precautions, or pitfalls	Emphasis on a particular waypoint

Scapula

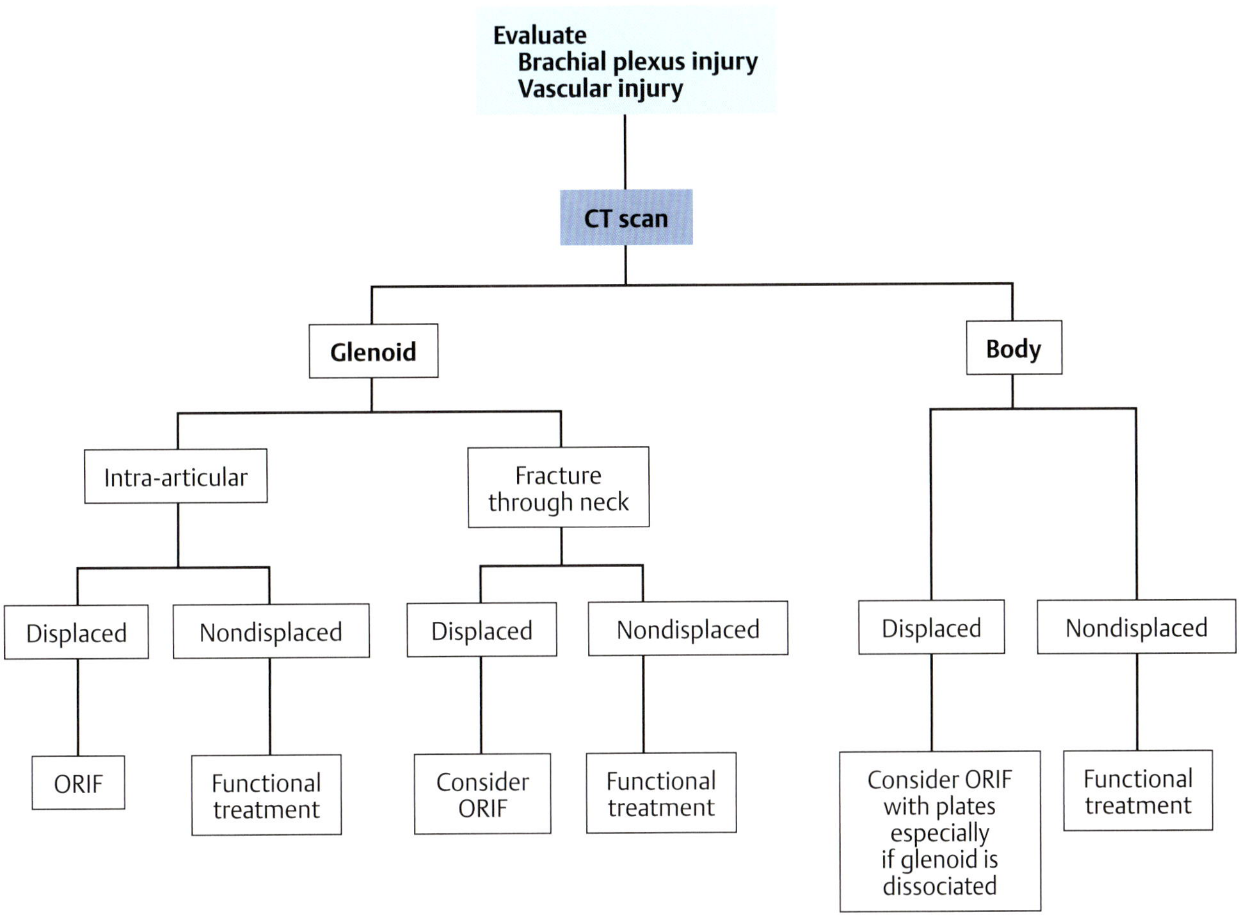

Algorithm 12.12

Parameters in decision-making	Additional options or guidelines	Warnings, precautions, or pitfalls	Emphasis on a particular waypoint

Chapter 13

Ligaments

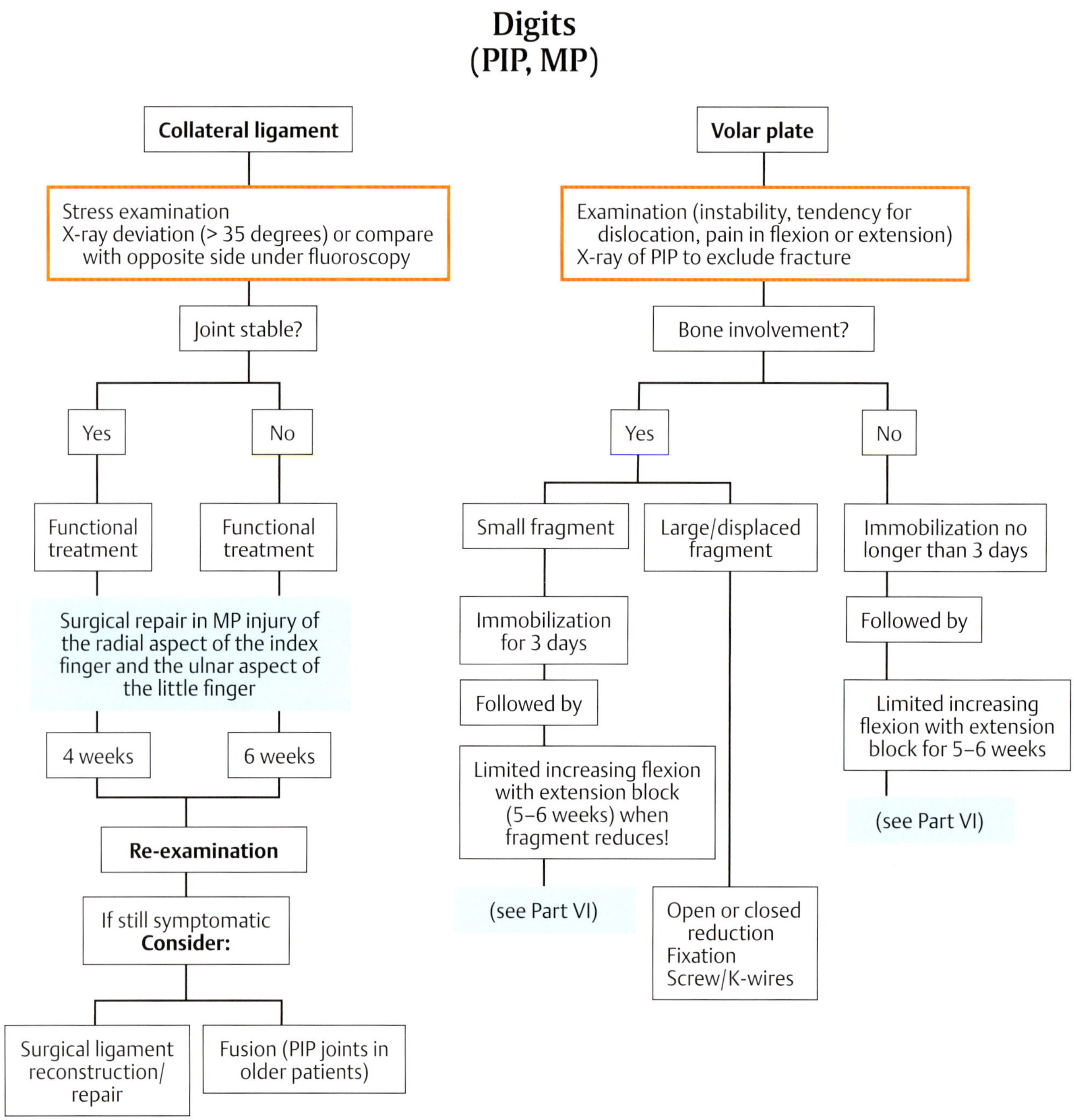

Algorithm 13.1

Parameters in decision-making	Additional options or guidelines	Warnings, precautions, or pitfalls	Emphasis on a particular waypoint

Thumb

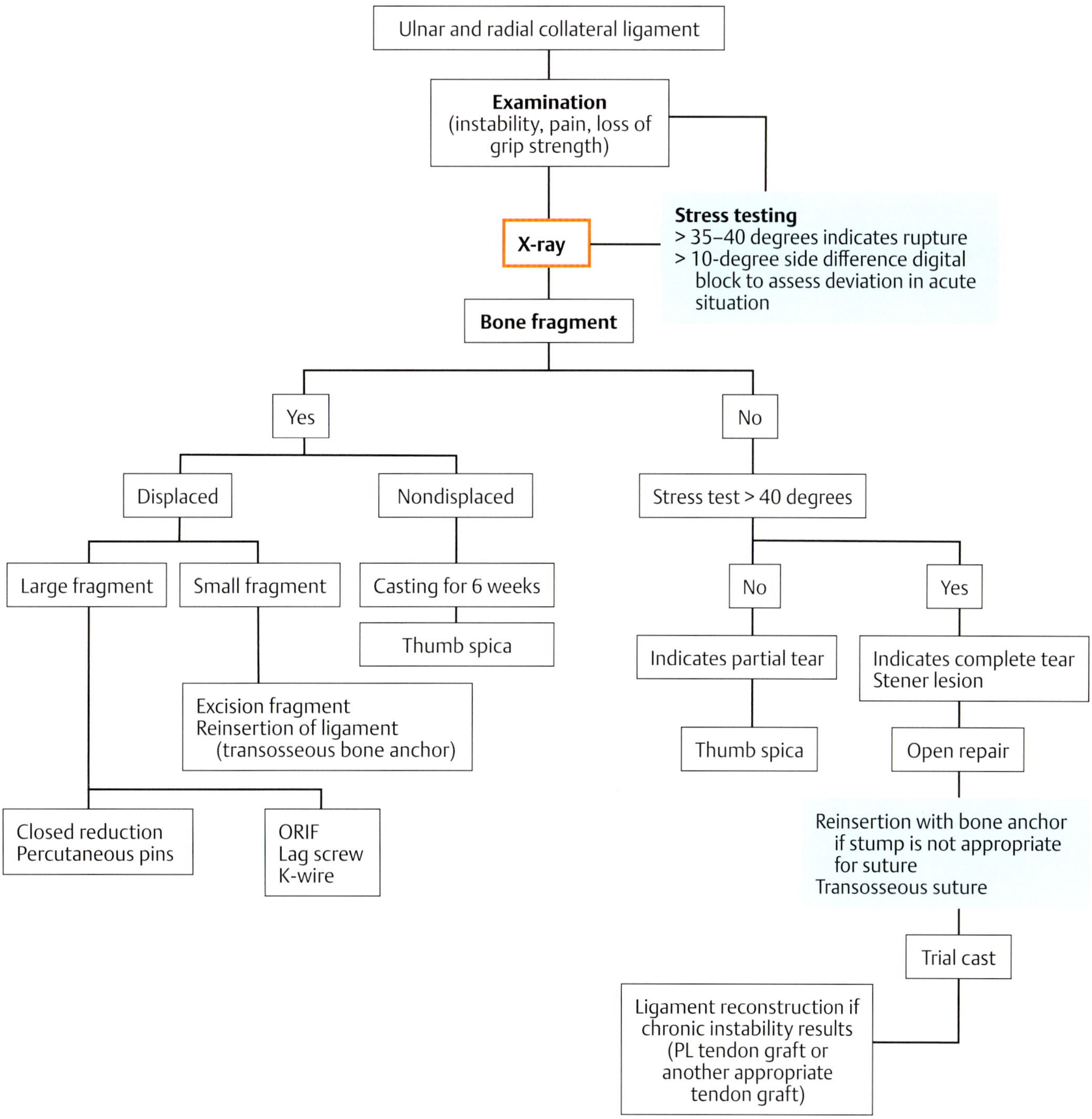

Algorithm 13.2

Parameters in decision-making	Additional options or guidelines	Warnings, precautions, or pitfalls	Emphasis on a particular waypoint

Wrist

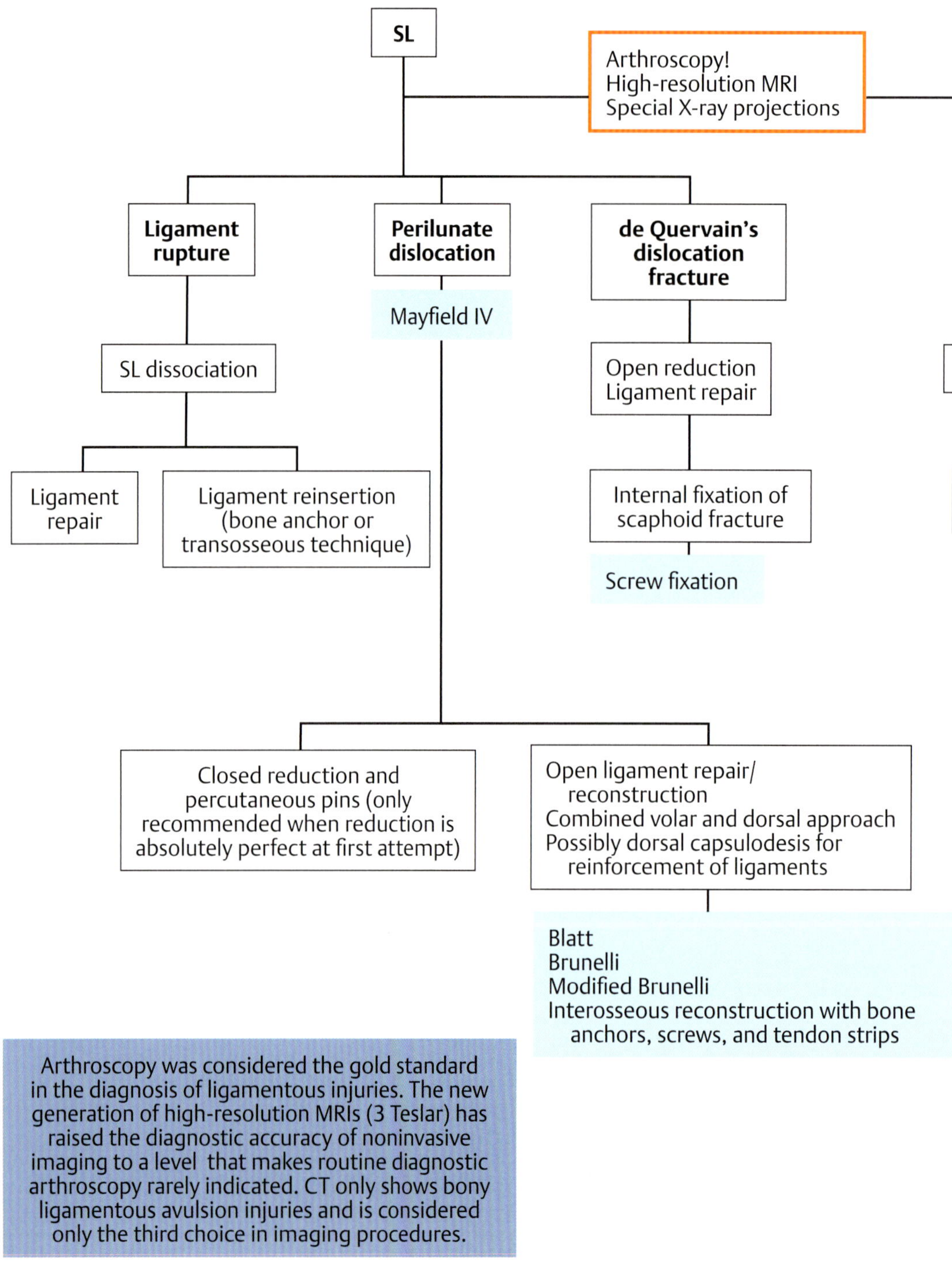

Algorithm 13.3

Parameters in decision-making	Additional options or guidelines	Warnings, precautions, or pitfalls	Emphasis on a particular waypoint

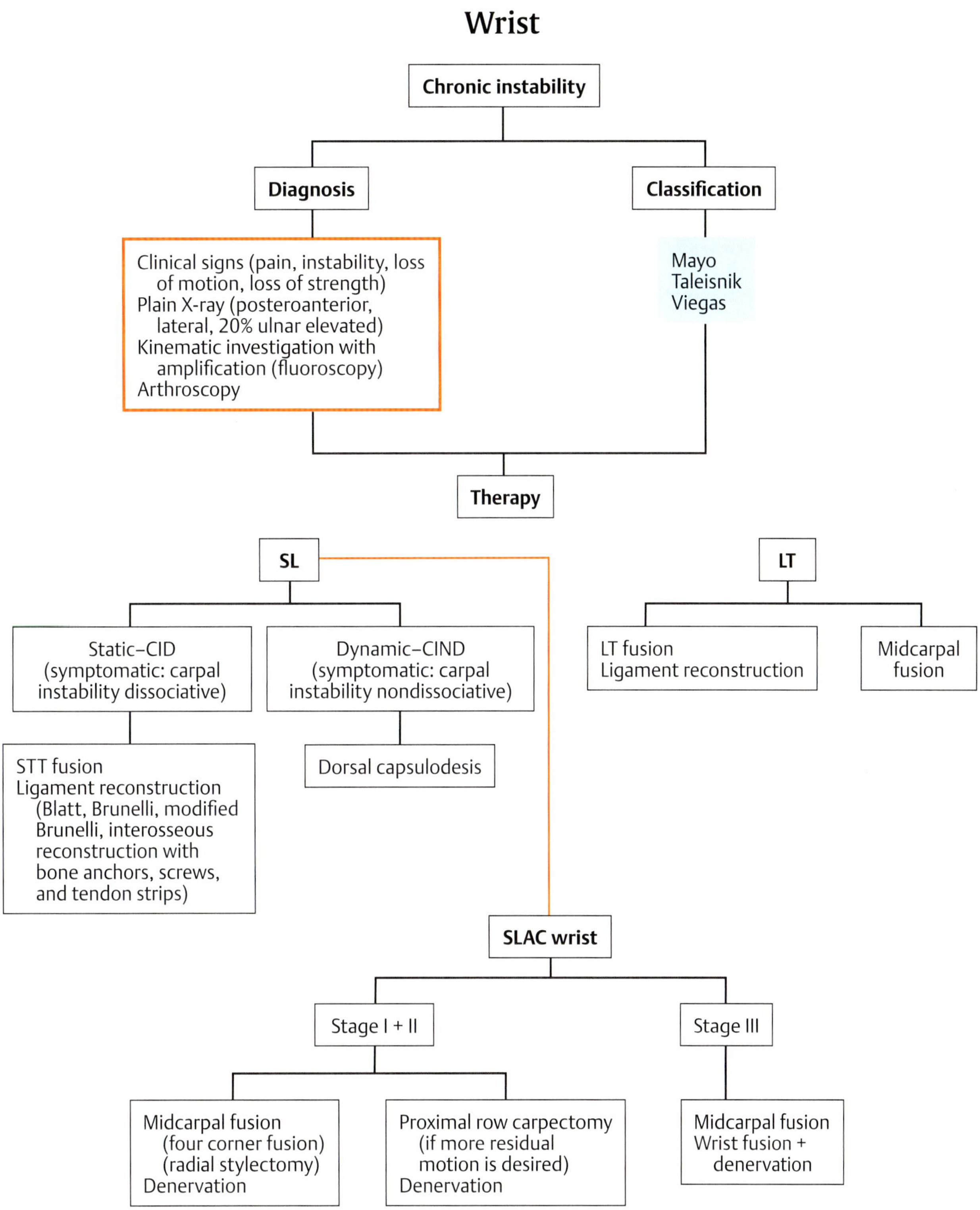

Algorithm 13.4

Parameters in decision-making	Additional options or guidelines	Warnings, precautions, or pitfalls	Emphasis on a particular waypoint

Chapter 14

Flexor Systems

Zones I and II

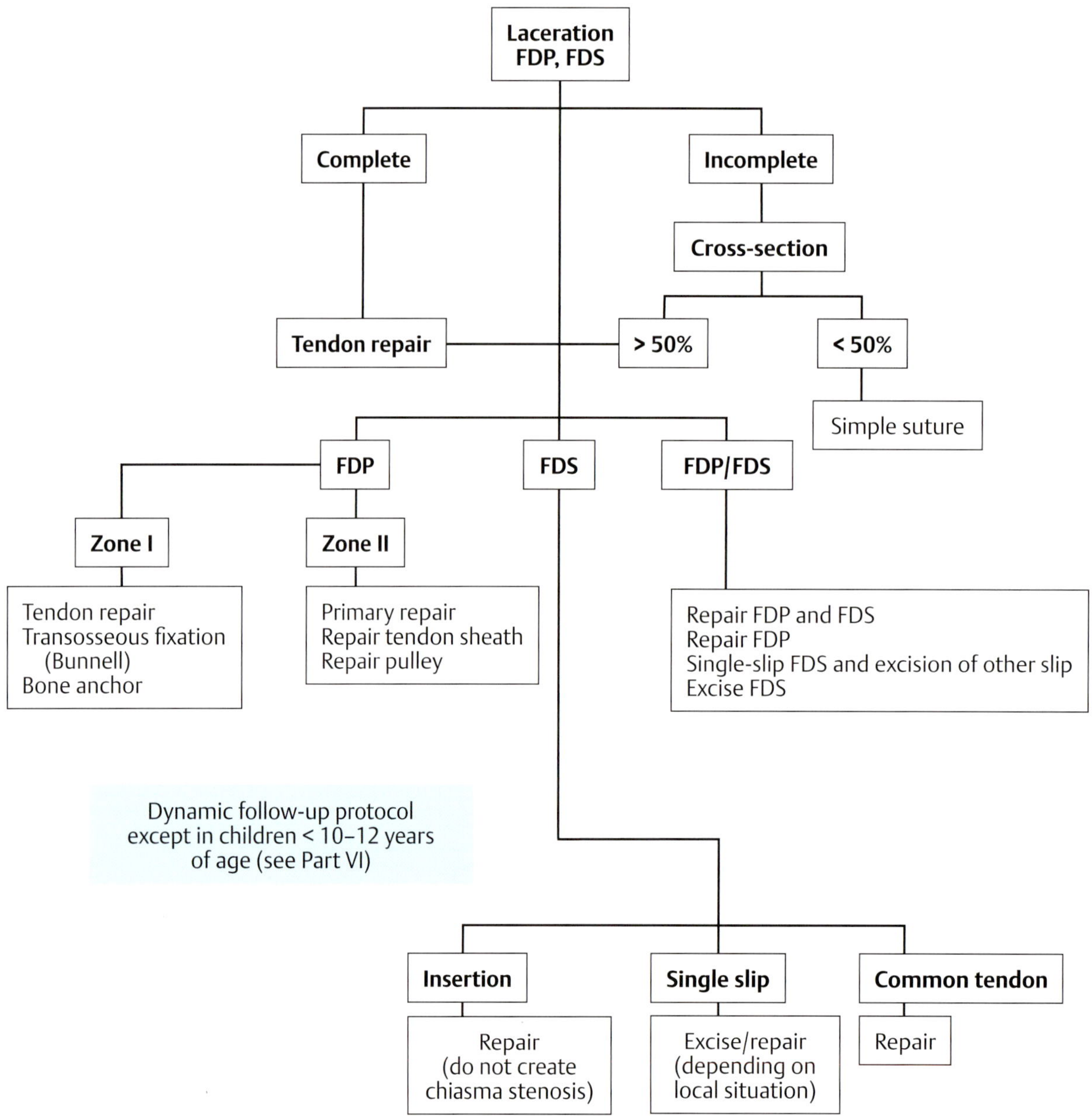

Algorithm 14.1

Parameters in decision-making	Additional options or guidelines	Warnings, precautions, or pitfalls	Emphasis on a particular waypoint

Tendon Loss, Rupture, Avulsion

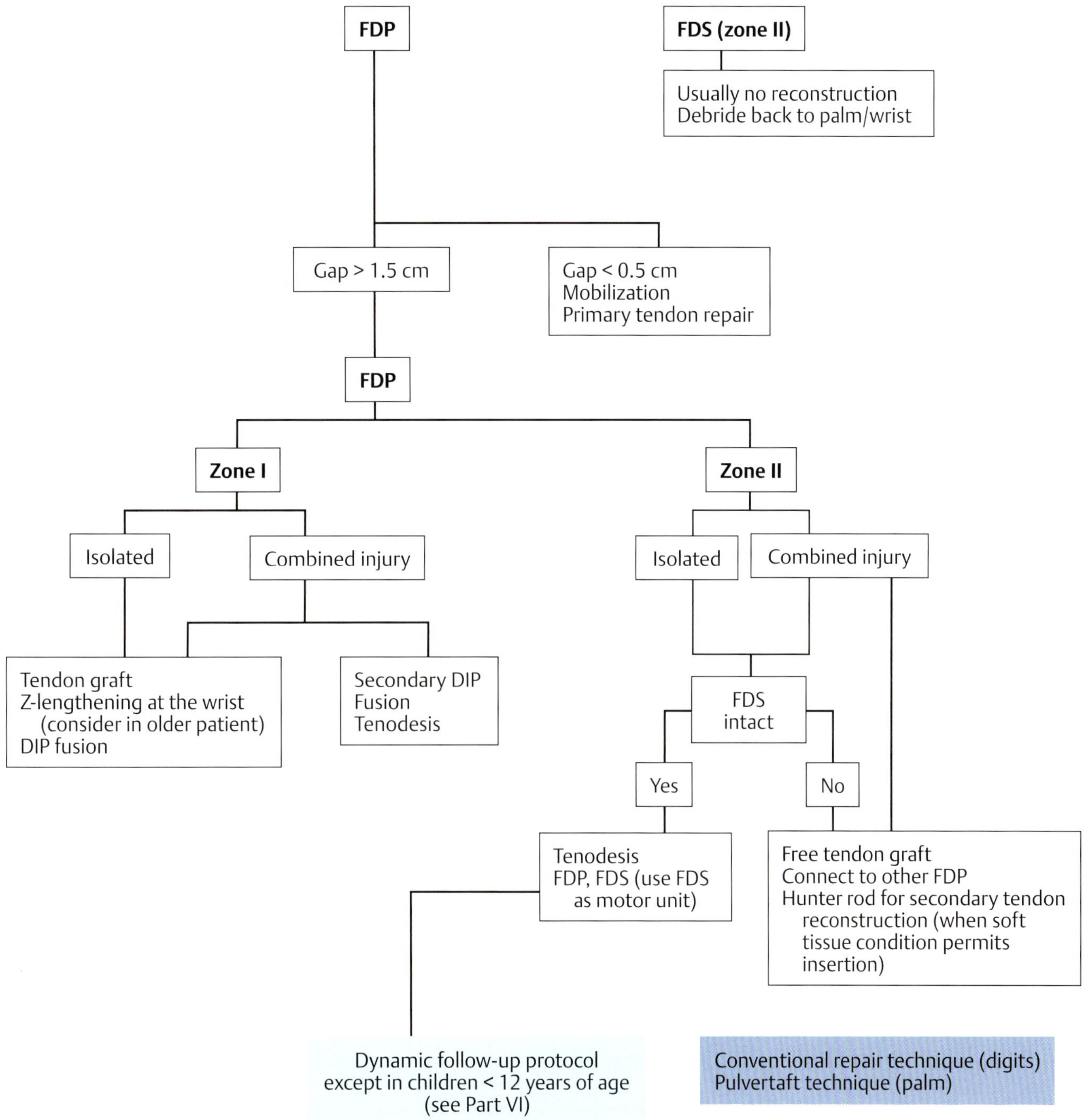

Algorithm 14.2

Parameters in decision-making	Additional options or guidelines	Warnings, precautions, or pitfalls	Emphasis on a particular waypoint

Zones III and IV

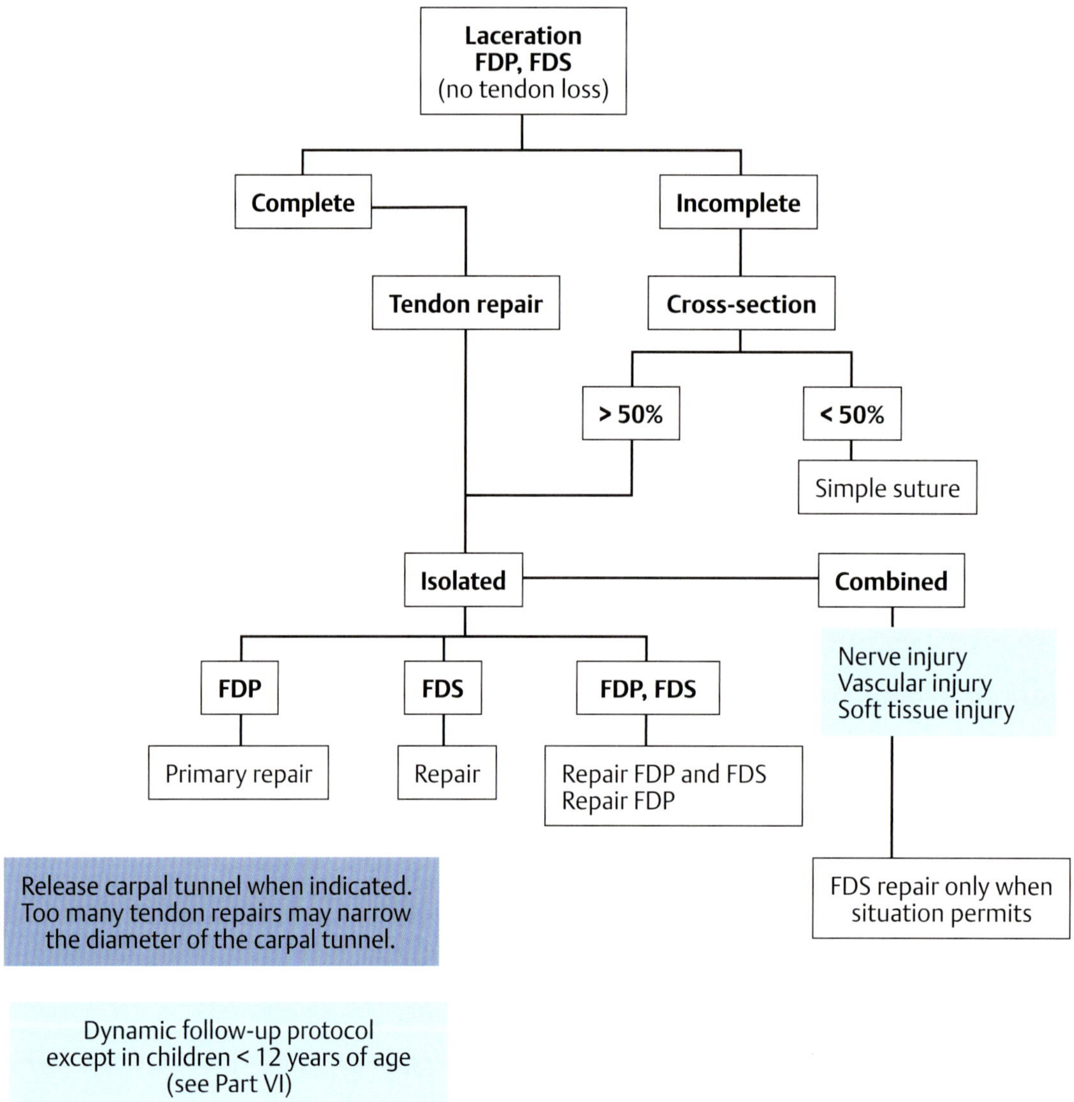

Algorithm 14.3

Parameters in decision-making	Additional options or guidelines	Warnings, precautions, or pitfalls	Emphasis on a particular waypoint

Zones III and IV

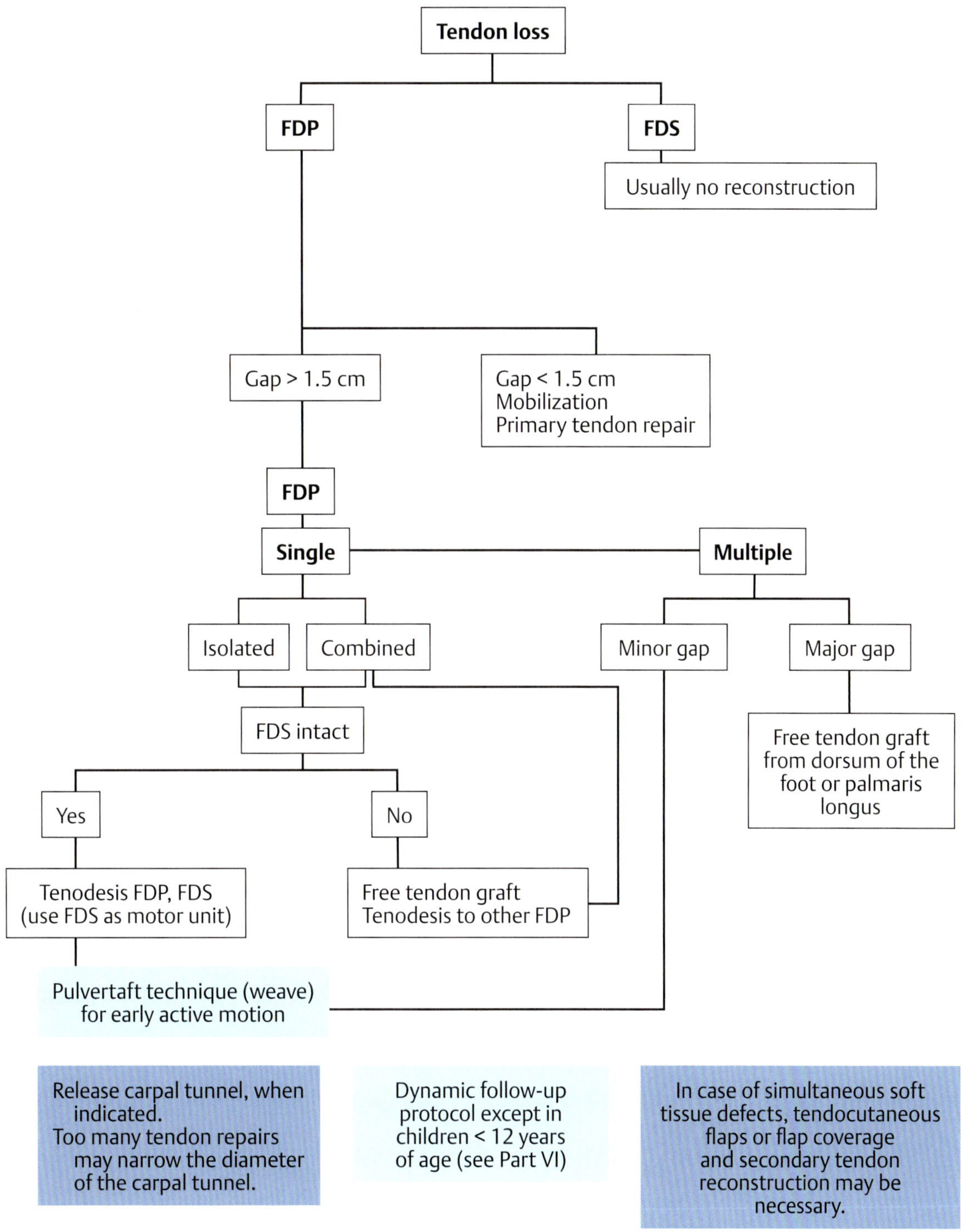

Algorithm 14.4

Parameters in decision-making	Additional options or guidelines	Warnings, precautions, or pitfalls	Emphasis on a particular waypoint

Zones V and VI (Wrist/Forearm)

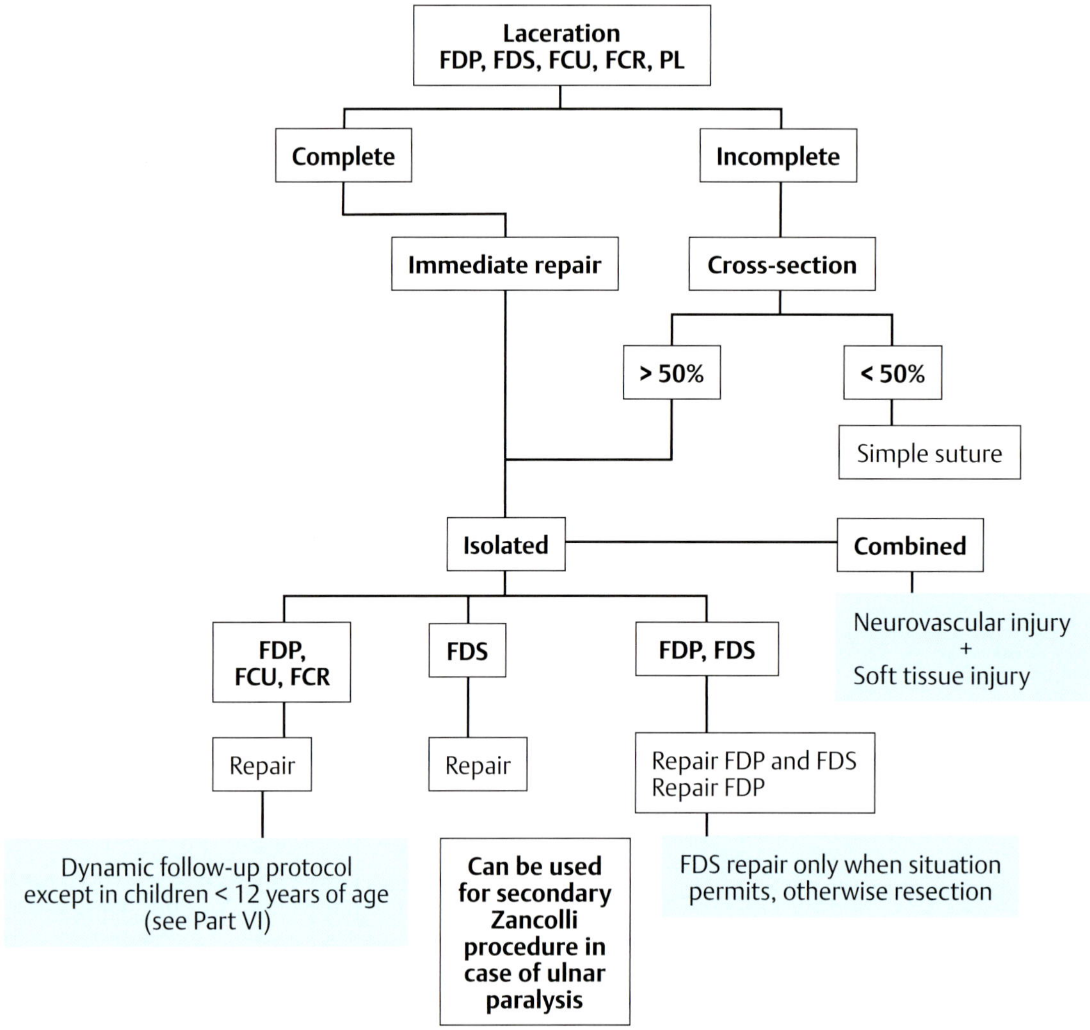

Algorithm 14.5

Parameters in decision-making	Additional options or guidelines	Warnings, precautions, or pitfalls	Emphasis on a particular waypoint

Zones V and VI (Wrist/Forearm)

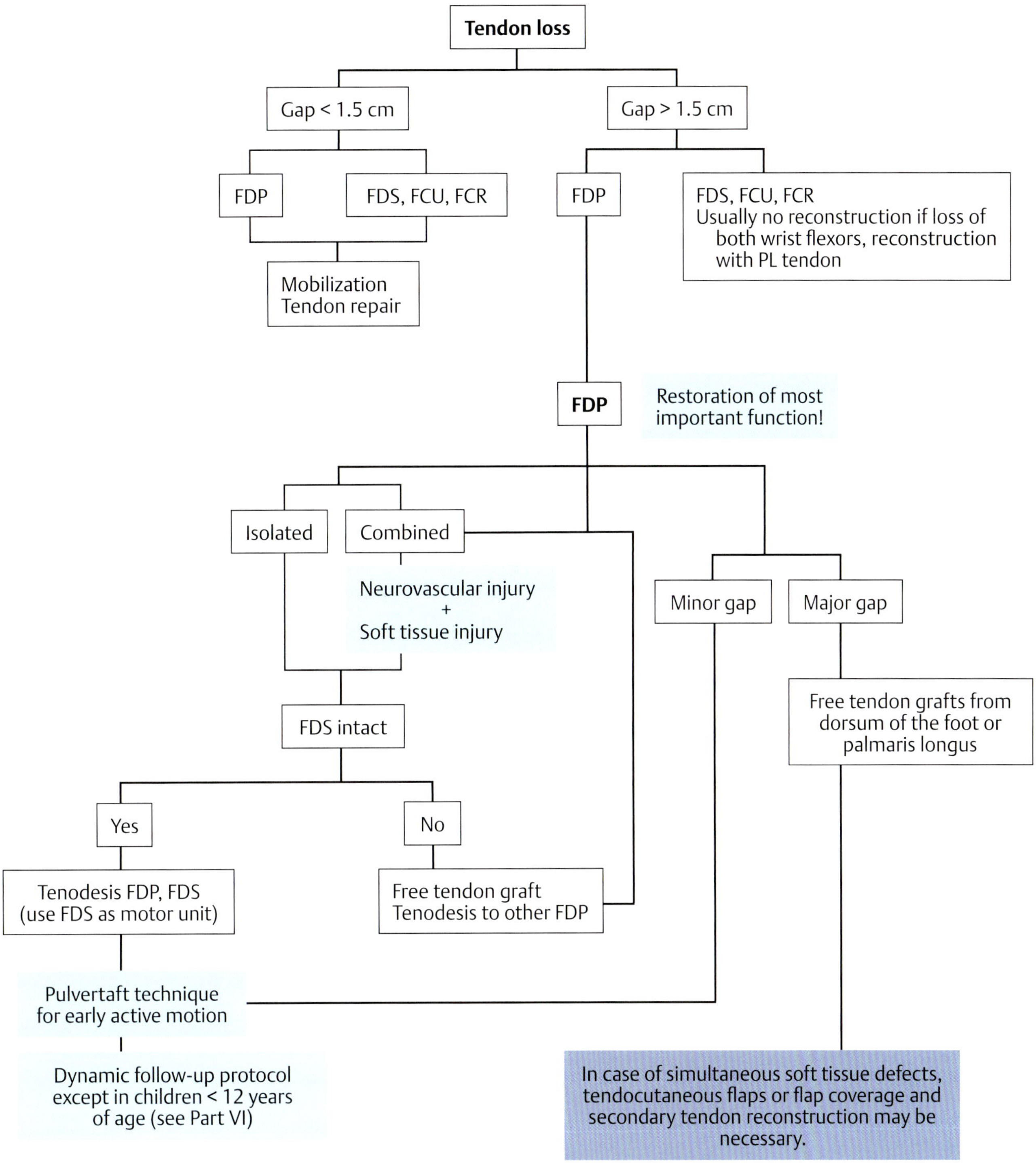

Algorithm 14.6

Parameters in decision-making	Additional options or guidelines	Warnings, precautions, or pitfalls	Emphasis on a particular waypoint

Zone VI (Musculotendinous Junction)

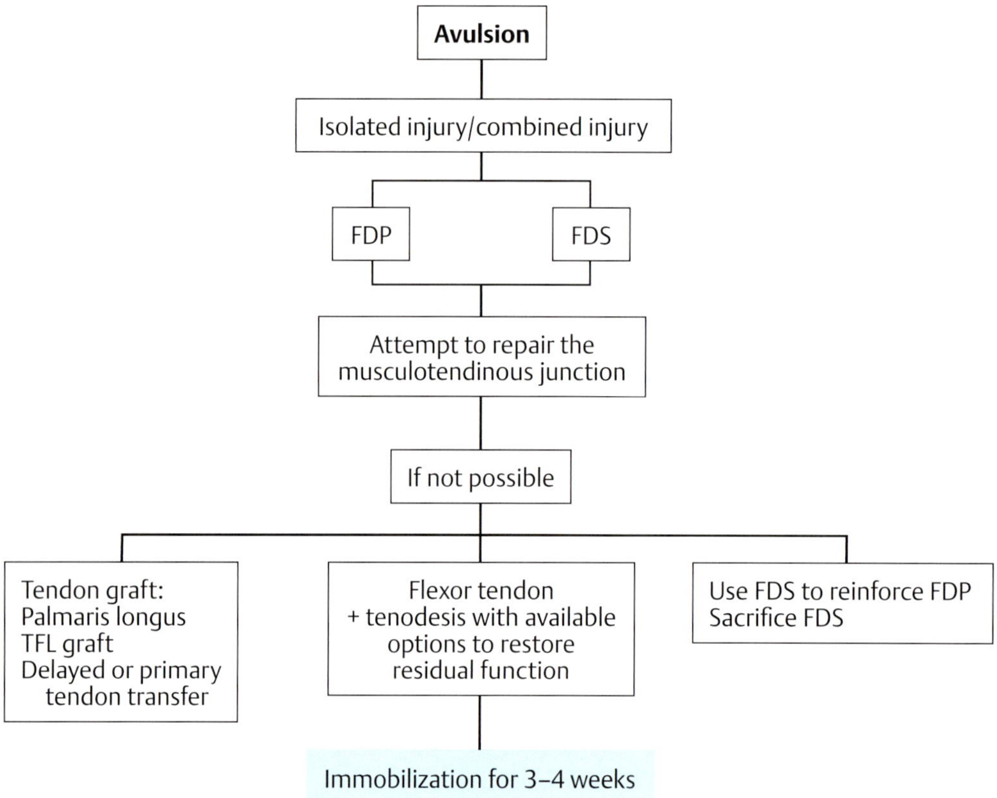

Algorithm 14.7

Parameters in decision-making	Additional options or guidelines	Warnings, precautions, or pitfalls	Emphasis on a particular waypoint

Forearm

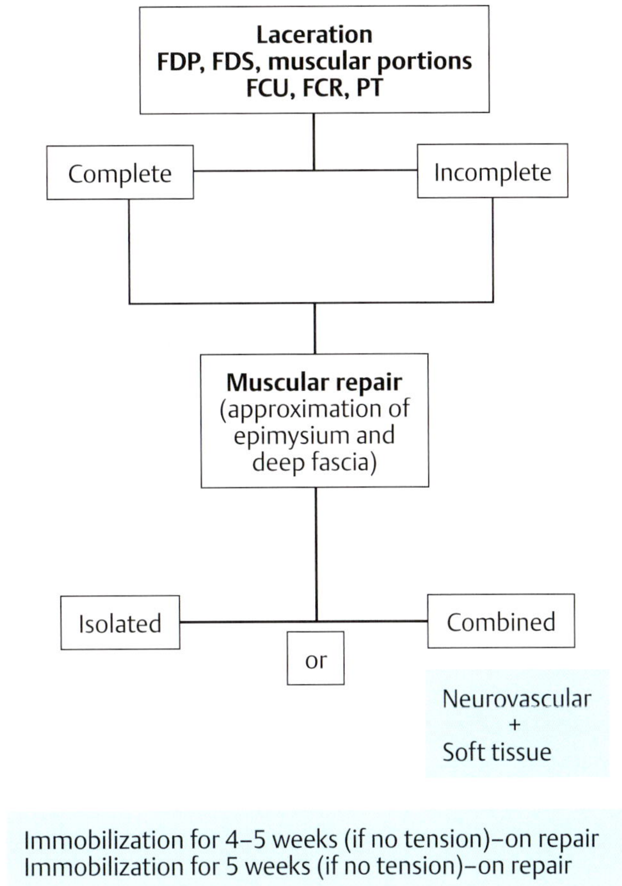

Algorithm 14.8

Parameters in decision-making	Additional options or guidelines	Warnings, precautions, or pitfalls	Emphasis on a particular waypoint

Forearm

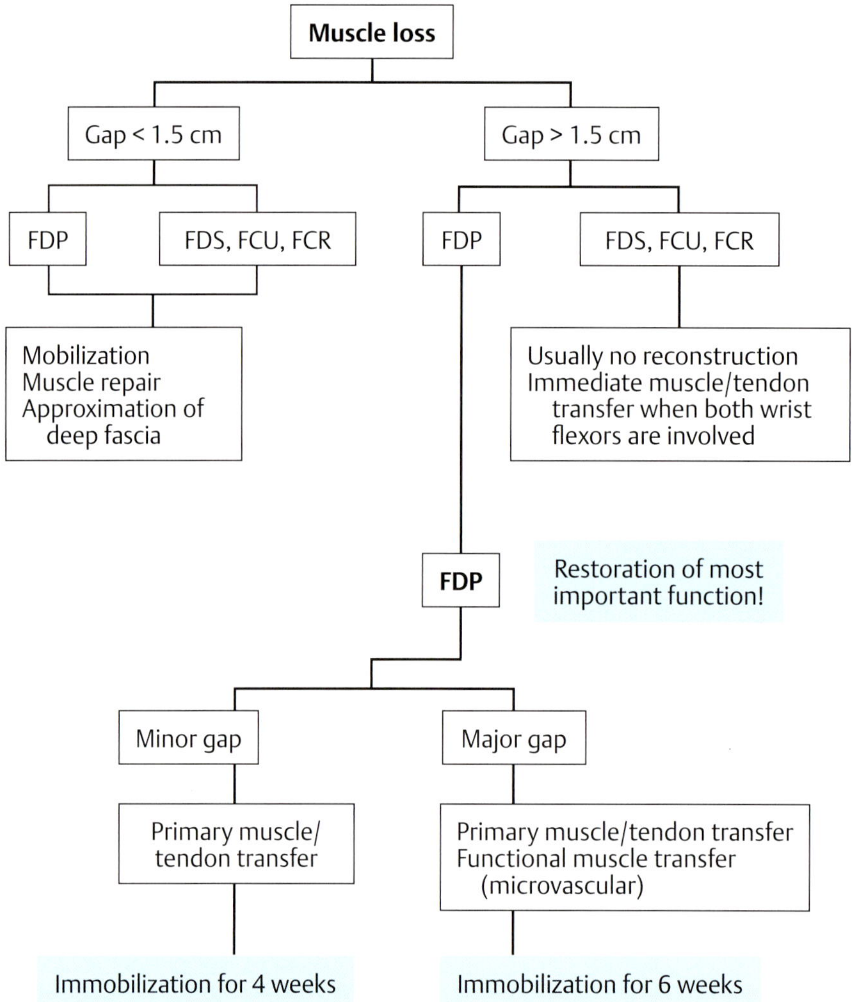

Algorithm 14.9

Parameters in decision-making	Additional options or guidelines	Warnings, precautions, or pitfalls	Emphasis on a particular waypoint

Forearm

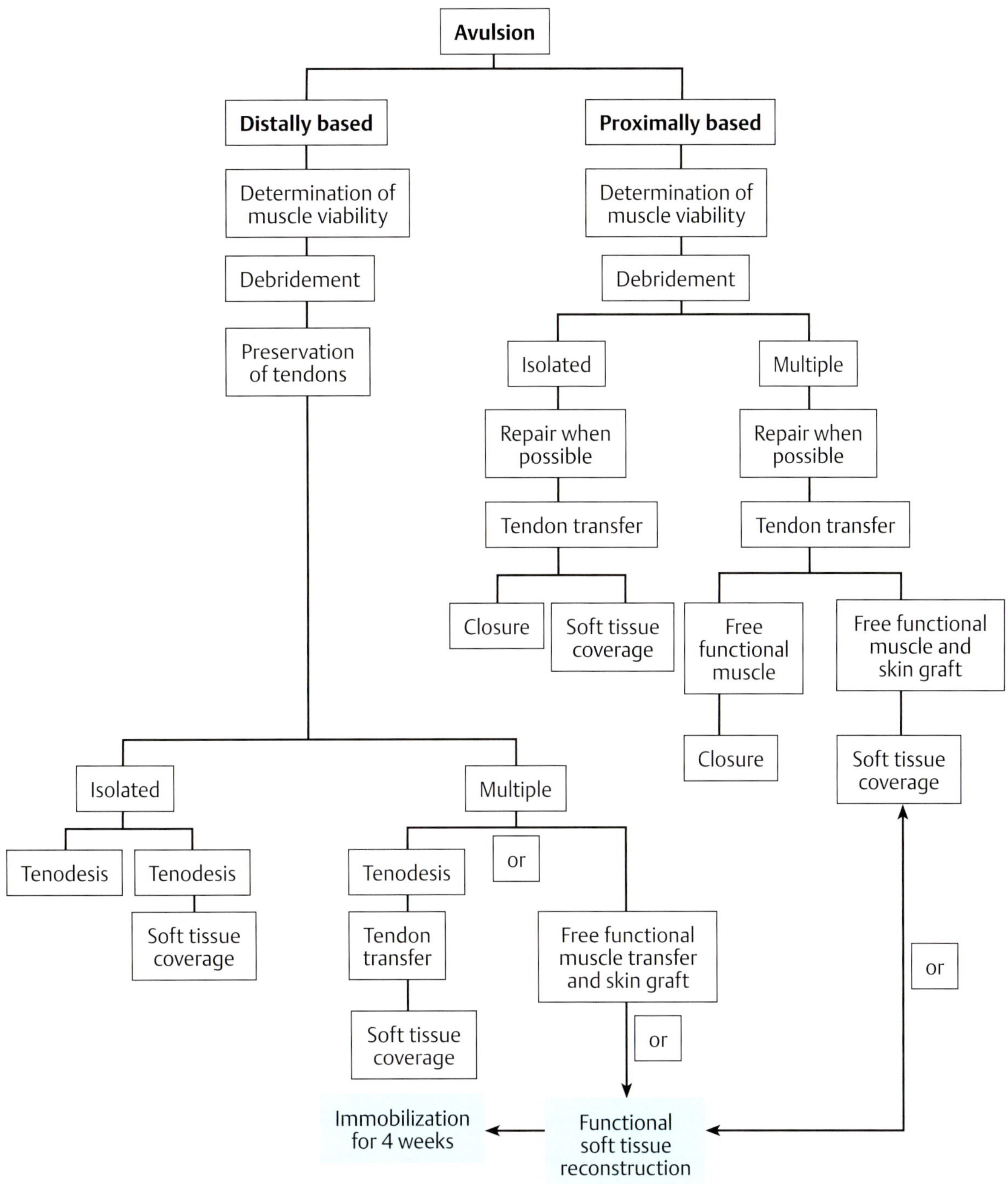

Algorithm 14.10

Parameters in decision-making	Additional options or guidelines	Warnings, precautions, or pitfalls	Emphasis on a particular waypoint

Brachium and Elbow

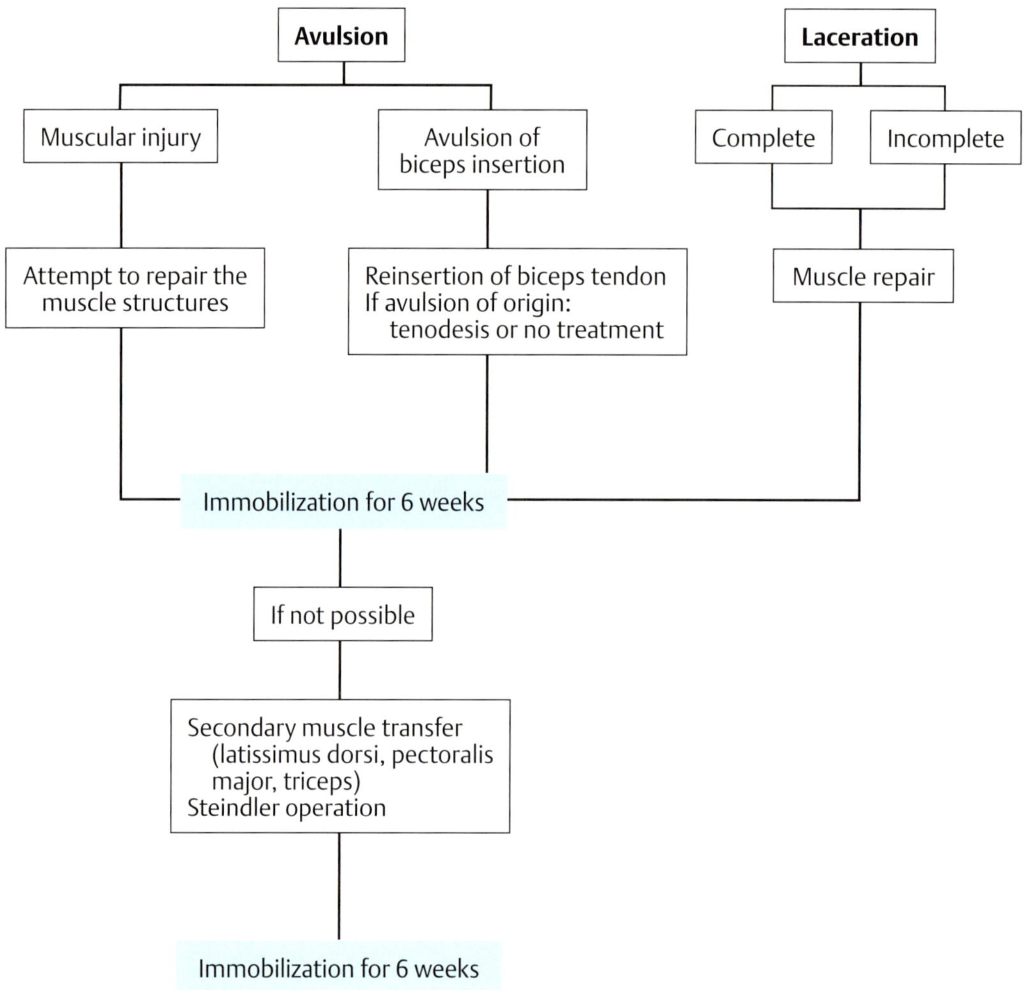

Algorithm 14.11

Parameters in decision-making	Additional options or guidelines	Warnings, precautions, or pitfalls	Emphasis on a particular waypoint

Flexor Tendon Reconstruction

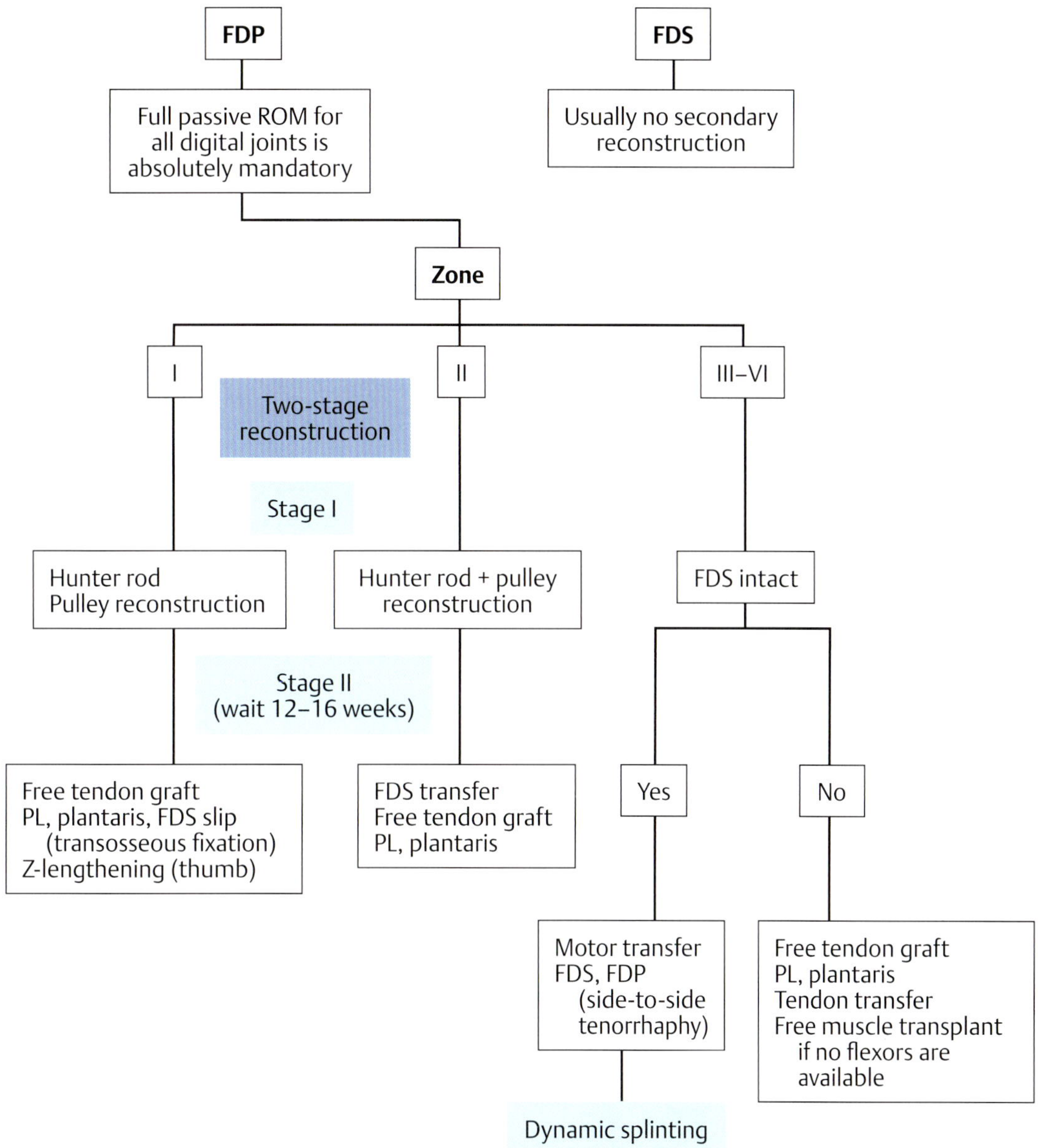

Algorithm 14.12

Parameters in decision-making	Additional options or guidelines	Warnings, precautions, or pitfalls	Emphasis on a particular waypoint

Chapter 15

Extensor Systems

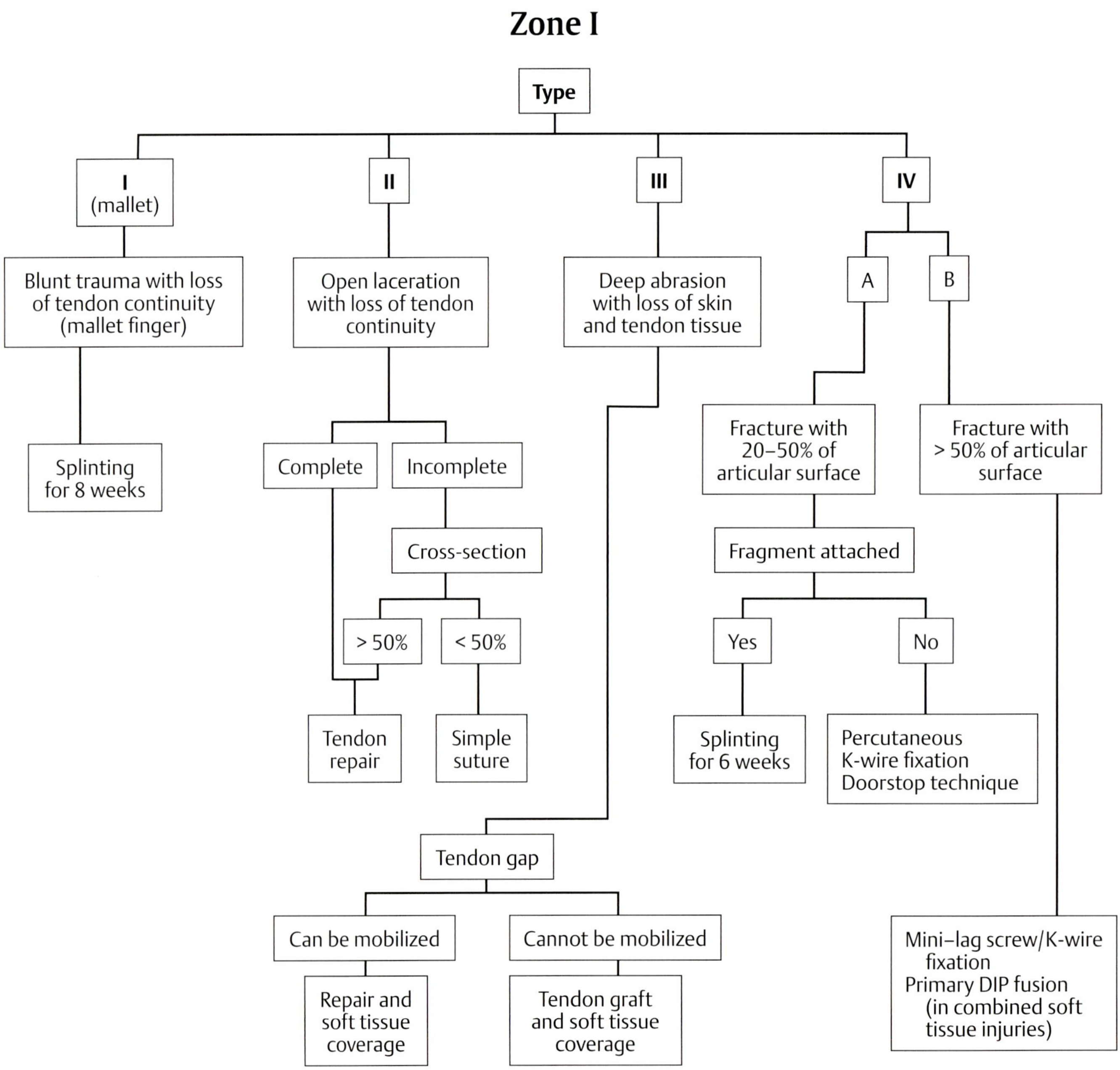

Algorithm 15.1

Zones II and IV–Thumb

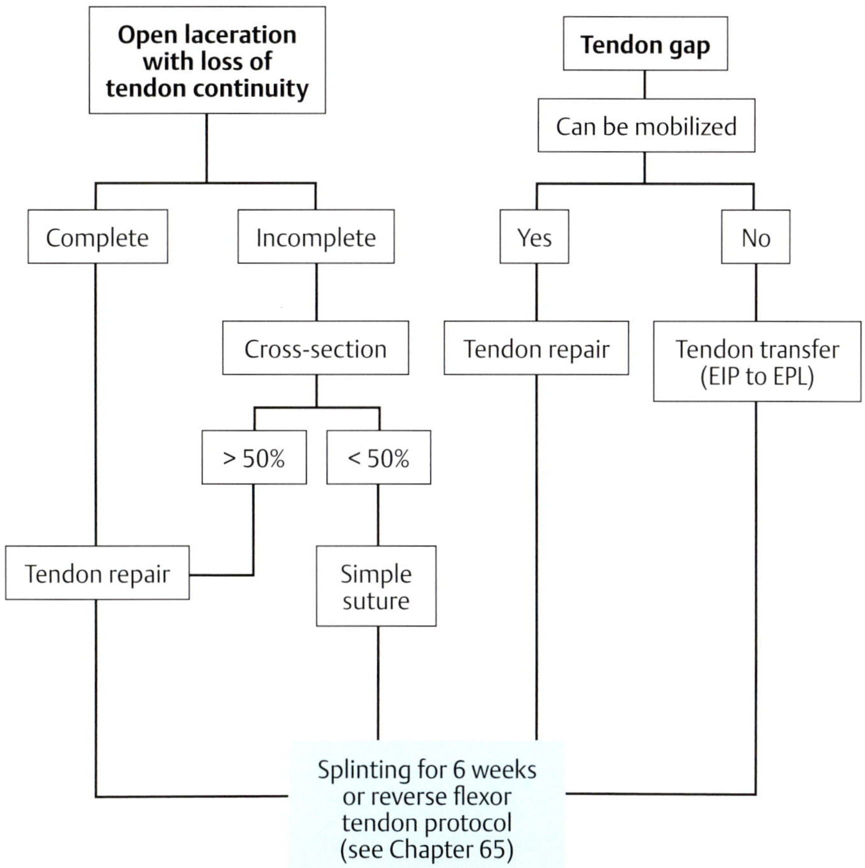

Algorithm 15.2

Parameters in decision-making	Additional options or guidelines	Warnings, precautions, or pitfalls	Emphasis on a particular waypoint

Zones III and IV–Central Slip

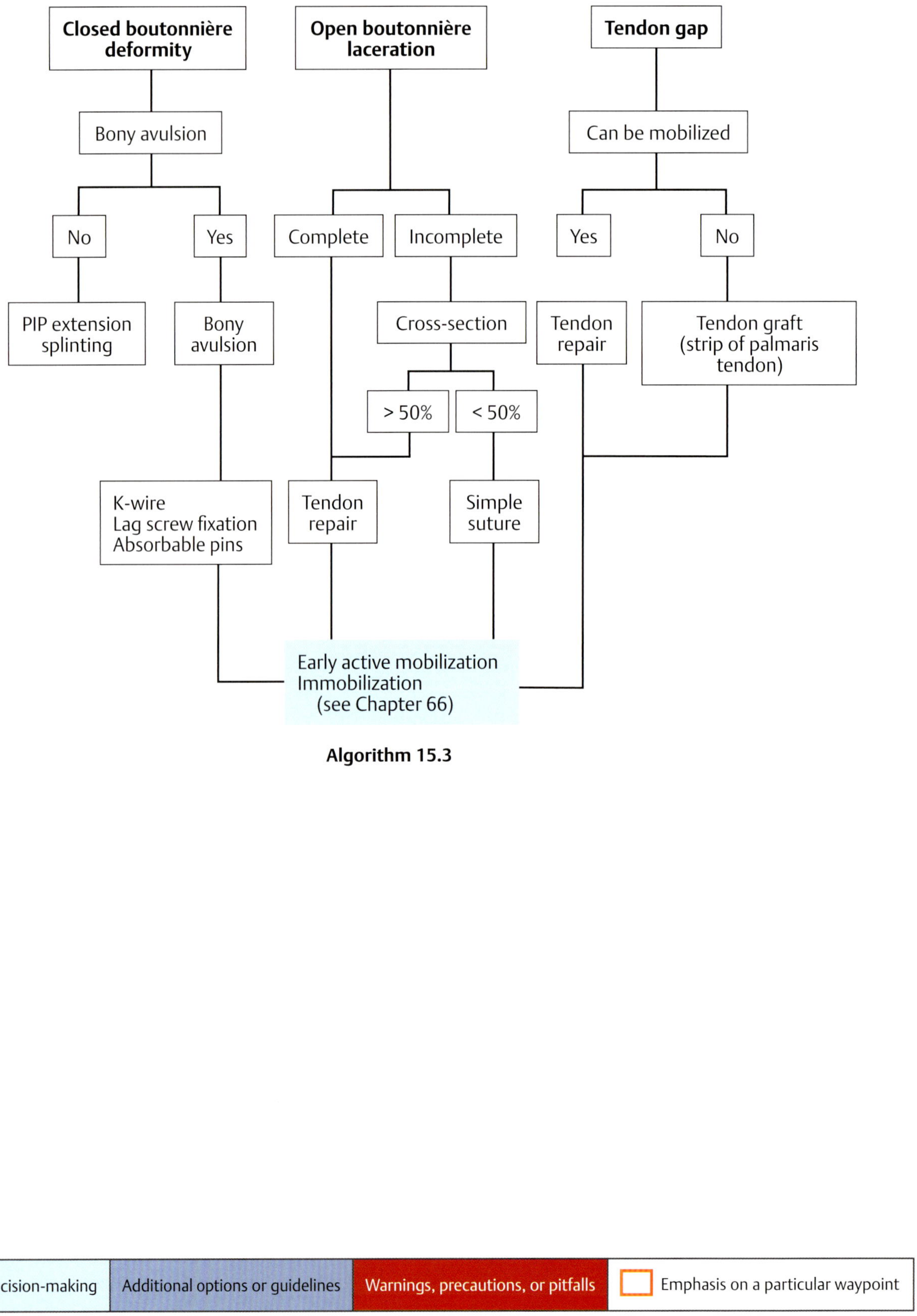

Algorithm 15.3

Zones V and VI–Thumb

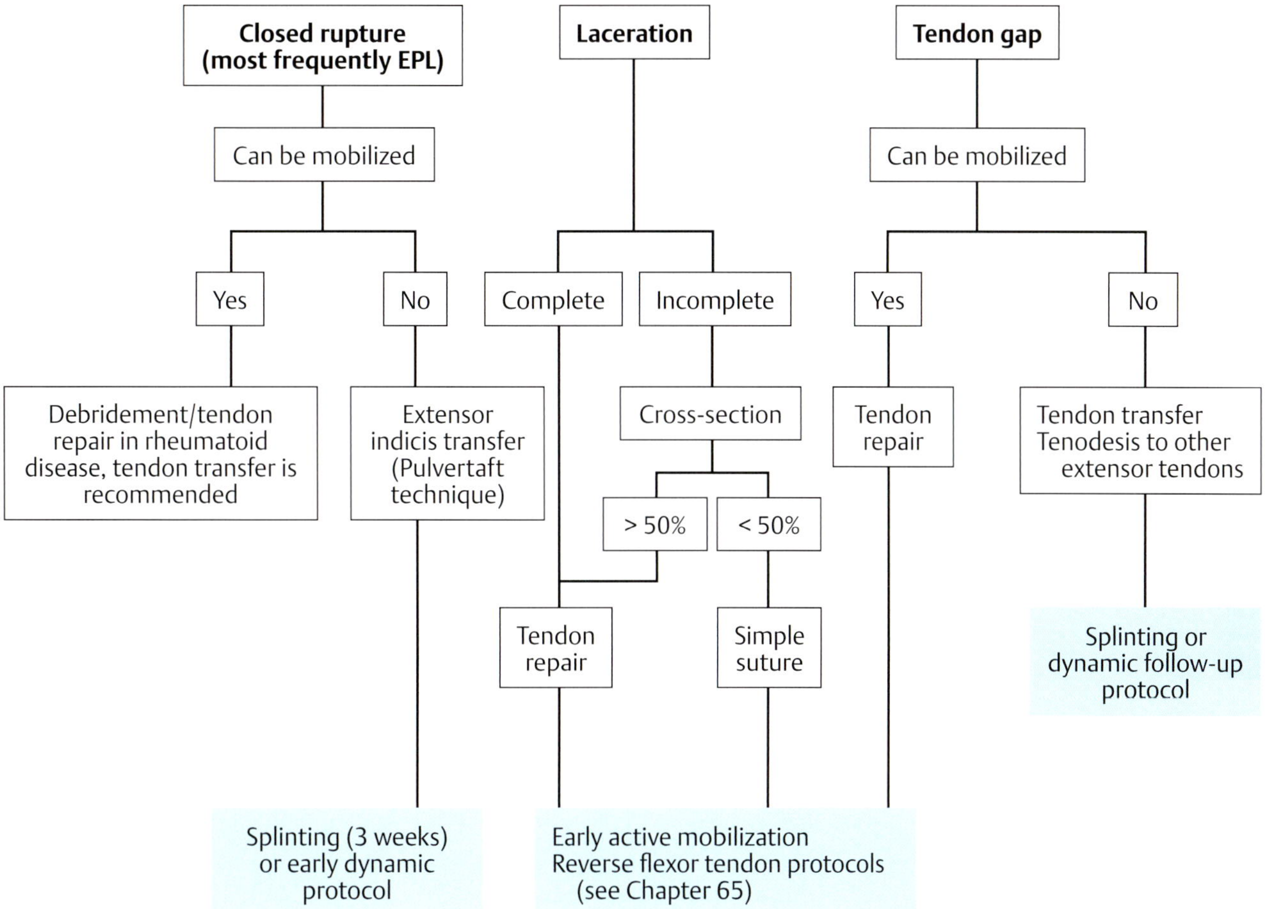

Algorithm 15.4

Parameters in decision-making	Additional options or guidelines	Warnings, precautions, or pitfalls	Emphasis on a particular waypoint

Zone VII

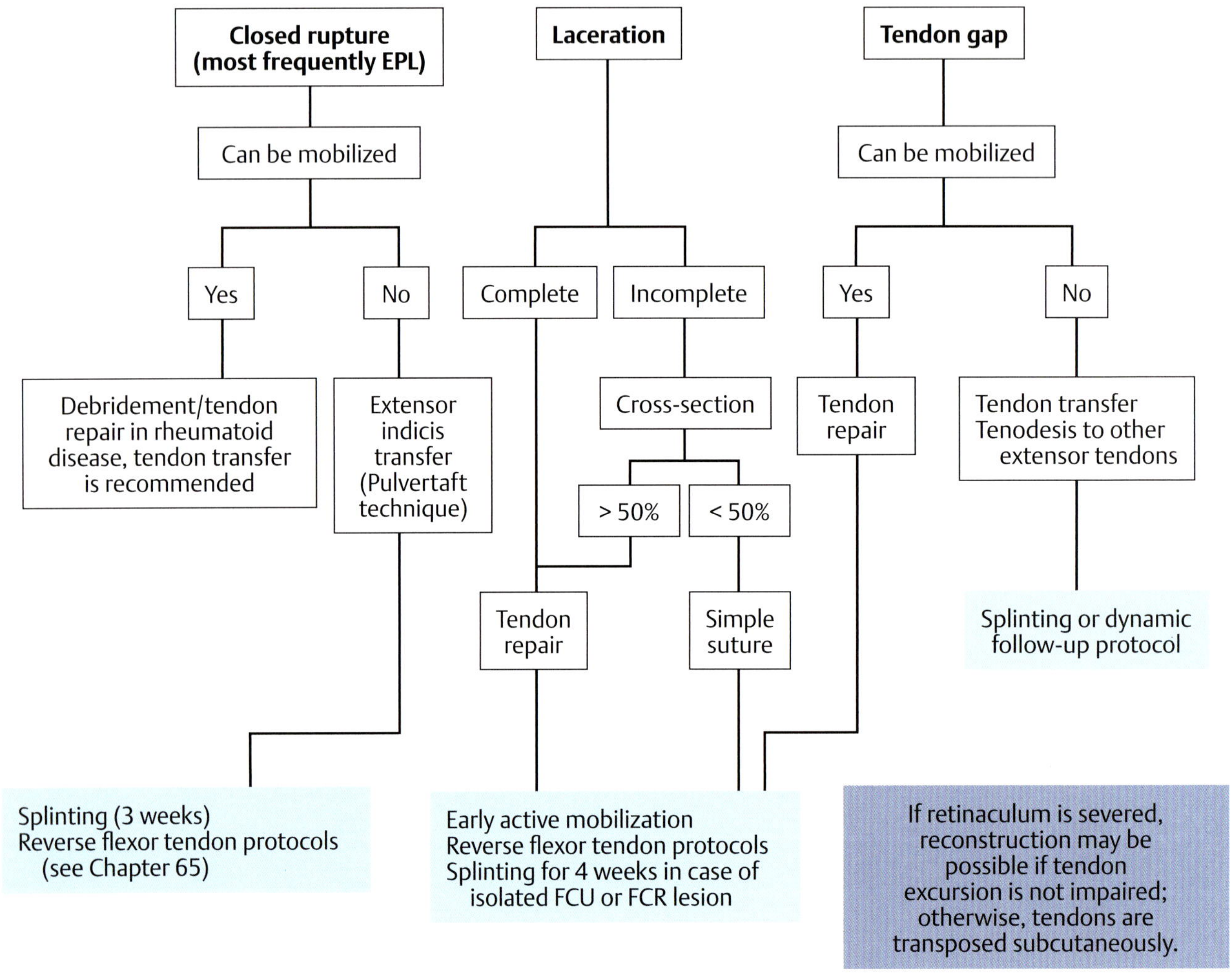

Algorithm 15.5

Parameters in decision-making	Additional options or guidelines	Warnings, precautions, or pitfalls	Emphasis on a particular waypoint

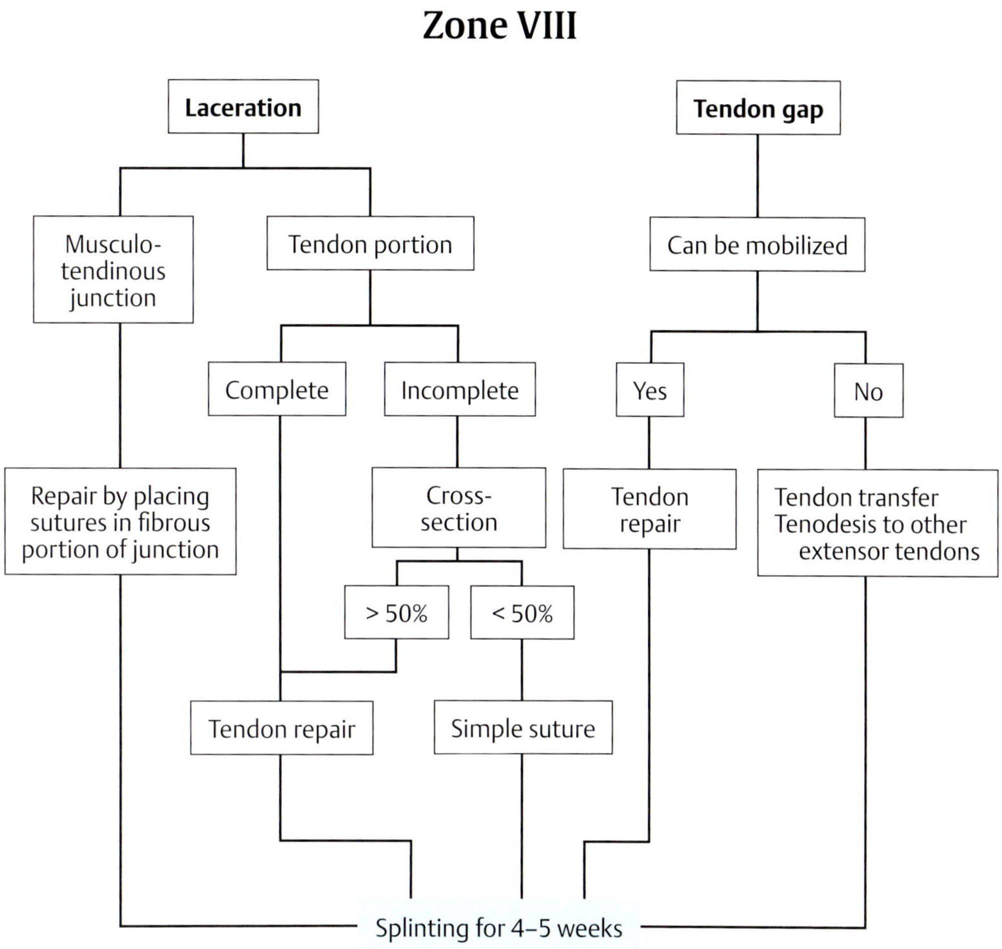

Algorithm 15.6

Zone VIII–Forearm

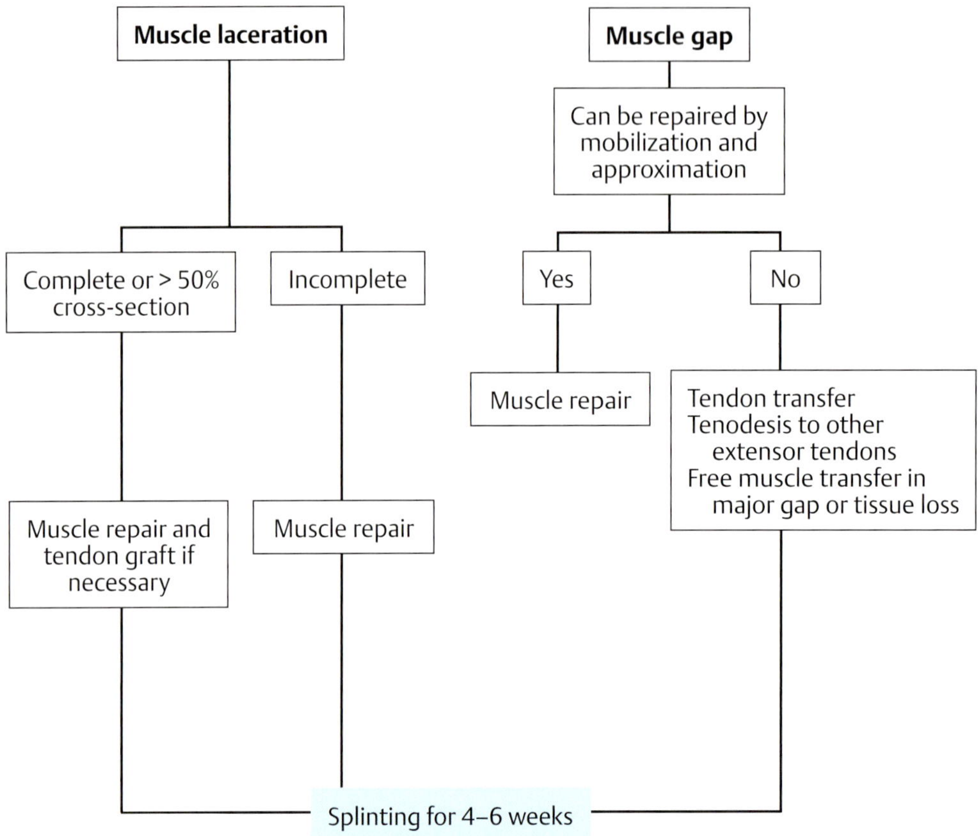

Algorithm 15.7

Parameters in decision-making | Additional options or guidelines | Warnings, precautions, or pitfalls | Emphasis on a particular waypoint

Forearm

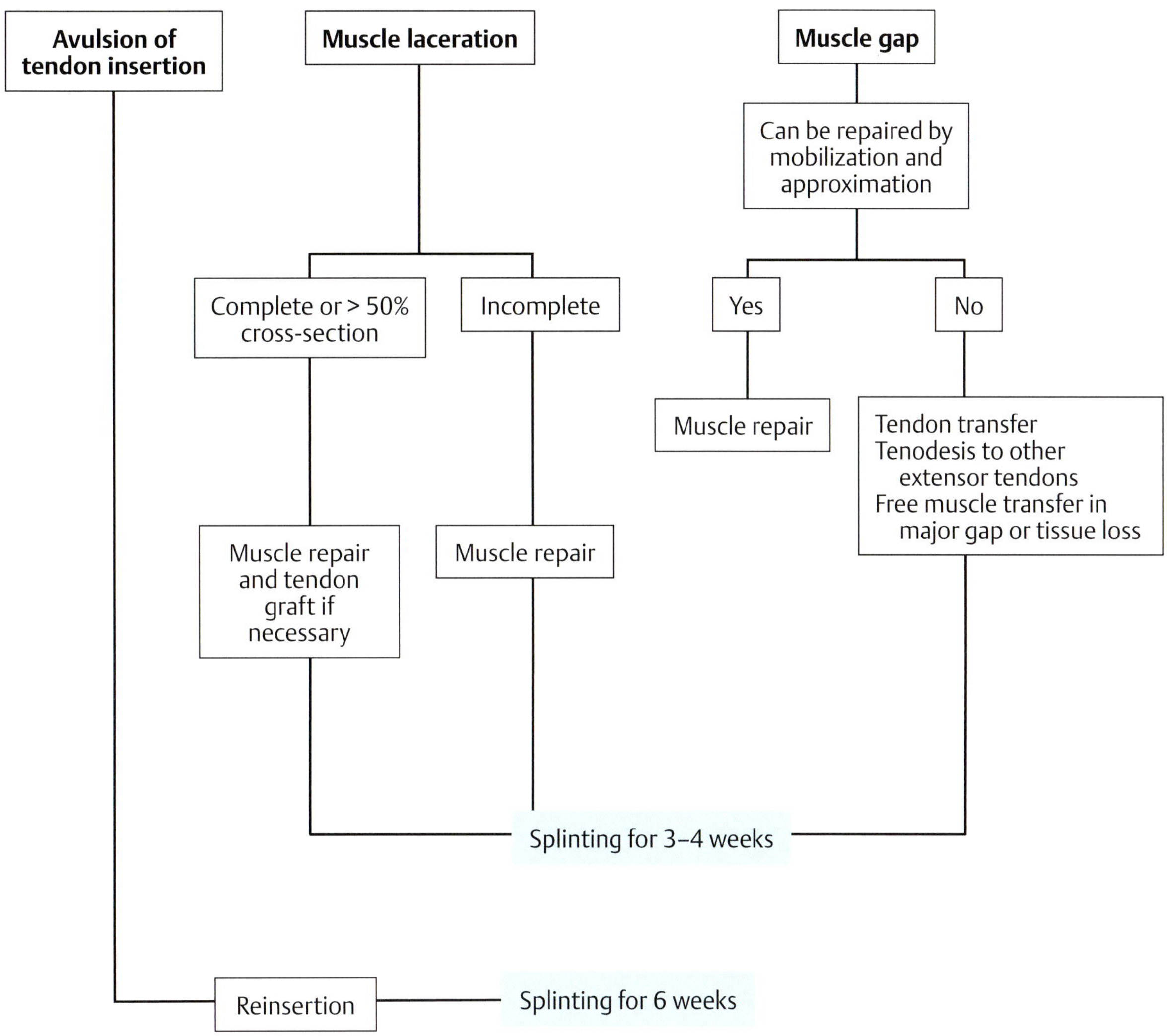

Algorithm 15.8

Parameters in decision-making	Additional options or guidelines	Warnings, precautions, or pitfalls	Emphasis on a particular waypoint

Brachium

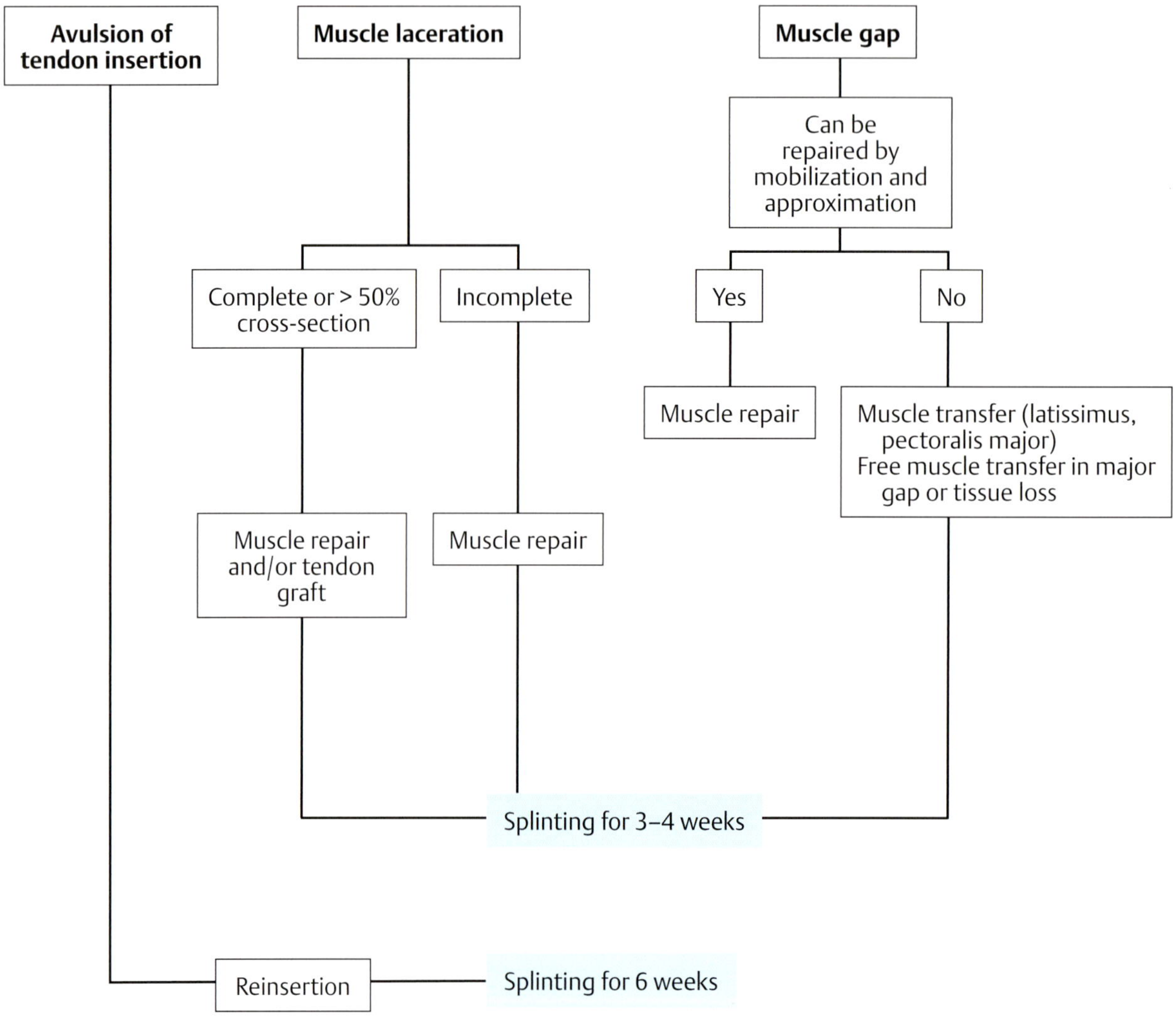

Algorithm 15.9

Parameters in decision-making | Additional options or guidelines | Warnings, precautions, or pitfalls | Emphasis on a particular waypoint

Chapter 16

Vessels

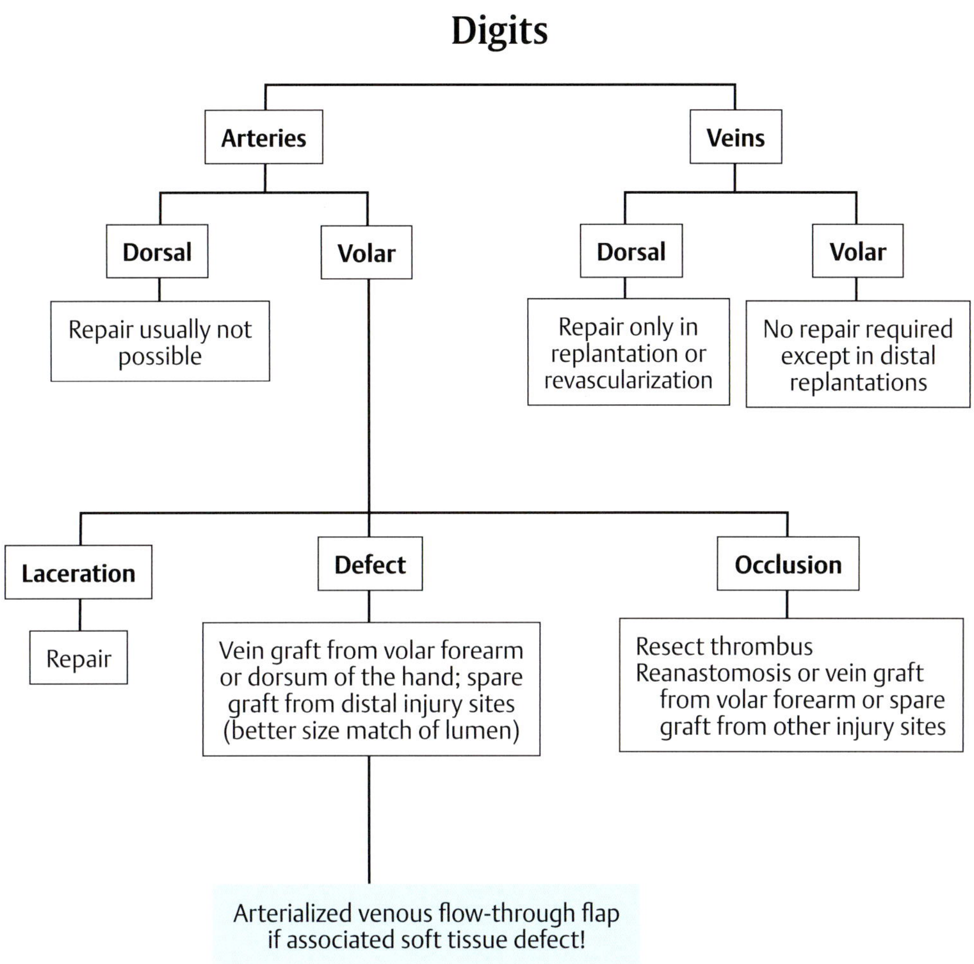

Algorithm 16.1

Parameters in decision-making	Additional options or guidelines	Warnings, precautions, or pitfalls	Emphasis on a particular waypoint

Palm and Dorsum of the Hand

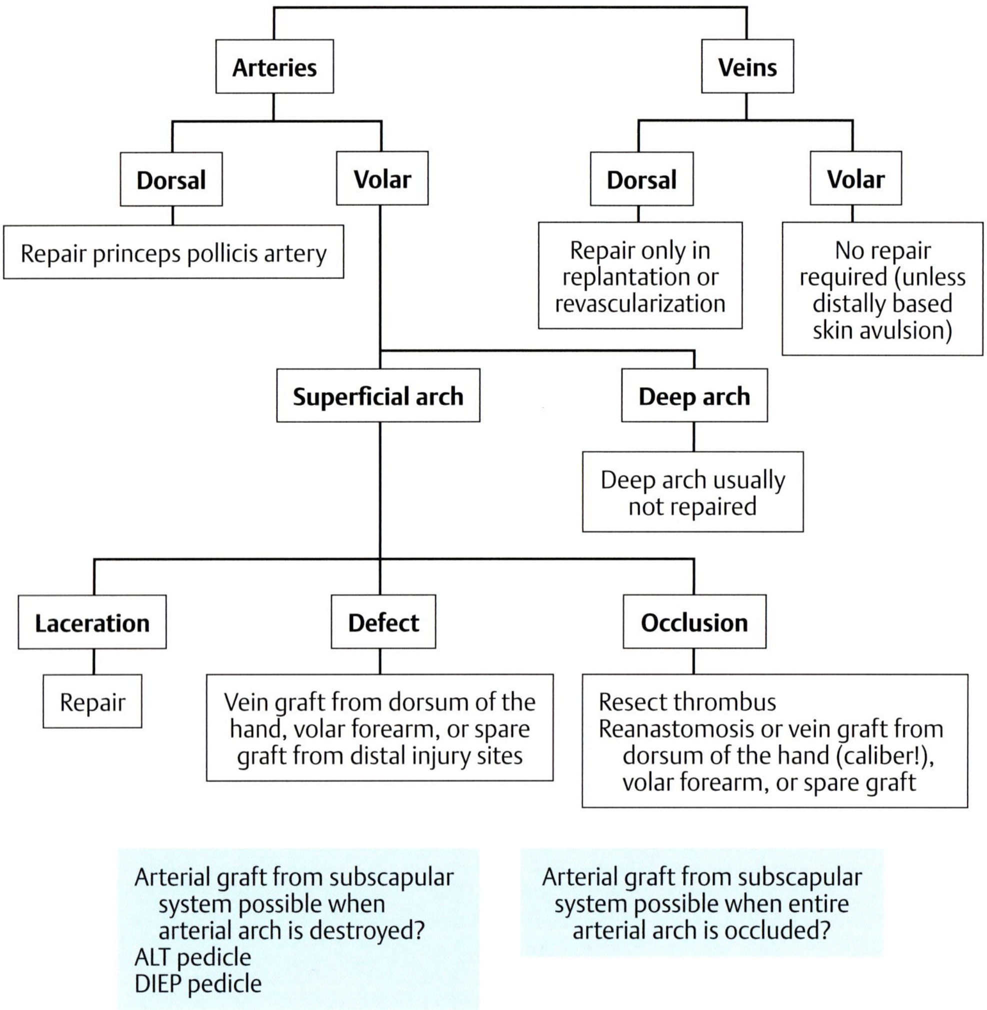

Algorithm 16.2

Parameters in decision-making	Additional options or guidelines	Warnings, precautions, or pitfalls	Emphasis on a particular waypoint

Forearm

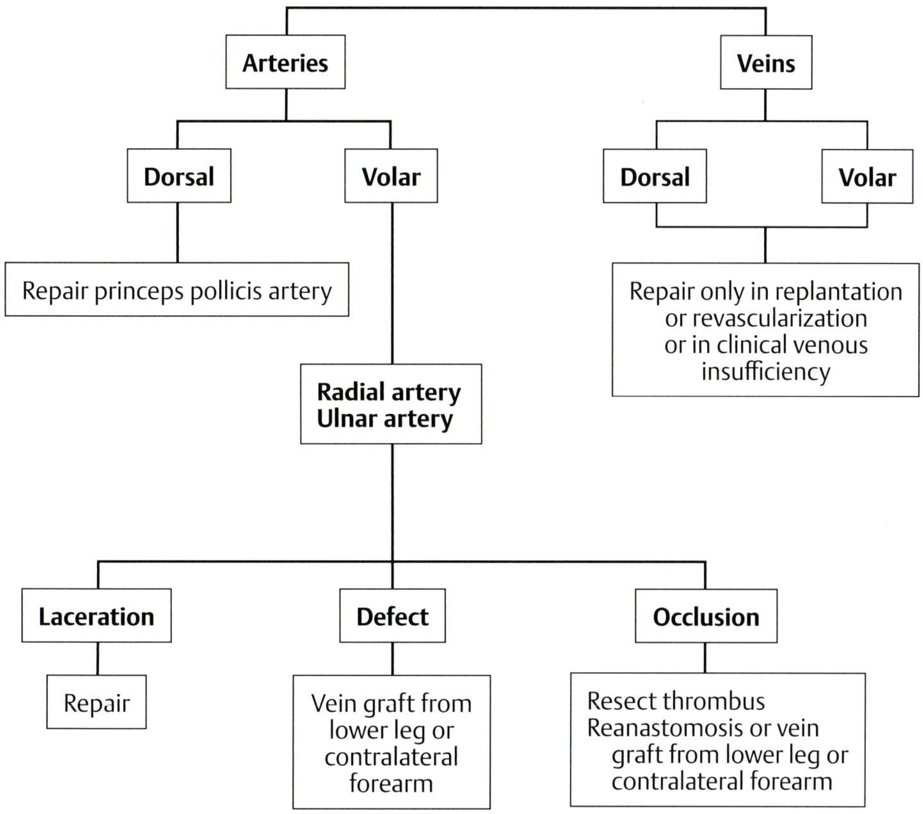

Always repair both arteries for the following reasons:
1. Reserve capacity
2. Possible secondary occlusion from sequelae of trauma
3. Reinjury later in life

Algorithm 16.3

Parameters in decision-making	Additional options or guidelines	Warnings, precautions, or pitfalls	Emphasis on a particular waypoint

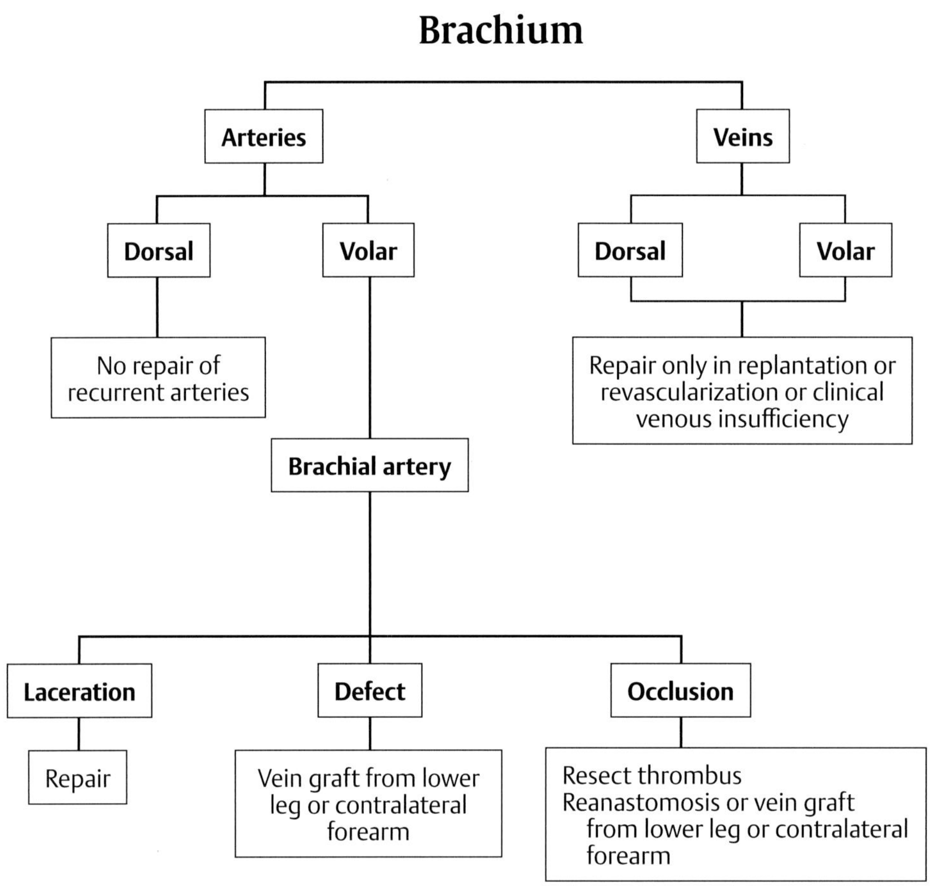

Algorithm 16.4

Chapter 17

Nerves

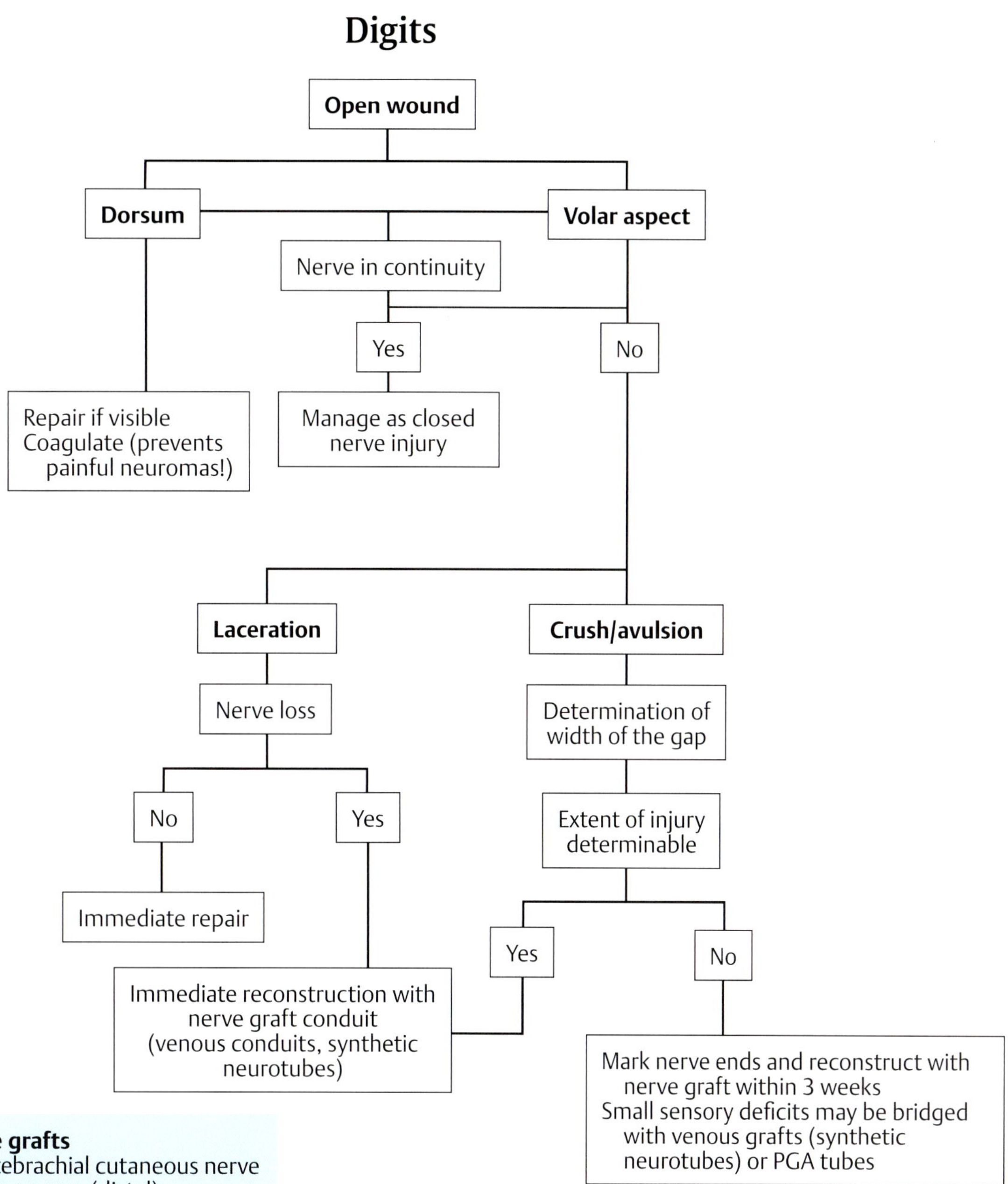

Spare parts for nerve grafts
Medial or lateral antebrachial cutaneous nerve
Posterior interosseous nerve (distal)
Repair small defects with venous conduit

Algorithm 17.1

Parameters in decision-making	Additional options or guidelines	Warnings, precautions, or pitfalls	Emphasis on a particular waypoint

Palm/Dorsum

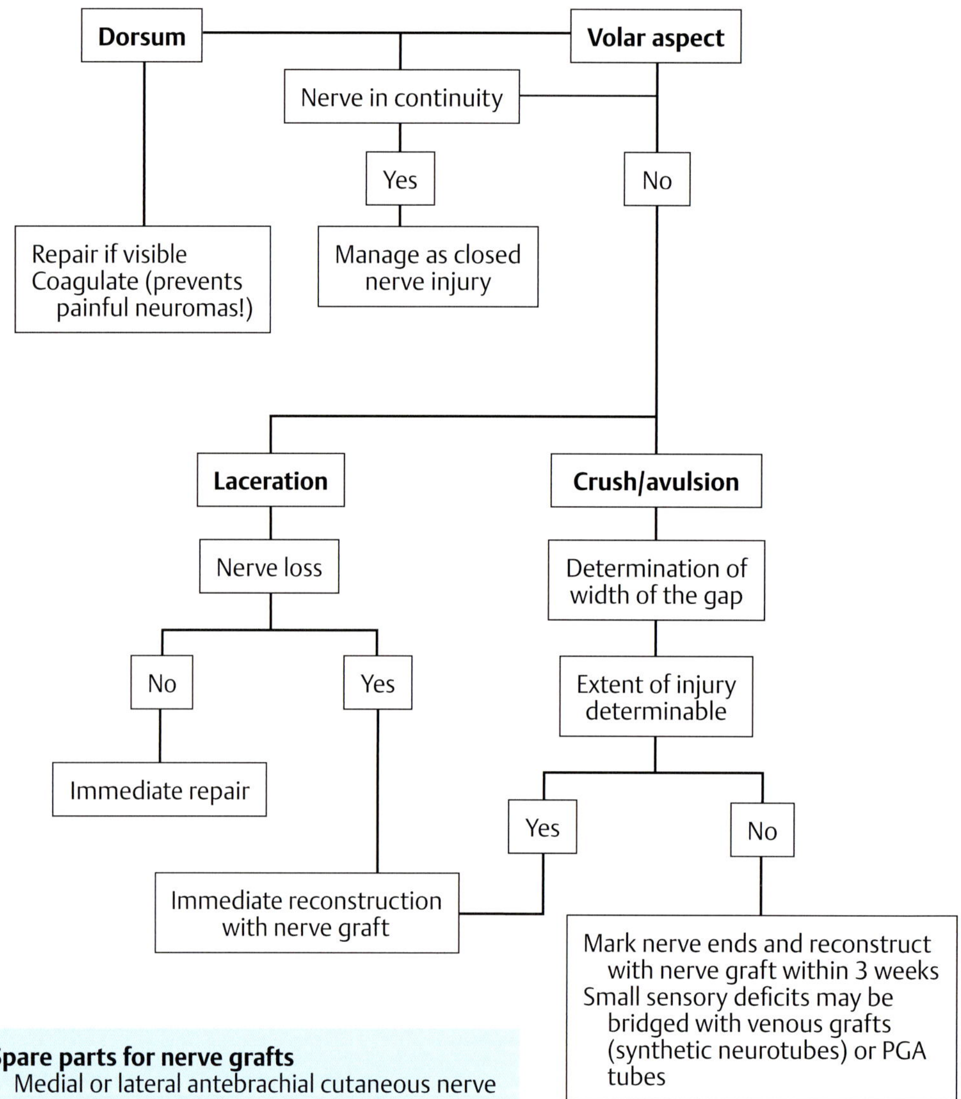

Spare parts for nerve grafts
- Medial or lateral antebrachial cutaneous nerve
- Posterior interosseous nerve (distal)
- Sural nerve
- Small defects with venous conduit

Algorithm 17.2

Parameters in decision-making	Additional options or guidelines	Warnings, precautions, or pitfalls	Emphasis on a particular waypoint

Wrist/Distal Forearm

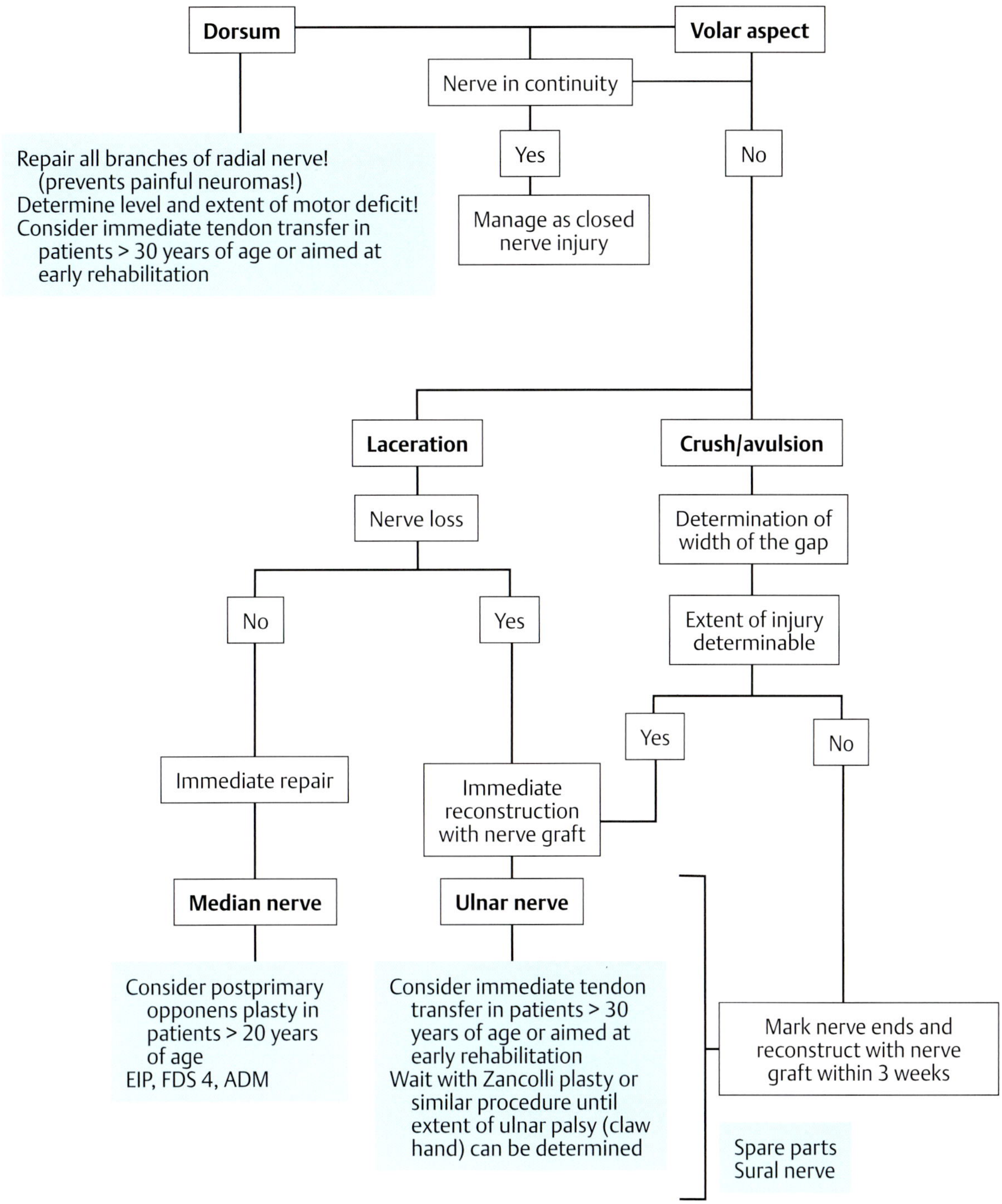

Algorithm 17.3

Parameters in decision-making	Additional options or guidelines	Warnings, precautions, or pitfalls	Emphasis on a particular waypoint

Brachium

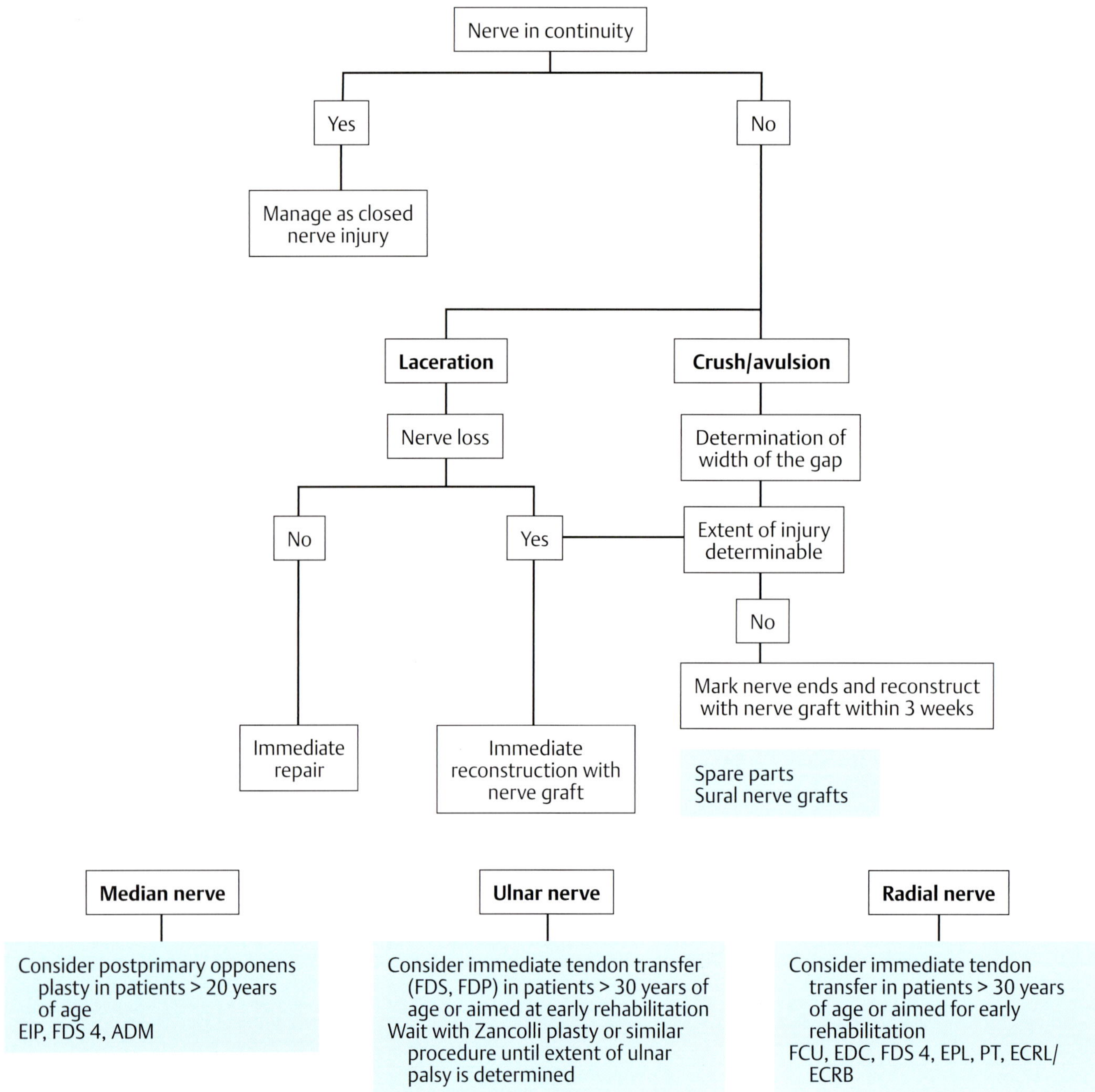

Algorithm 17.4

Parameters in decision-making	Additional options or guidelines	Warnings, precautions, or pitfalls	Emphasis on a particular waypoint

Closed Nerve Injury

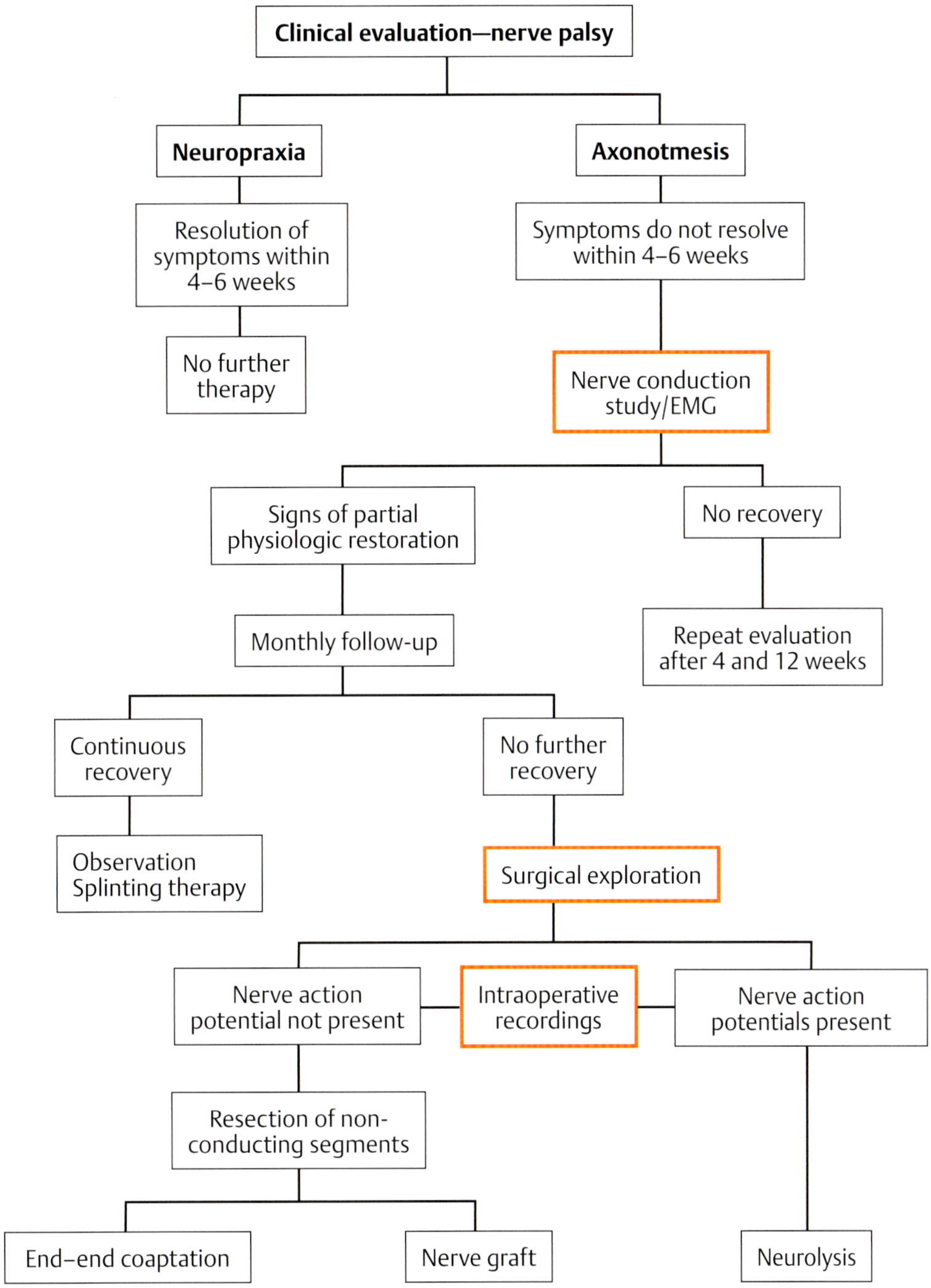

Algorithm 17.5

Parameters in decision-making	Additional options or guidelines	Warnings, precautions, or pitfalls	Emphasis on a particular waypoint

Closed Brachial Plexus Injury with Complete Palsy

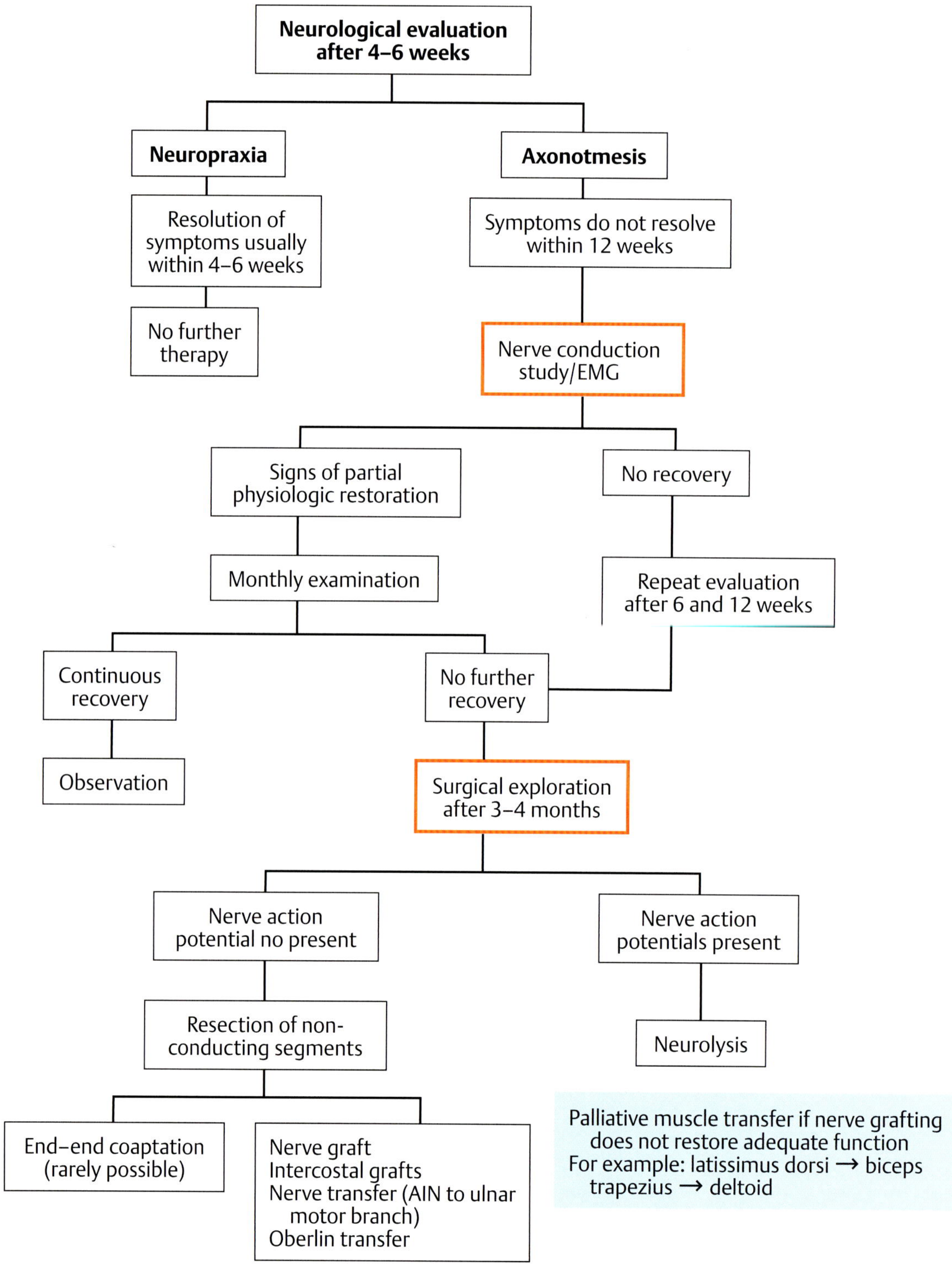

Algorithm 17.6

Parameters in decision-making	Additional options or guidelines	Warnings, precautions, or pitfalls	Emphasis on a particular waypoint

Secondary Nerve Reconstruction

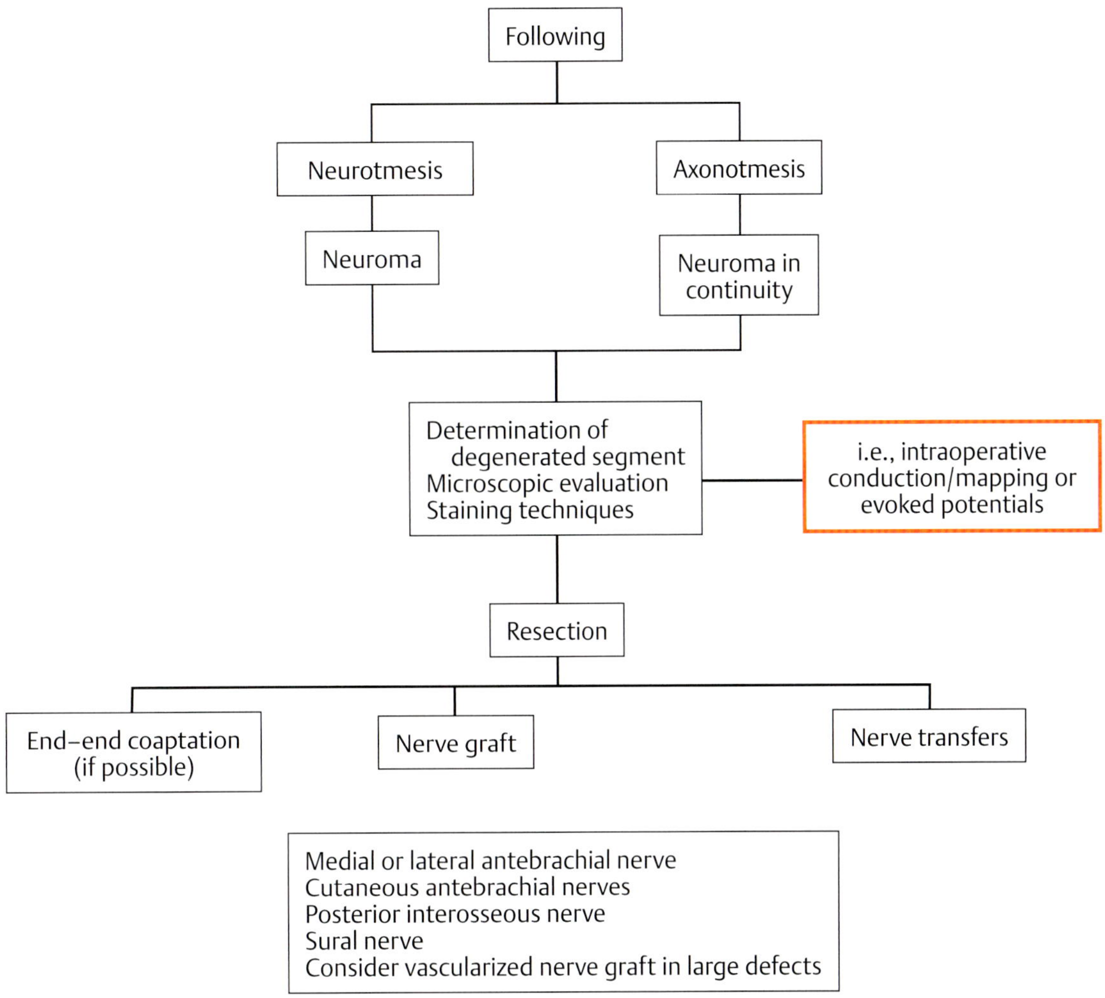

Algorithm 17.7

Parameters in decision-making	Additional options or guidelines	Warnings, precautions, or pitfalls	Emphasis on a particular waypoint

Neuroma

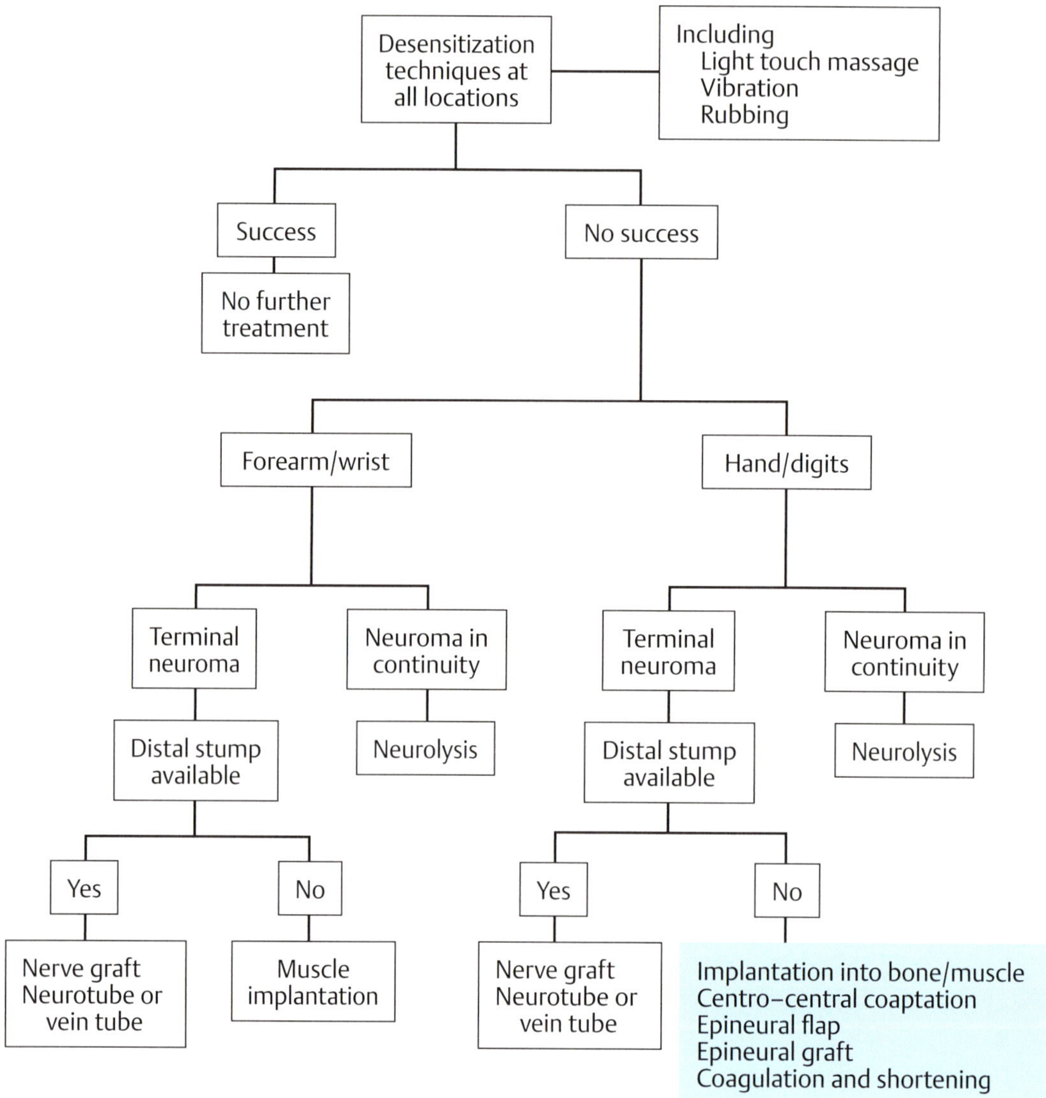

Algorithm 17.8

Parameters in decision-making	Additional options or guidelines	Warnings, precautions, or pitfalls	Emphasis on a particular waypoint

Chapter 18

Skin and Soft Tissue

Injuries to the Nail Complex—Nail Plate and Germinal Matrix

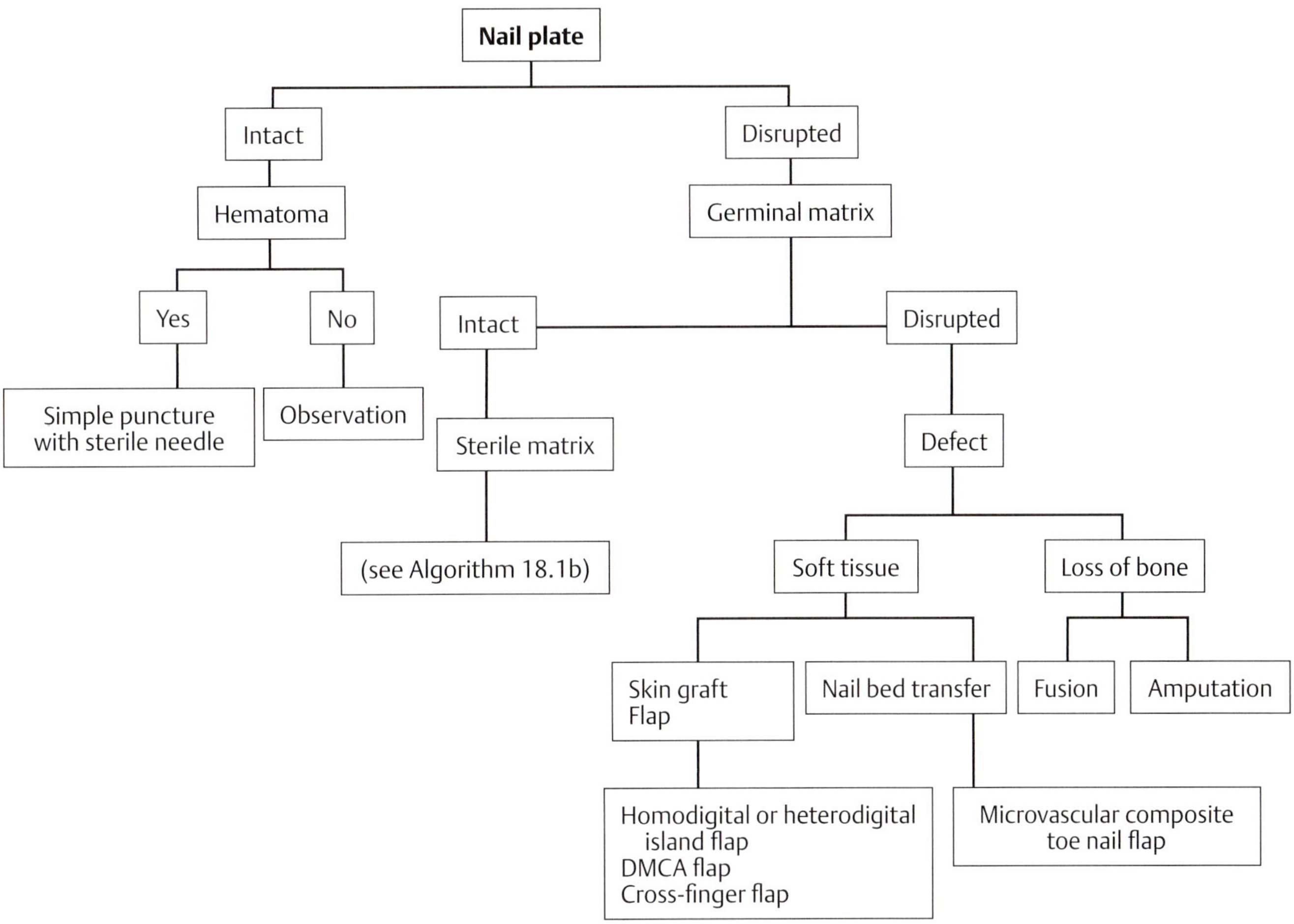

Algorithm 18.1a

Injuries to the Nail Complex—Sterile Matrix

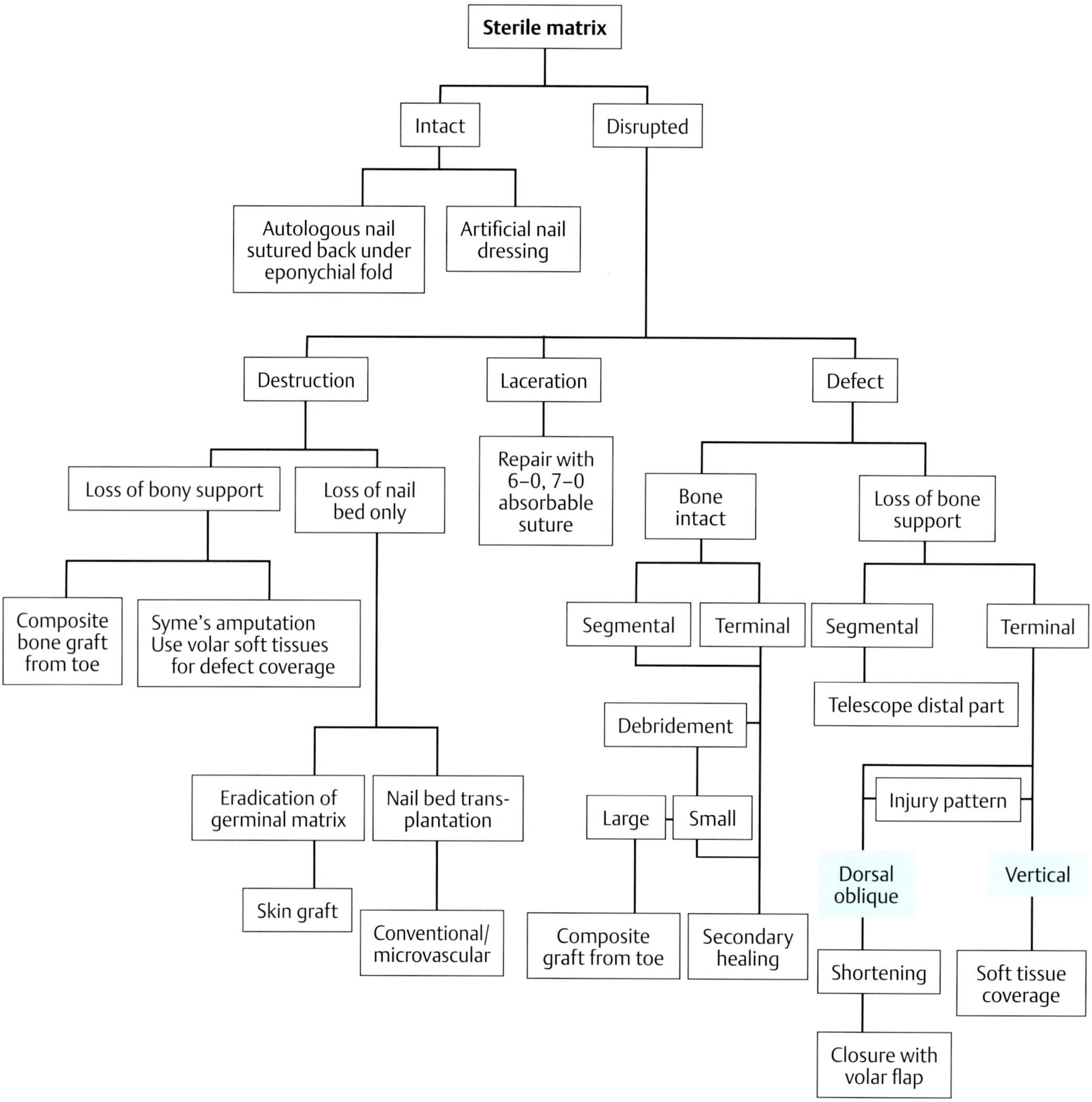

Algorithm 18.1b

Parameters in decision-making	Additional options or guidelines	Warnings, precautions, or pitfalls	Emphasis on a particular waypoint

Fingertips

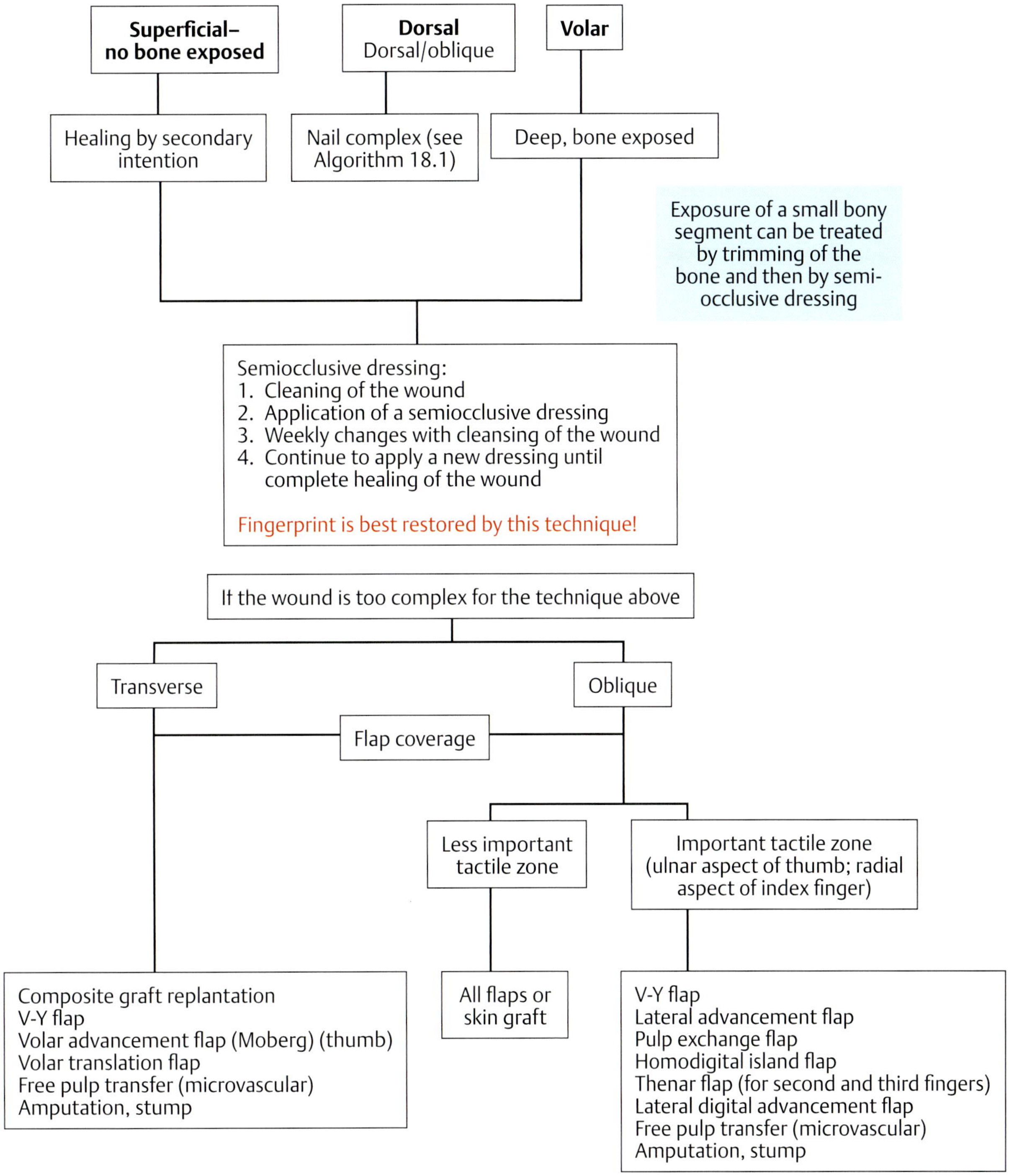

Algorithm 18.2

Parameters in decision-making	Additional options or guidelines	Warnings, precautions, or pitfalls	Emphasis on a particular waypoint

Thumb

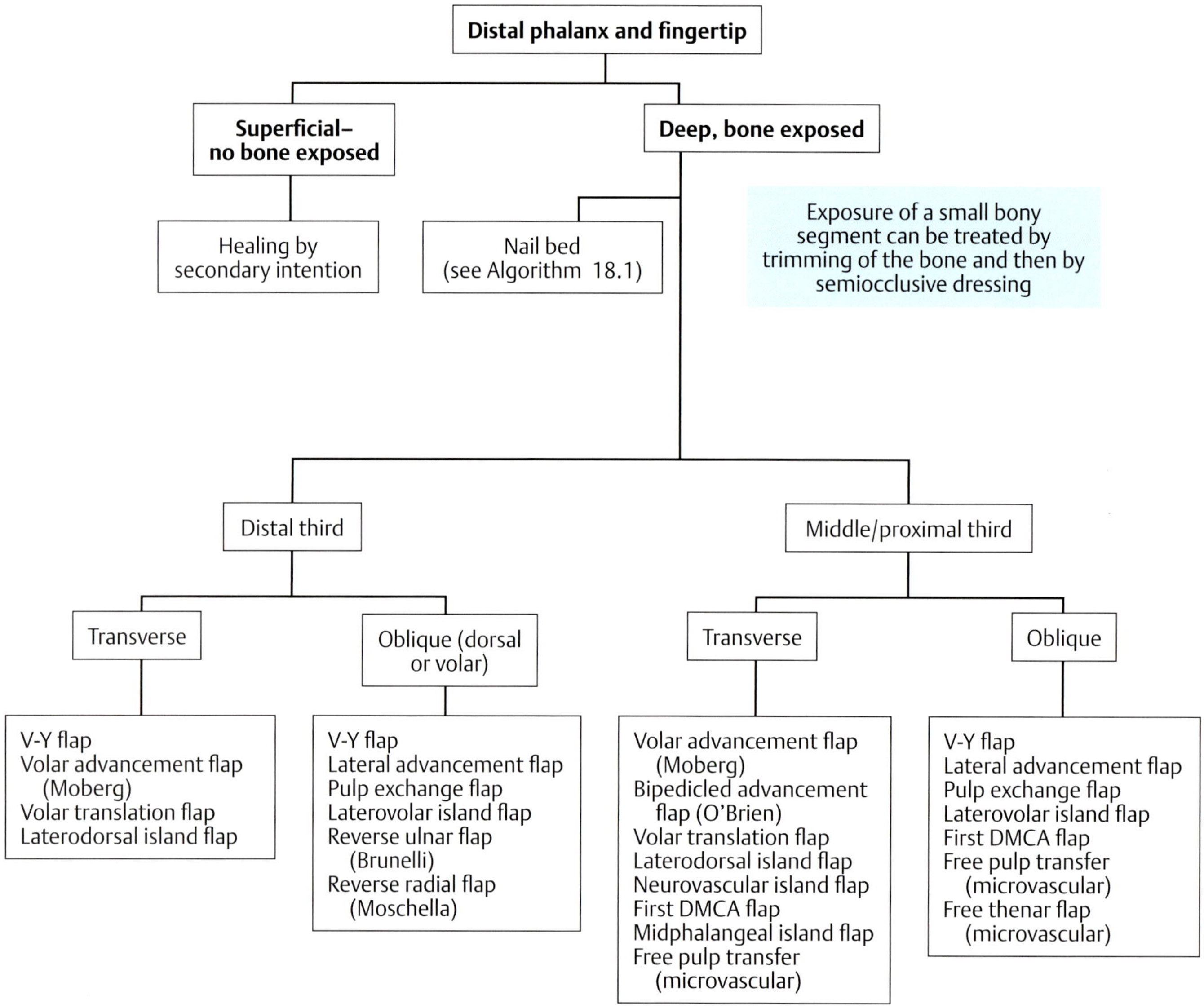

Algorithm 18.3

Parameters in decision-making	Additional options or guidelines	Warnings, precautions, or pitfalls	Emphasis on a particular waypoint

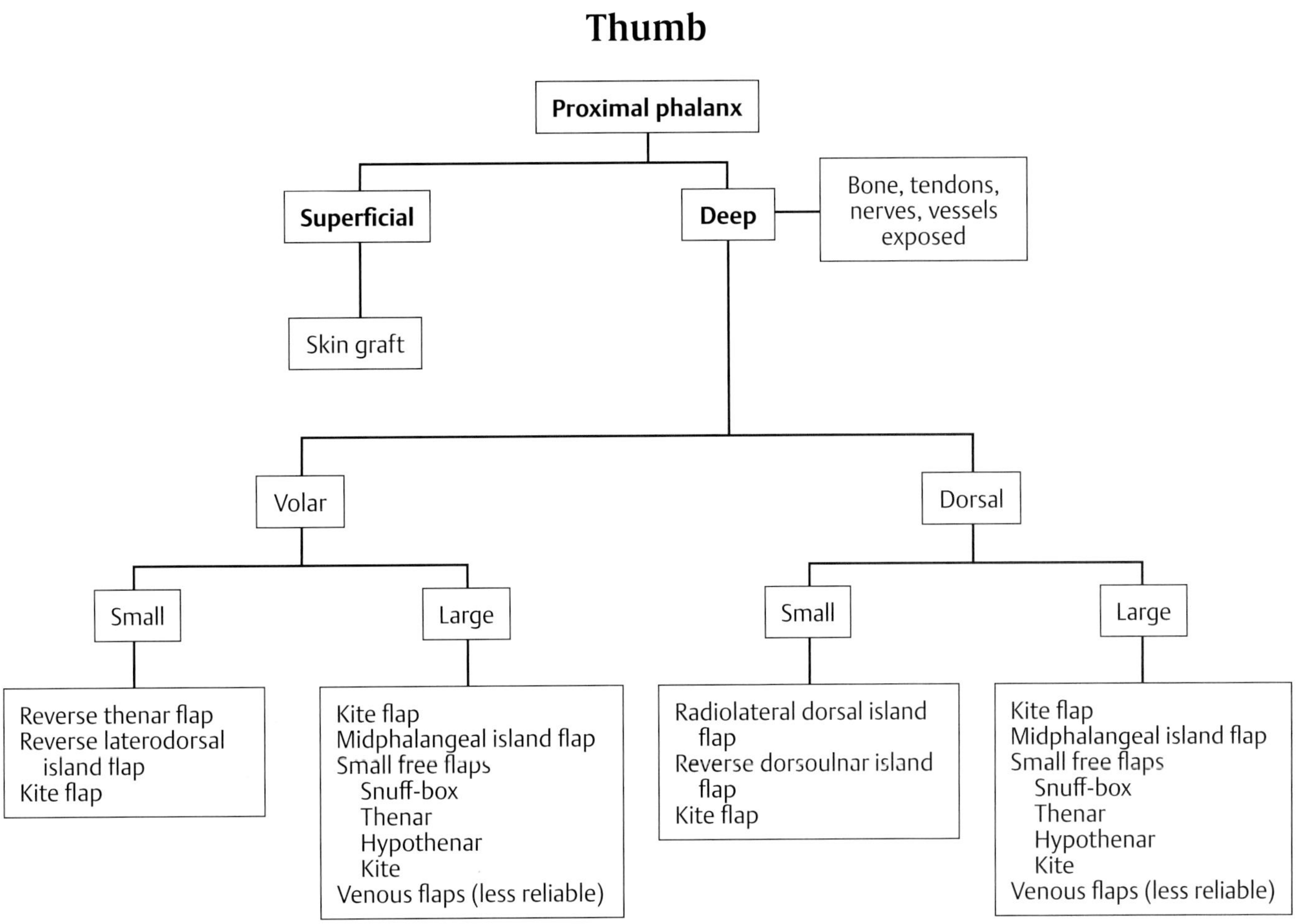

Algorithm 18.4

Thumb

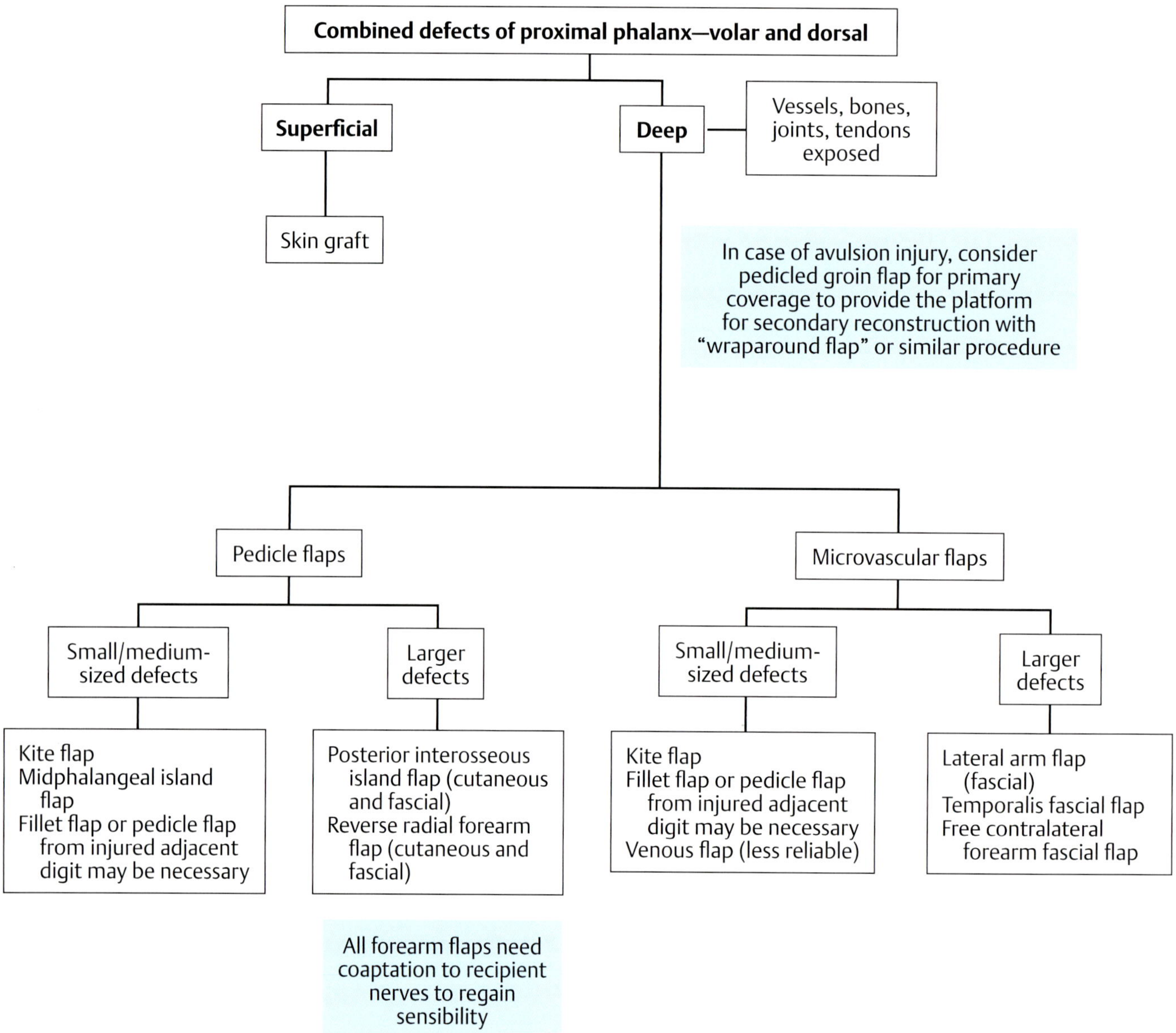

Algorithm 18.5

Parameters in decision-making	Additional options or guidelines	Warnings, precautions, or pitfalls	Emphasis on a particular waypoint

Compound Defects of Proximal and Distal Phalanx of Thumb

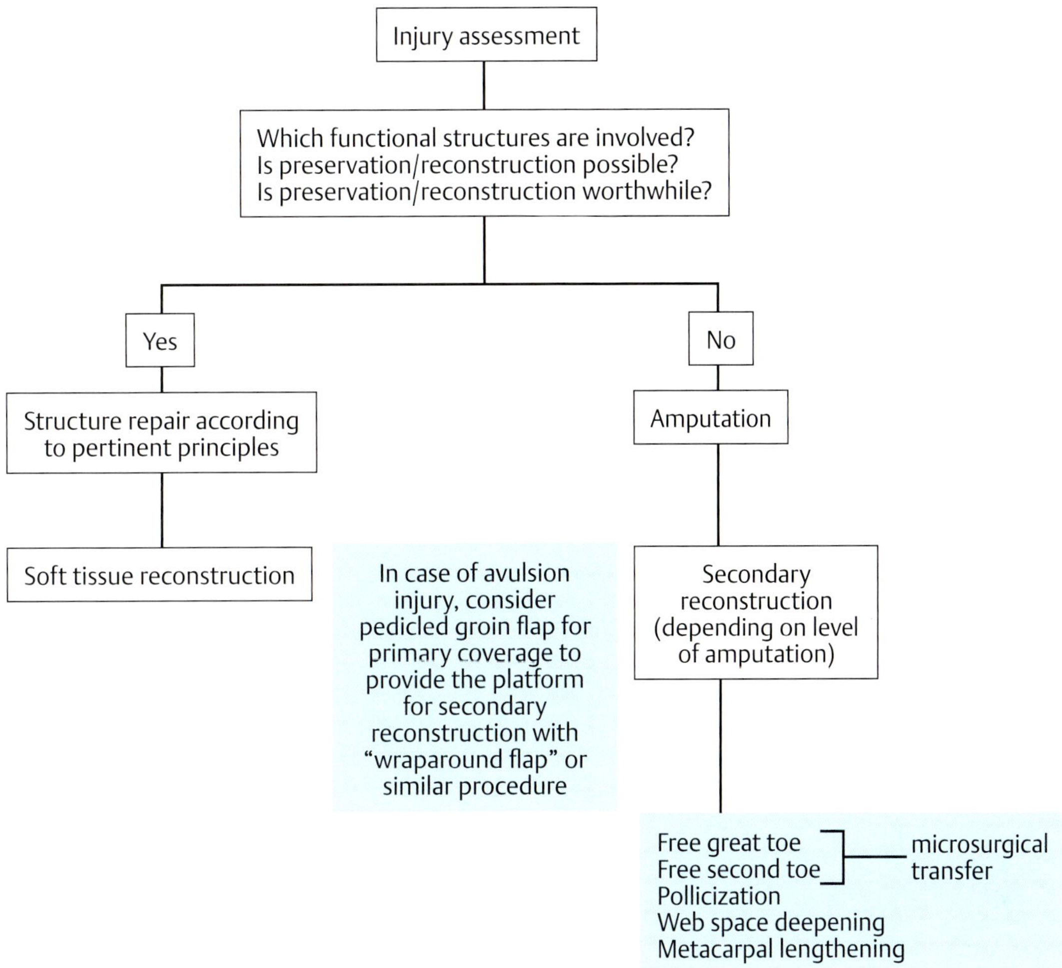

Algorithm 18.6

Parameters in decision-making	Additional options or guidelines	Warnings, precautions, or pitfalls	Emphasis on a particular waypoint

Thumb Reconstruction

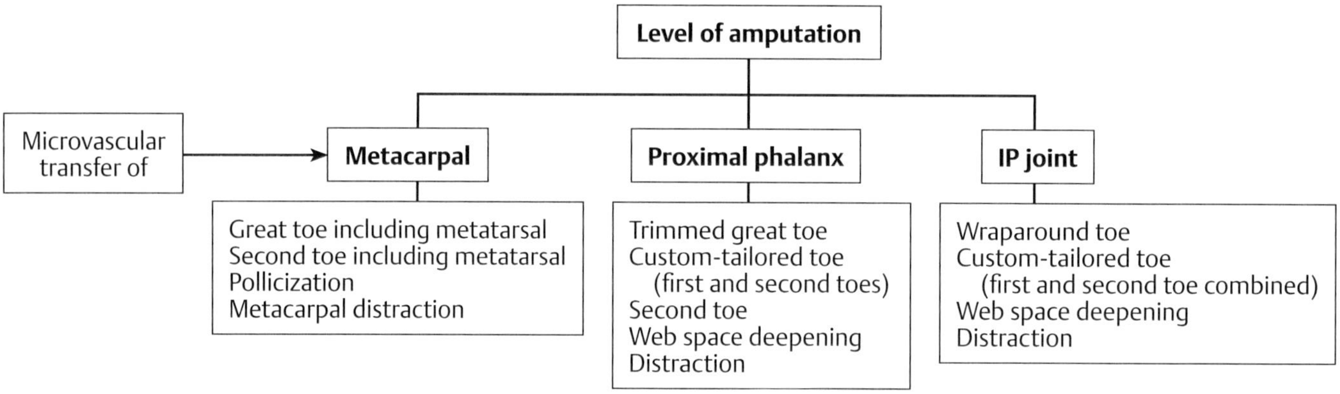

Algorithm 18.7

Digits

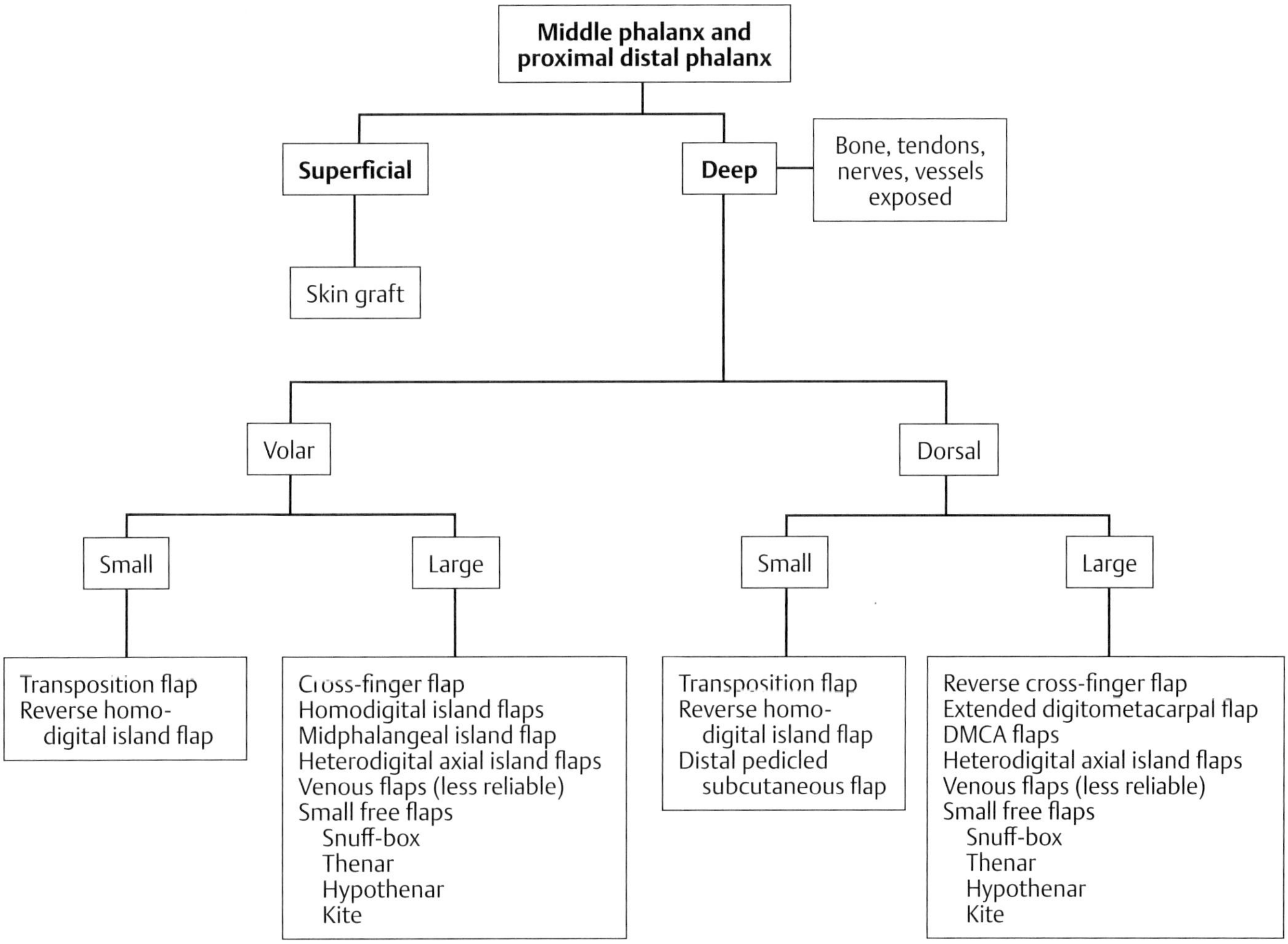

Algorithm 18.8

Digits

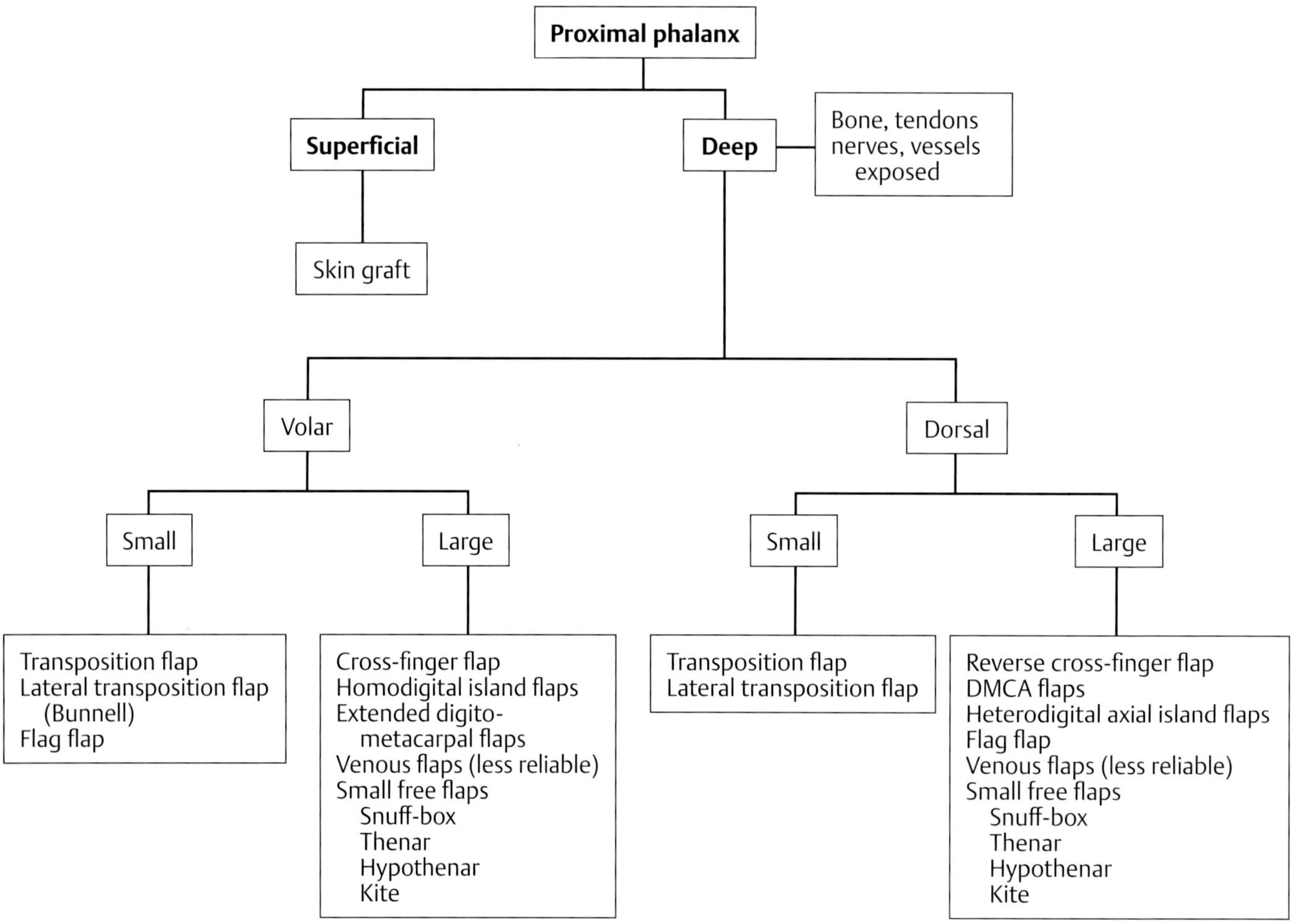

Algorithm 18.9

Digits

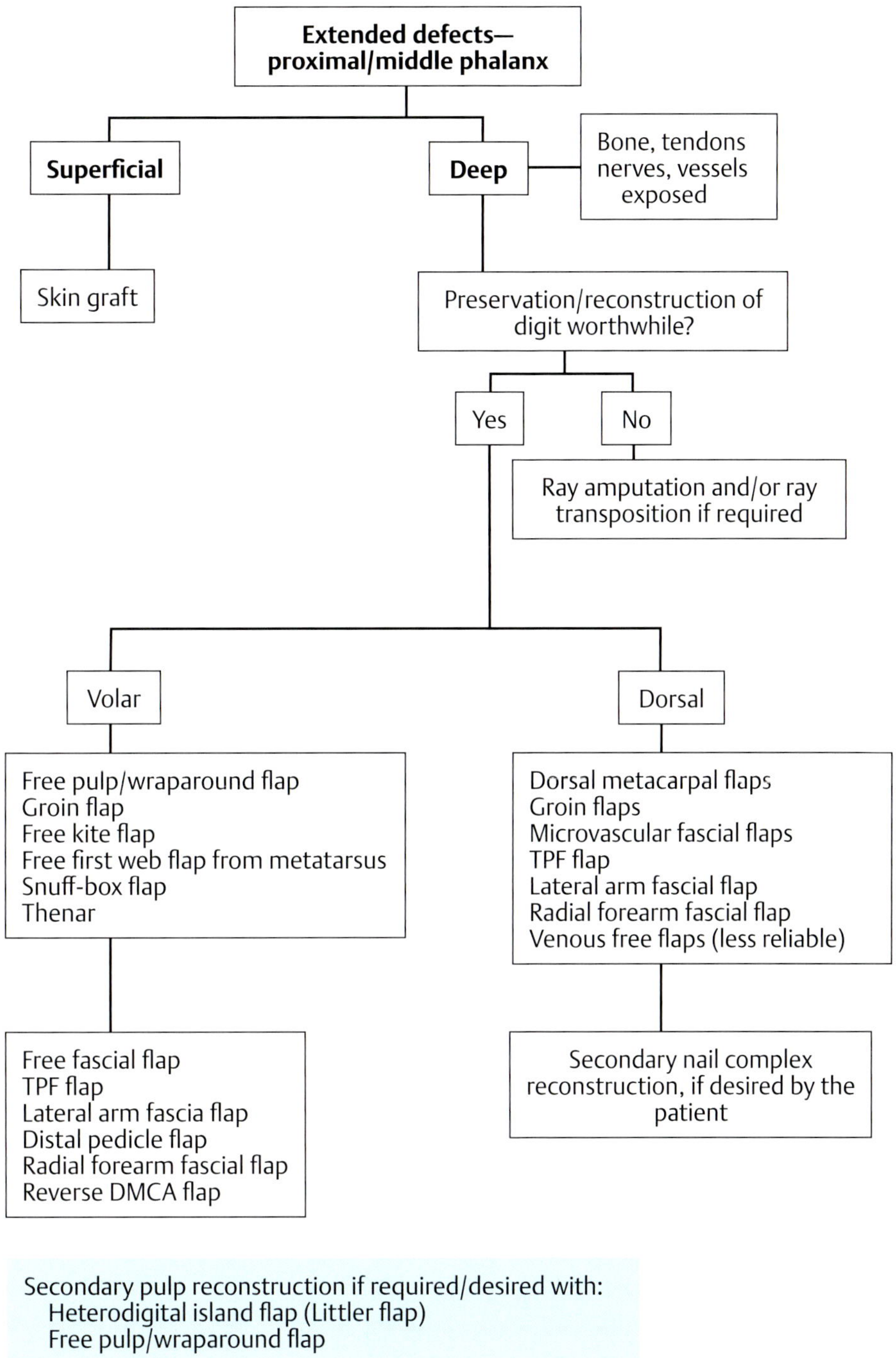

Algorithm 18.10

Parameters in decision-making	Additional options or guidelines	Warnings, precautions, or pitfalls	Emphasis on a particular waypoint

Multidigital Injuries

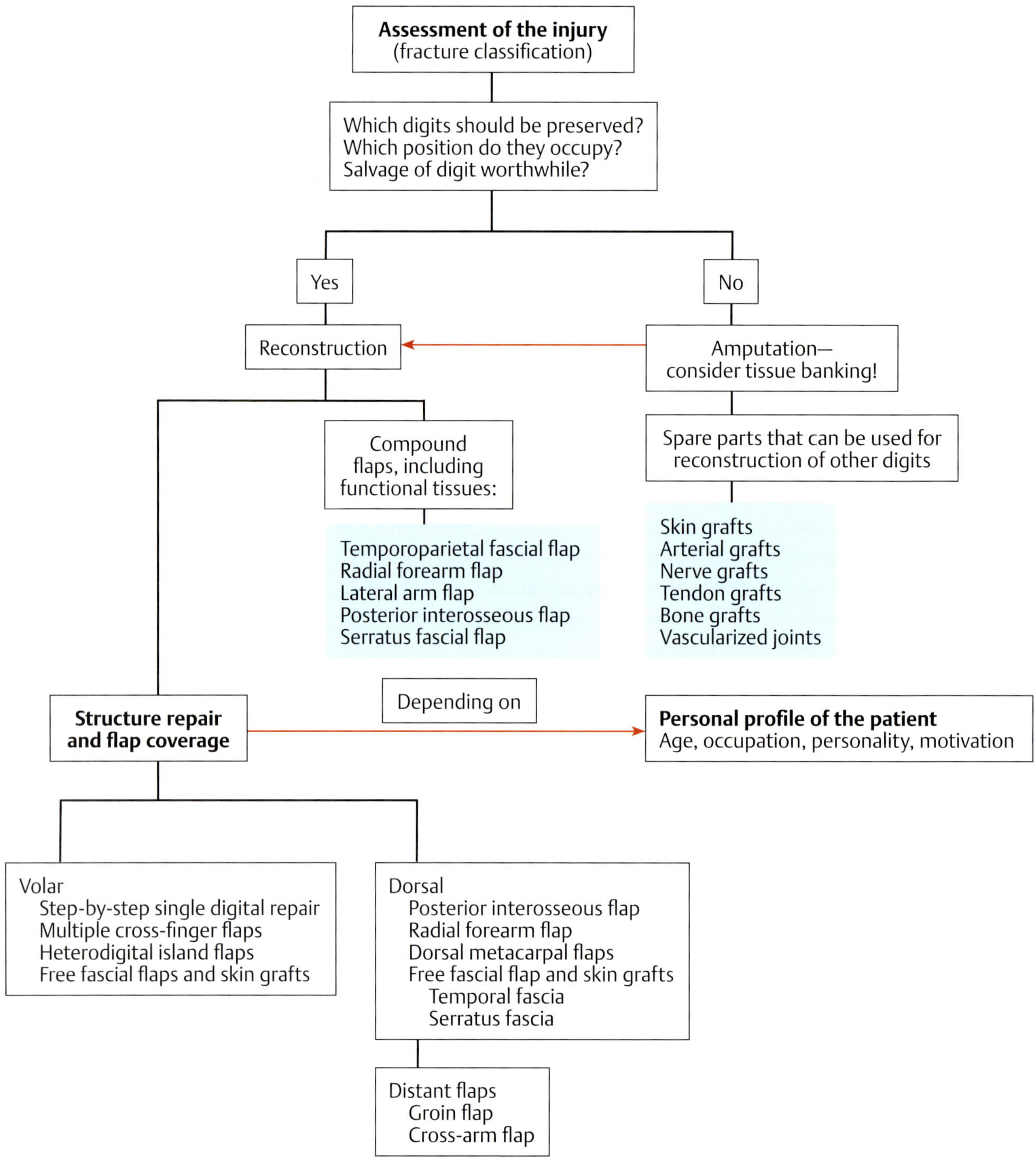

Algorithm 18.11

Parameters in decision-making	Additional options or guidelines	Warnings, precautions, or pitfalls	Emphasis on a particular waypoint

Palm

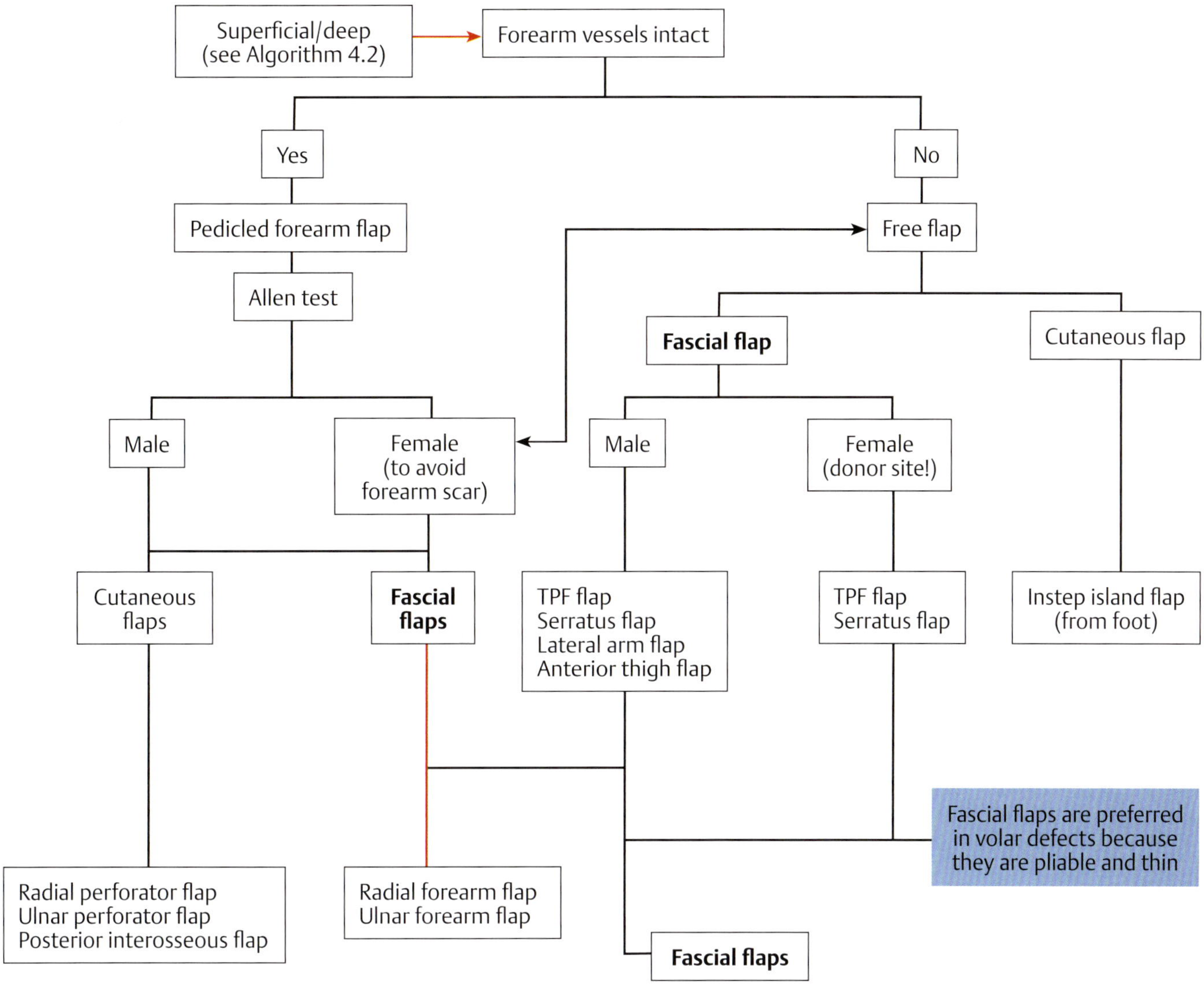

Partial flap necrosis has been reported in all types of pedicled fascial flaps so that delayed skin grafting should be considered if there are signs of questionable flap viability!
Increased capillary bleeding may also been seen in fascial flaps. In these cases secondary grafting is also recommended!

Tip: Harvest skin graft at primary operation
Storage in refrigerator
Leave catheter in brachial plexus for analgesia
Skin grafting after 2–3 days as “dressing room” procedure

Algorithm 18.12

Parameters in decision-making	Additional options or guidelines	Warnings, precautions, or pitfalls	Emphasis on a particular waypoint

Dorsal Hand Defects

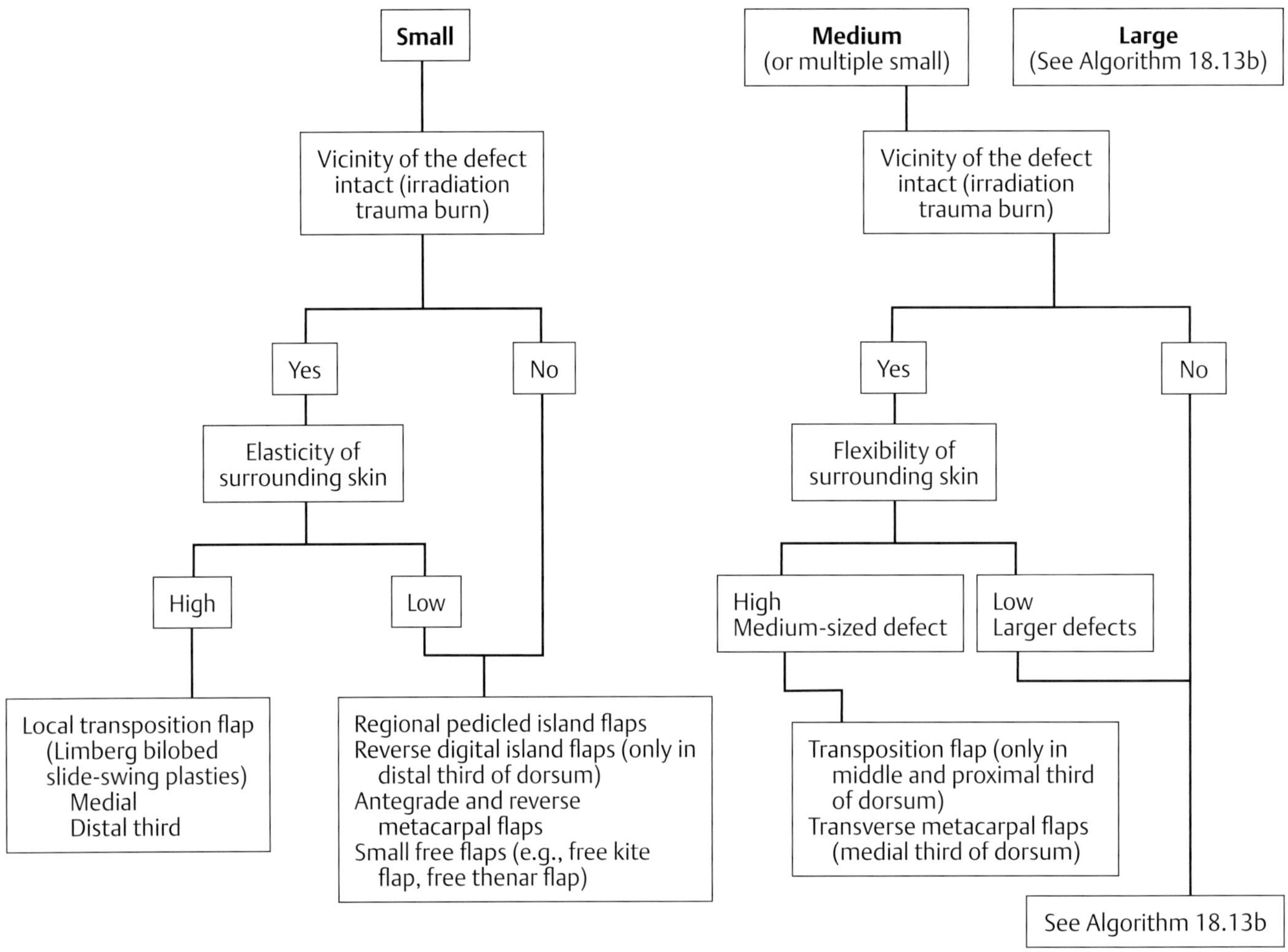

Algorithm 18.13a

Dorsal Hand Defects

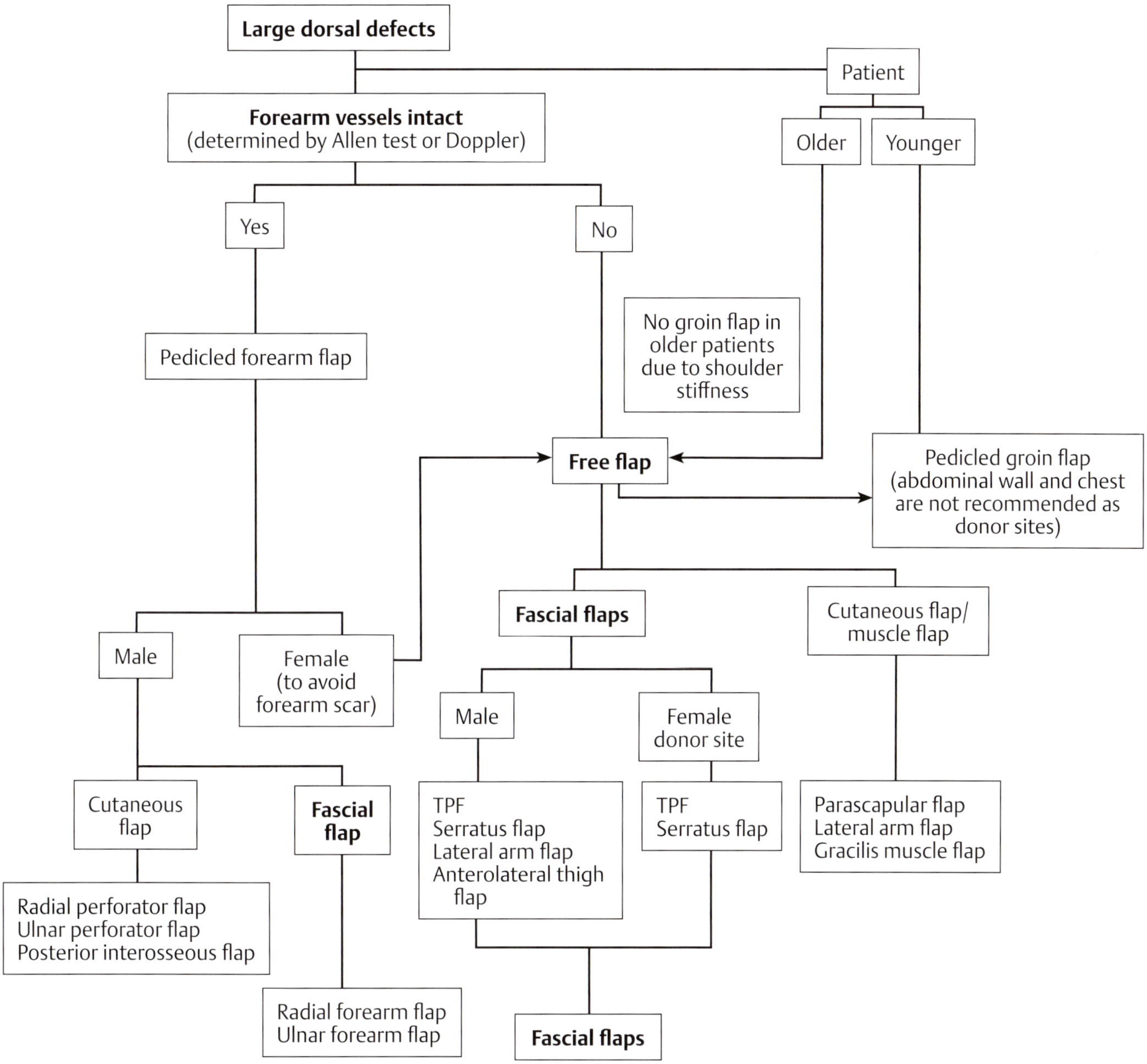

Partial flap necrosis has been reported in all types of pedicled fascial flaps so that delayed skin grafting should be considered if there are signs of questionable flap viability!
Increased capillary bleeding may also been seen in fascial flaps.
In these cases secondary grafting is also recommended!

Tip: Harvest skin graft at primary operation
Store in refrigerator
Leave catheter in brachial plexus
Skin grafting after 2–3 days as "dressing room" procedure

Algorithm 18.13b

Parameters in decision-making	Additional options or guidelines	Warnings, precautions, or pitfalls	Emphasis on a particular waypoint

Complex Volar and Dorsal Defects

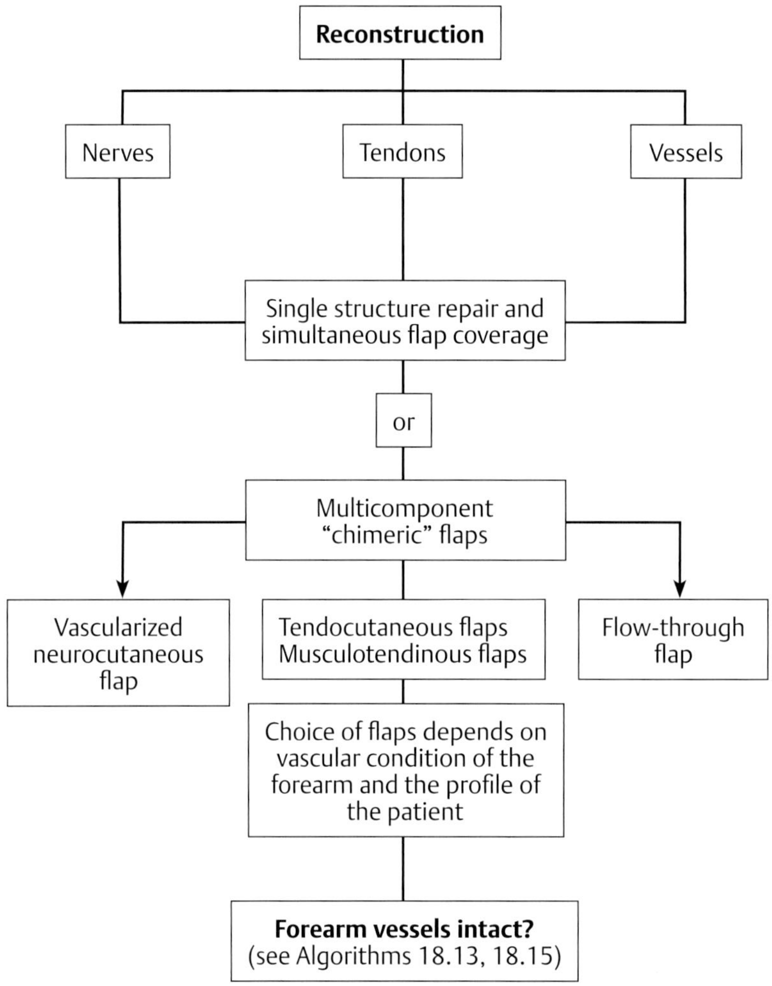

Algorithm 18.14

Forearm—Distal Third and Wrist

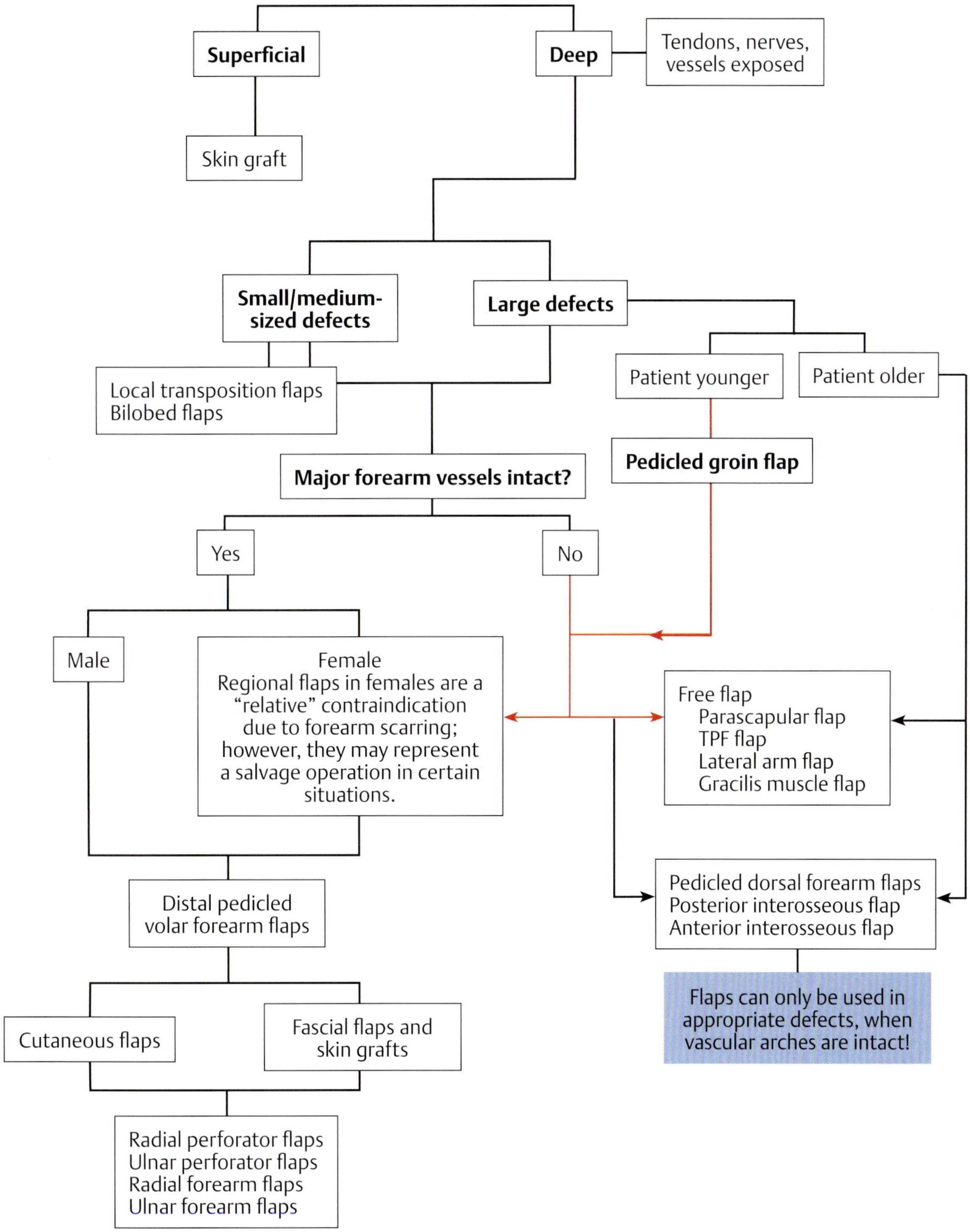

Algorithm 18.15

Parameters in decision-making	Additional options or guidelines	Warnings, precautions, or pitfalls	Emphasis on a particular waypoint

Forearm—Middle Third

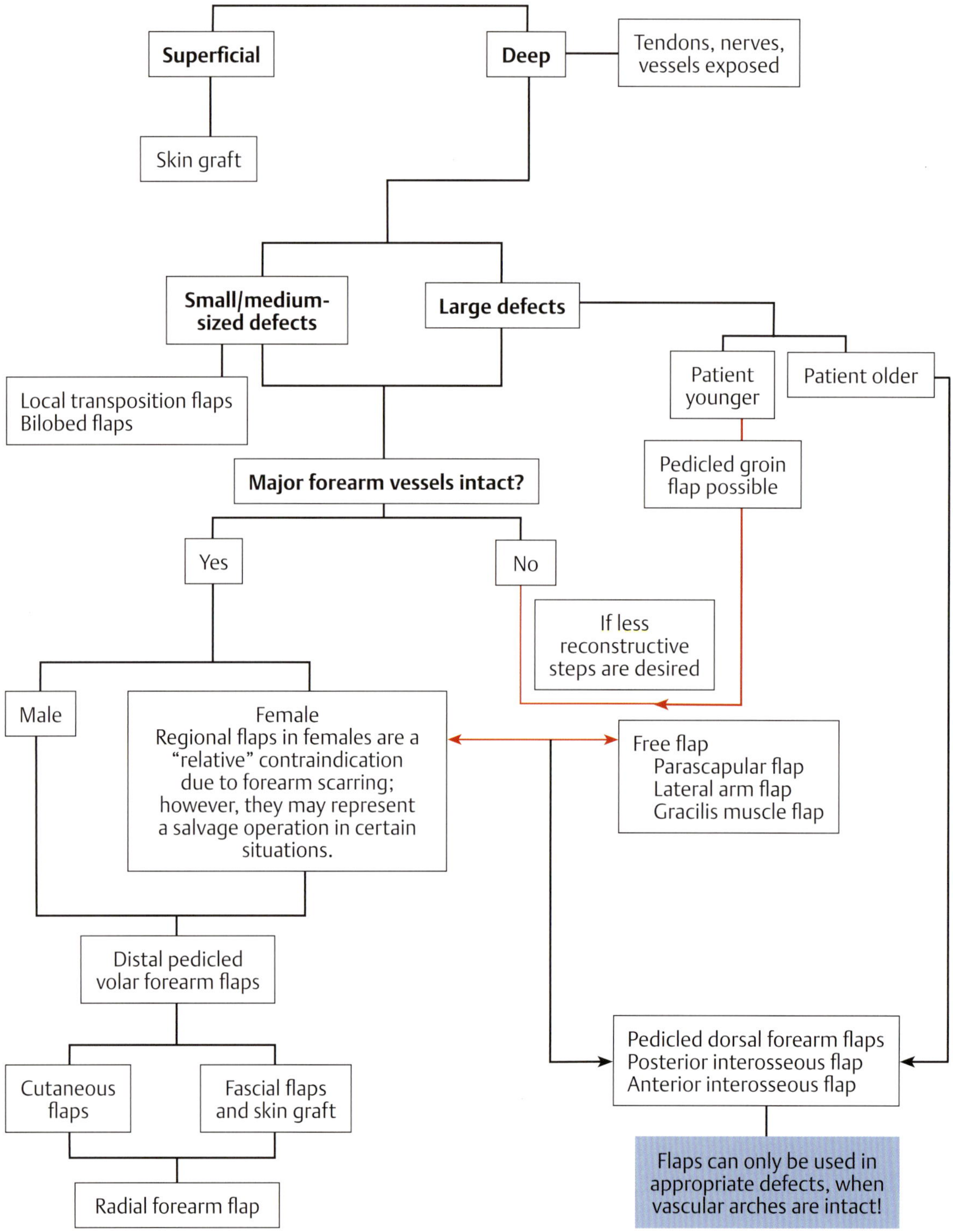

Algorithm 18.16

Parameters in decision-making	Additional options or guidelines	Warnings, precautions, or pitfalls	Emphasis on a particular waypoint

Complex Forearm Defects

Combined multistructural defects

Nerves | Vessels | Bones | Muscles

Reconstruction

Single structure repair and simultaneous flap coverage

or

Chimeric flaps

Free flap
Vascularized neurocutaneous flap
Flow-through flap

Osteocutaneous flaps
Fibular flap
Parascapular flap
Iliac crest flap
Osteocutaneous medial geniculate flap

Vascularized tendon transfer
Free muscle transfer (gracilis, latissimus dorsi)

Pedicle flap
Osteocutaneous posterior interosseous flap
Osteocutaneous radial forearm flap
Distal pedicled osteocutaneous lateral arm flap
Tendocutaneous lateral arm flap

Use of these flaps depends on volar versus dorsal injury zones.

Decision criteria
(see Algorithms 18.12 through 18.16)

Algorithm 18.17

Parameters in decision-making | Additional options or guidelines | Warnings, precautions, or pitfalls | Emphasis on a particular waypoint

Ventral Elbow and Proximal Forearm

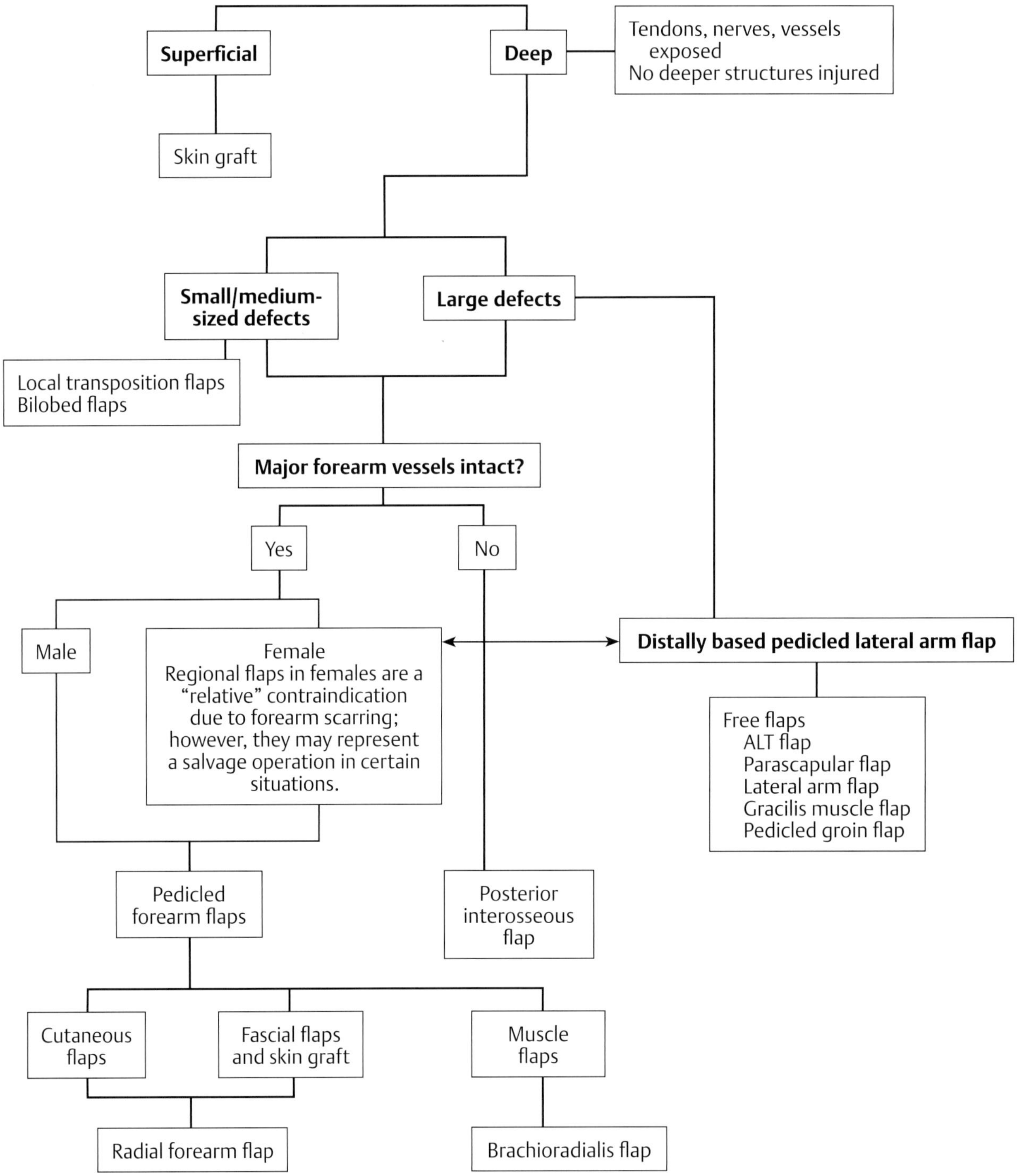

Algorithm 18.18

Elbow and Proximal Forearm

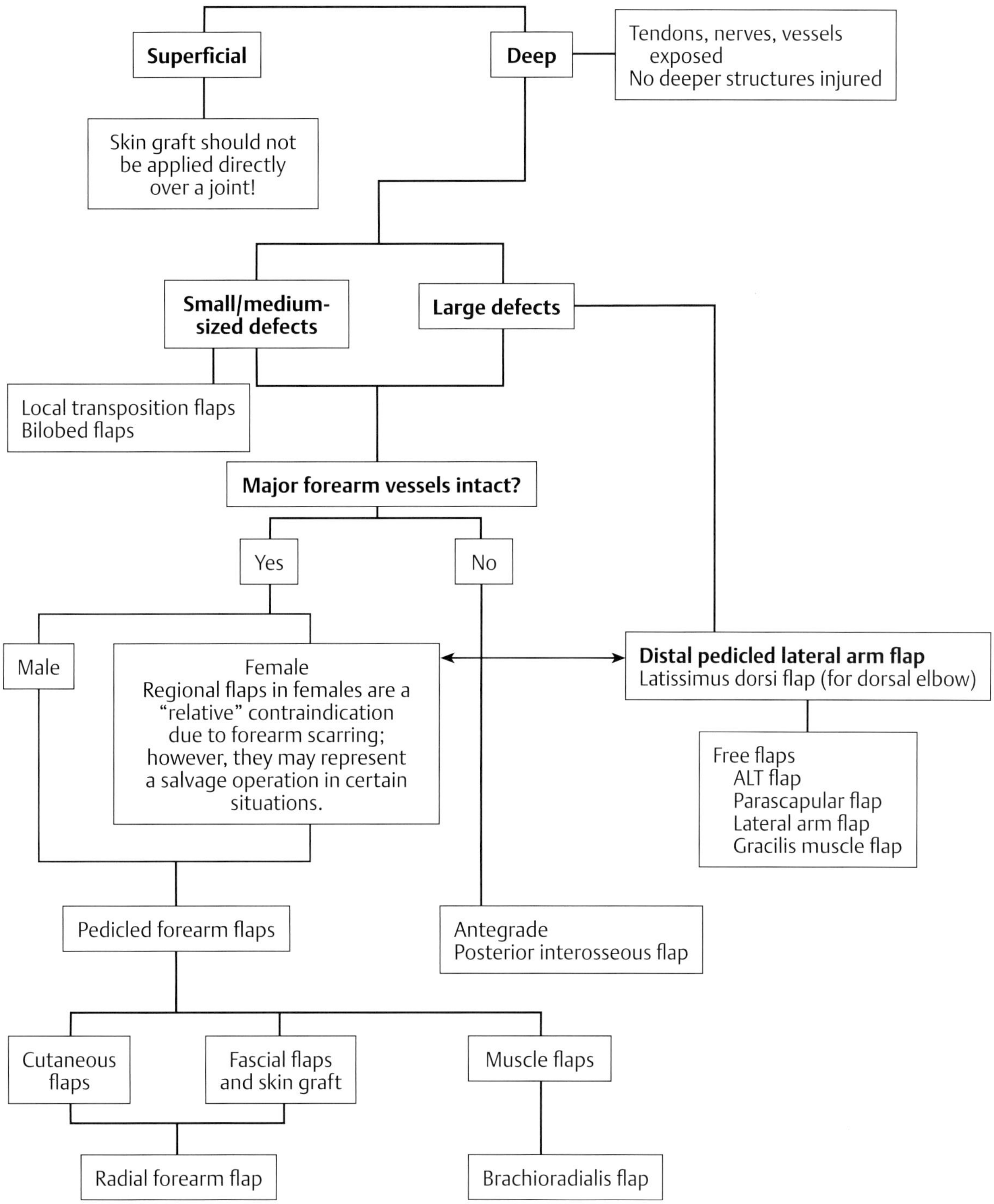

Algorithm 18.19

Brachium

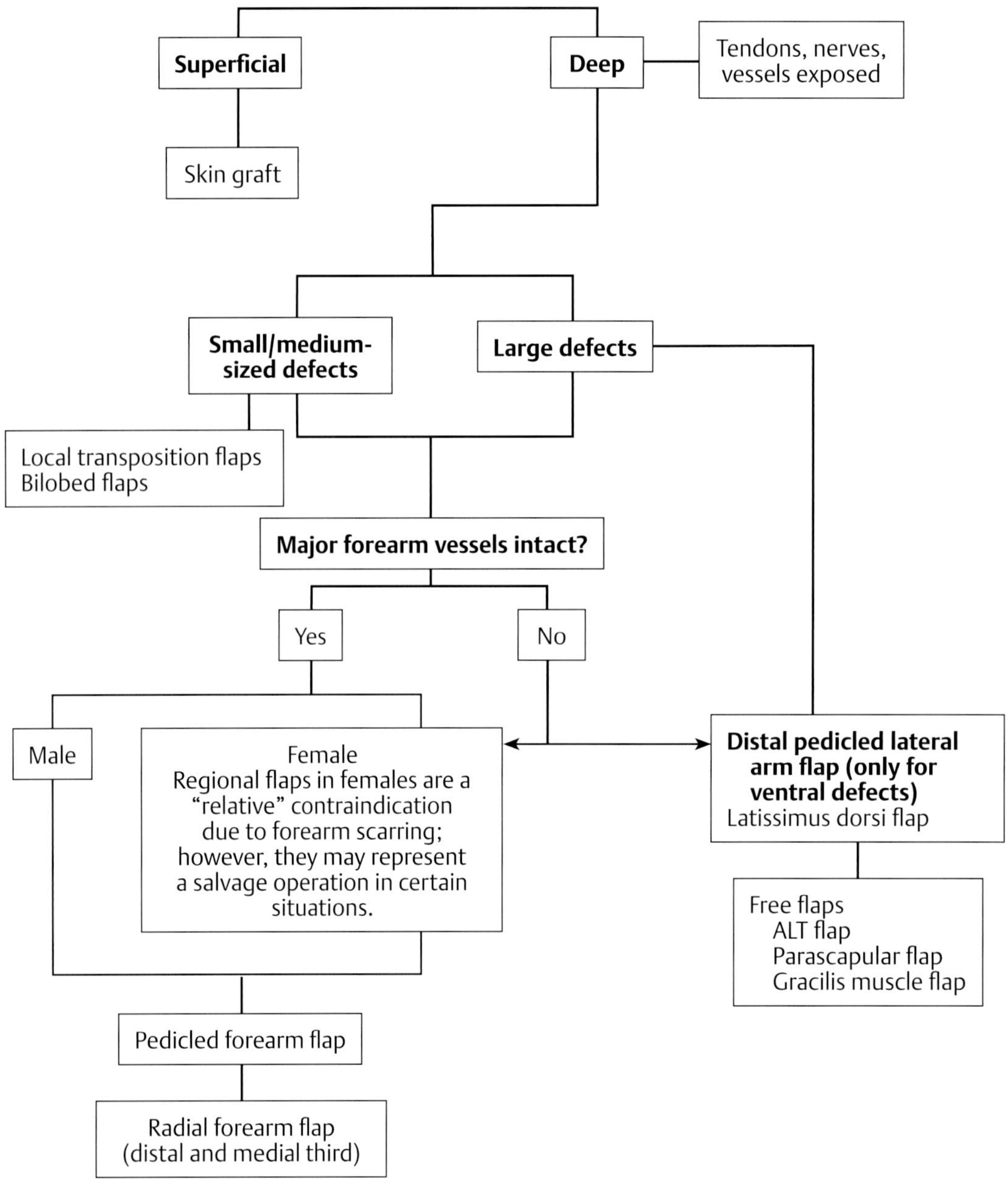

Algorithm 18.20

Shoulder and Proximal Brachium

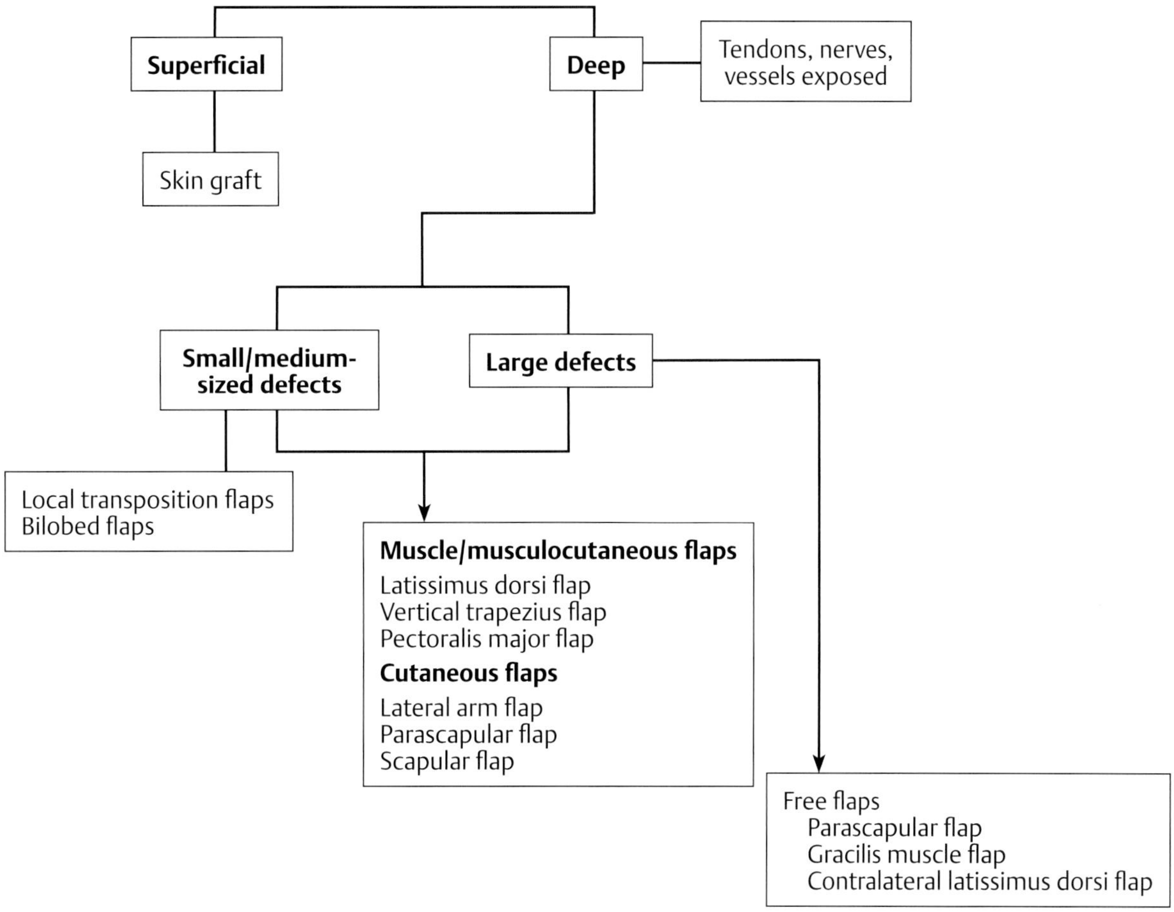

Algorithm 18.21

Complex Defects of the Upper Arm

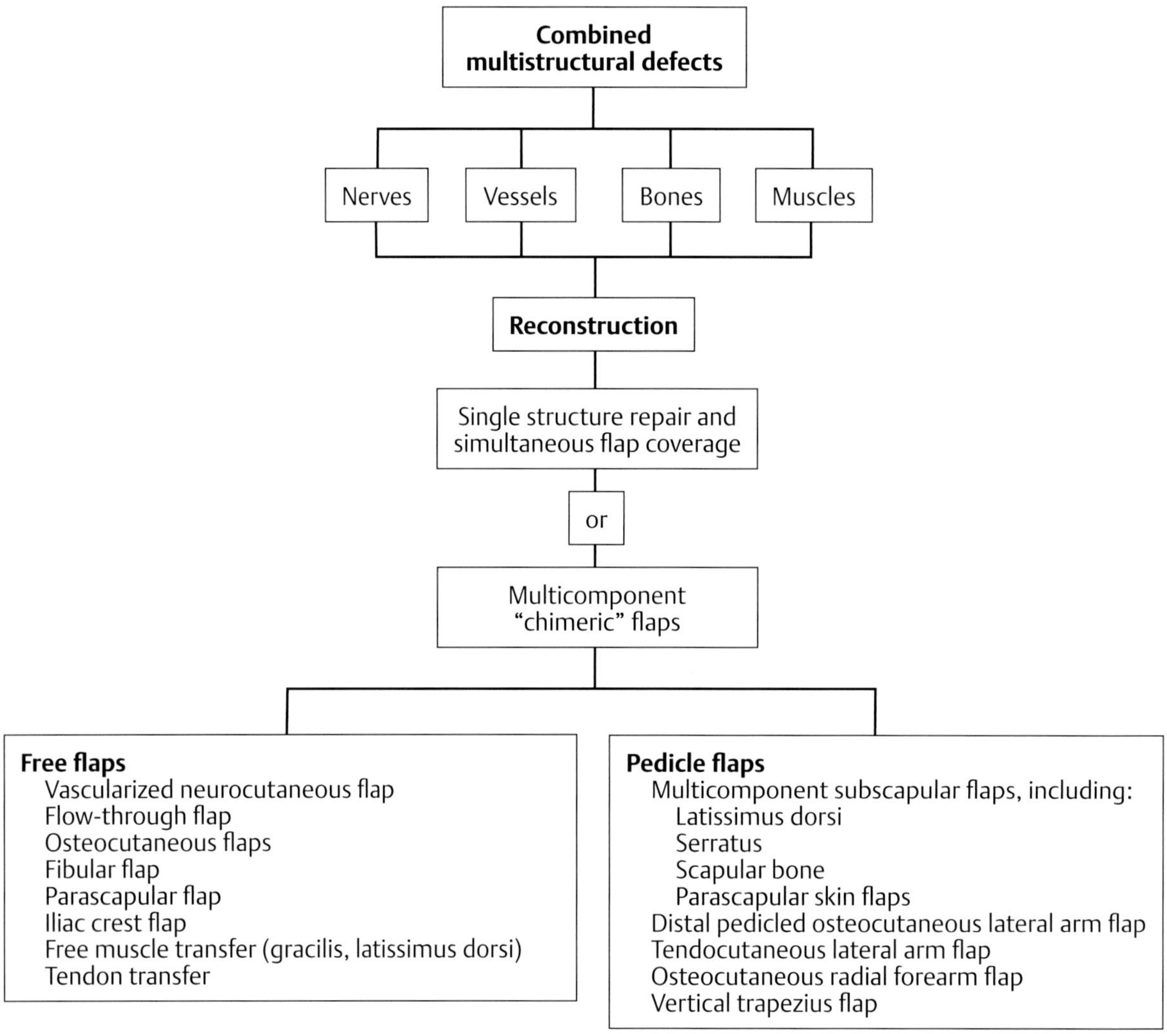

Algorithm 18.22

Part IV

Clinical Examples

Chapter 19

Gunshot Wound

Case history: 23-year-old man with a gunshot wound to the hand.

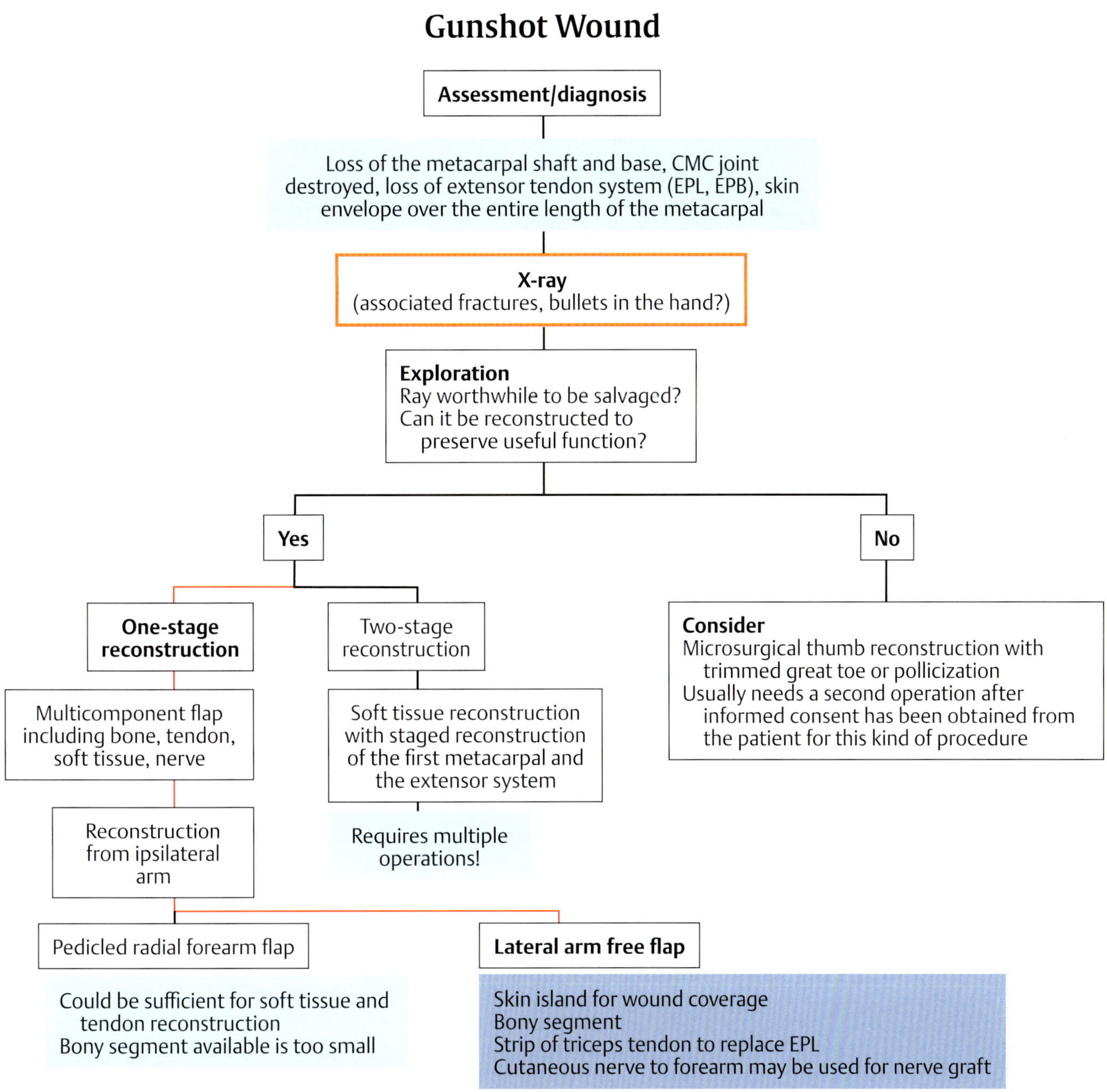

Algorithm 19.1

Parameters in decision-making	Additional options or guidelines	Warnings, precautions, or pitfalls	Emphasis on a particular waypoint

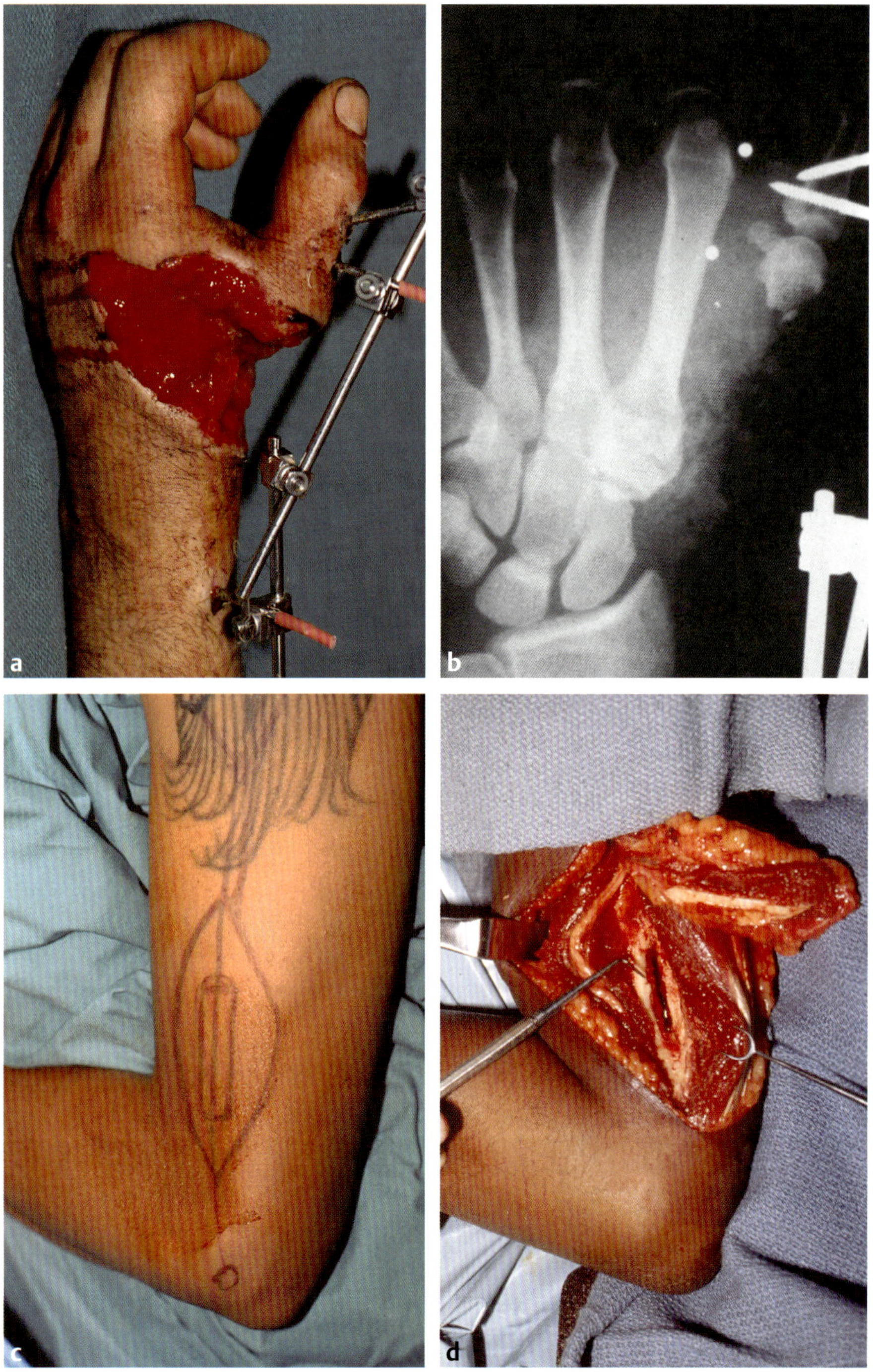

Fig. 19.1 (a) This patient has sustained a gunshot wound to the hand, with loss of the metacarpal and concomitant soft tissue injury. **(b)** A spanning external fixator is used to stabilize the thumb remnant and to maintain the thumb-index web space. **(c)** The design of the osteocutaneous flap includes a segment of the humeral corticalis. **(d)** The flap is elevated on the posterior radial collateral artery. This composite flap includes skin, subcutaneous tissue, and vascularized bone (*continued*).

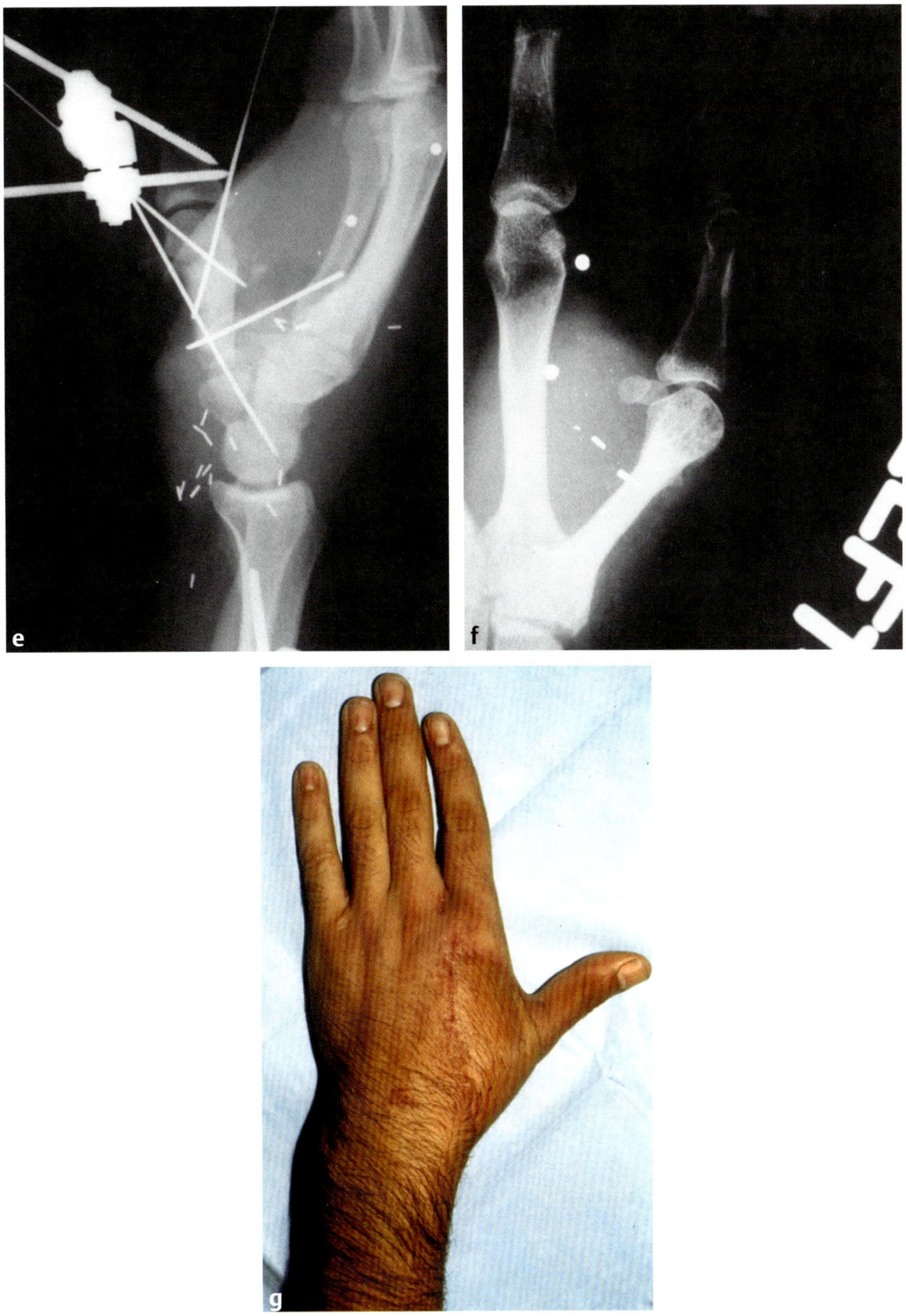

Fig. 19.1 (*continued*) **(e,f)** The metacarpal graft is fixated during the healing of vascularized bone to create a metacarpal shaft. **(g)** The final appearance of the patient's reconstructed hand is shown; thumb function and the thumb-index web space have been maintained. EPL was reconstructed with a second-stage free tendon graft.

Chapter 20

Burn

Case history: 22-year-old woman with a third-degree friction burn to the dorsum of her hand. Second-degree burns on the left leg and thigh will spontaneously heal.

Friction Burn

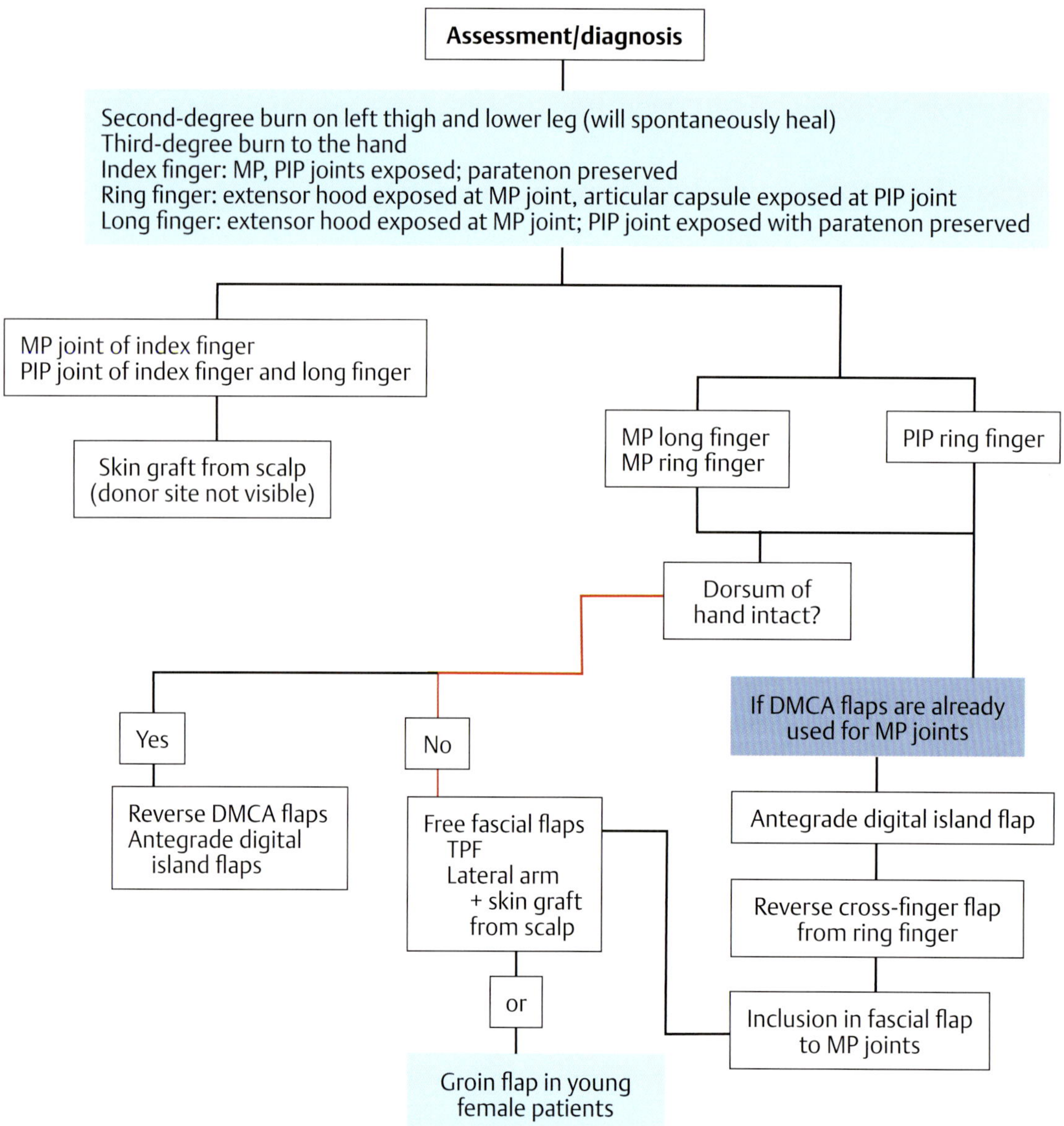

Algorithm 20.1

Parameters in decision-making	Additional options or guidelines	Warnings, precautions, or pitfalls	Emphasis on a particular waypoint

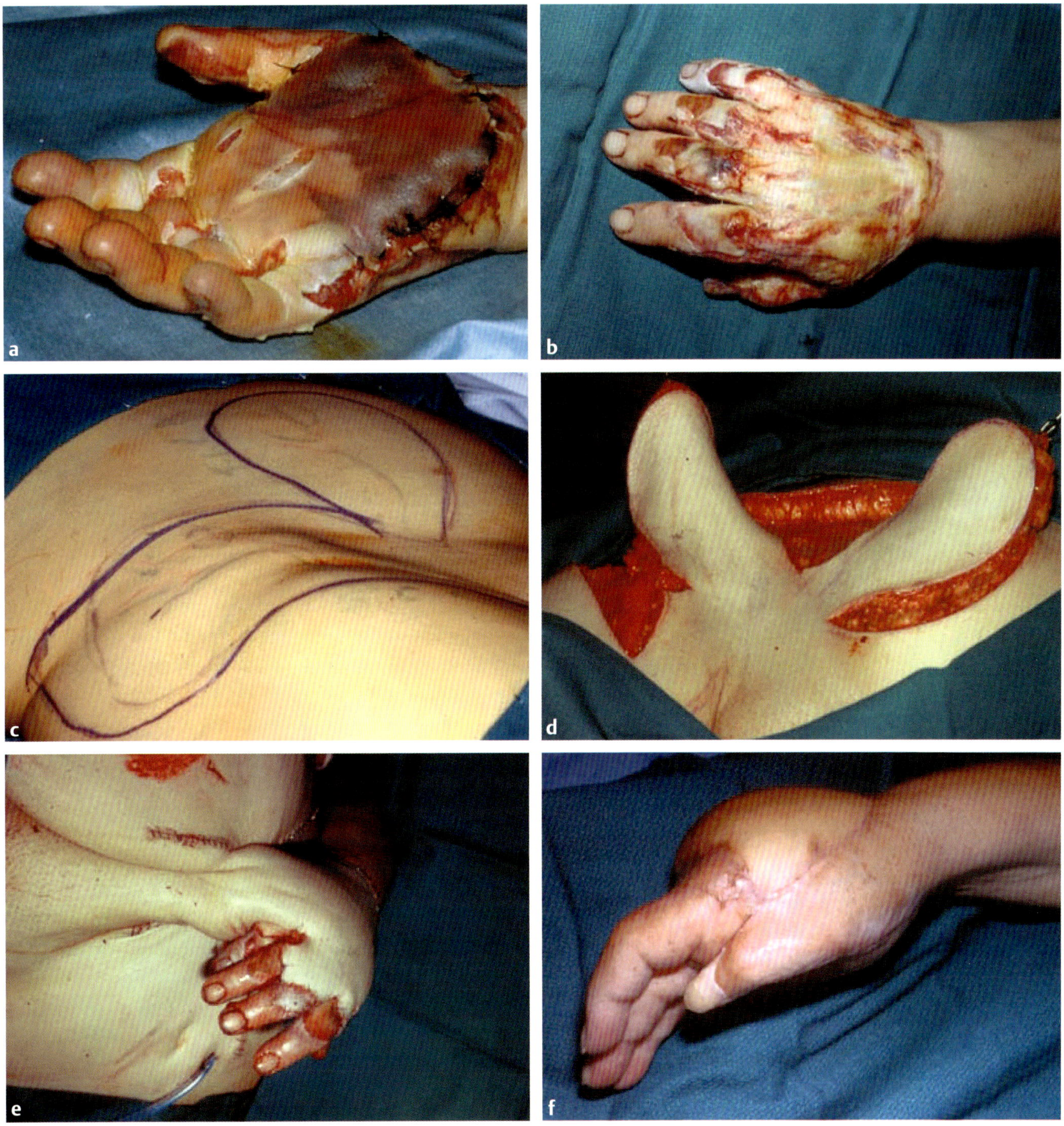

Fig. 20.1 (a) This patient had a crush/burn injury in a hot press machine. The palm was avulsed and a portion of this did not survive. **(b)** She also had third-degree burns to the dorsum of the hand. **(c)** Markings for deep circumflex iliac artery and superficial circumflex iliac artery flaps. **(d)** The flaps were raised. **(e)** Both flaps were attached to the hand. **(f)** The hand is shown before tissue expansion for the thumb-index web contracture (*continued*).

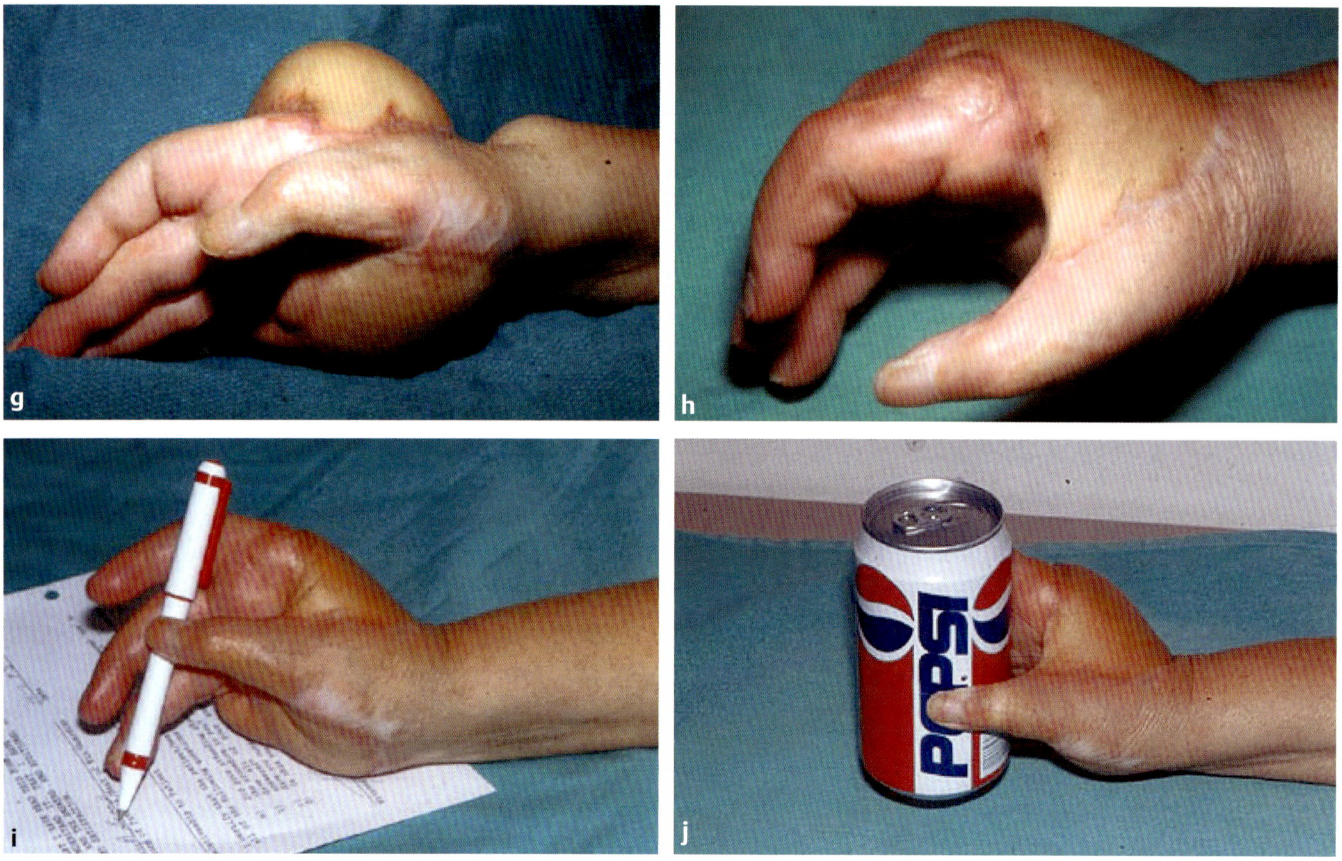

Fig. 20.1 (*continued*) **(g)** A tissue expander was placed under the groin flap. **(h)** Web space was improved after expansion of the dorsal flap and transposition. **(i)** Writing. **(j)** Opposition.

Chapter 21

Carpal Injury

Case history: 42-year-old man with an open carpal injury from an MVA (convertible), with overlying soft tissue loss.

Open Carpal Injury

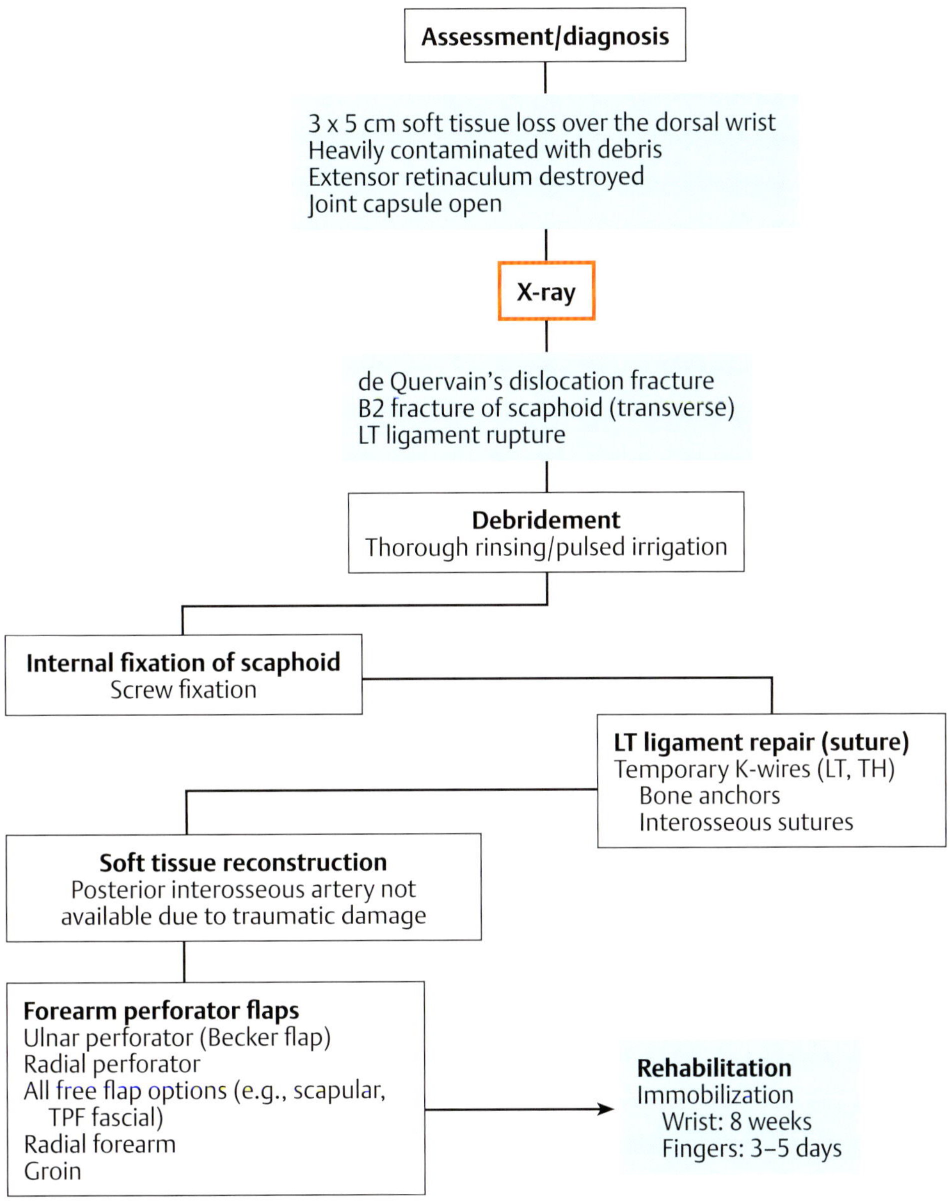

Algorithm 21.1

Parameters in decision-making | Additional options or guidelines | Warnings, precautions, or pitfalls | Emphasis on a particular waypoint

Chapter 22

Crush Injury

Case history: 34-year-old man with an occupational crush injury to the distal phalanx of the long finger.

Crush Injury to Long Finger

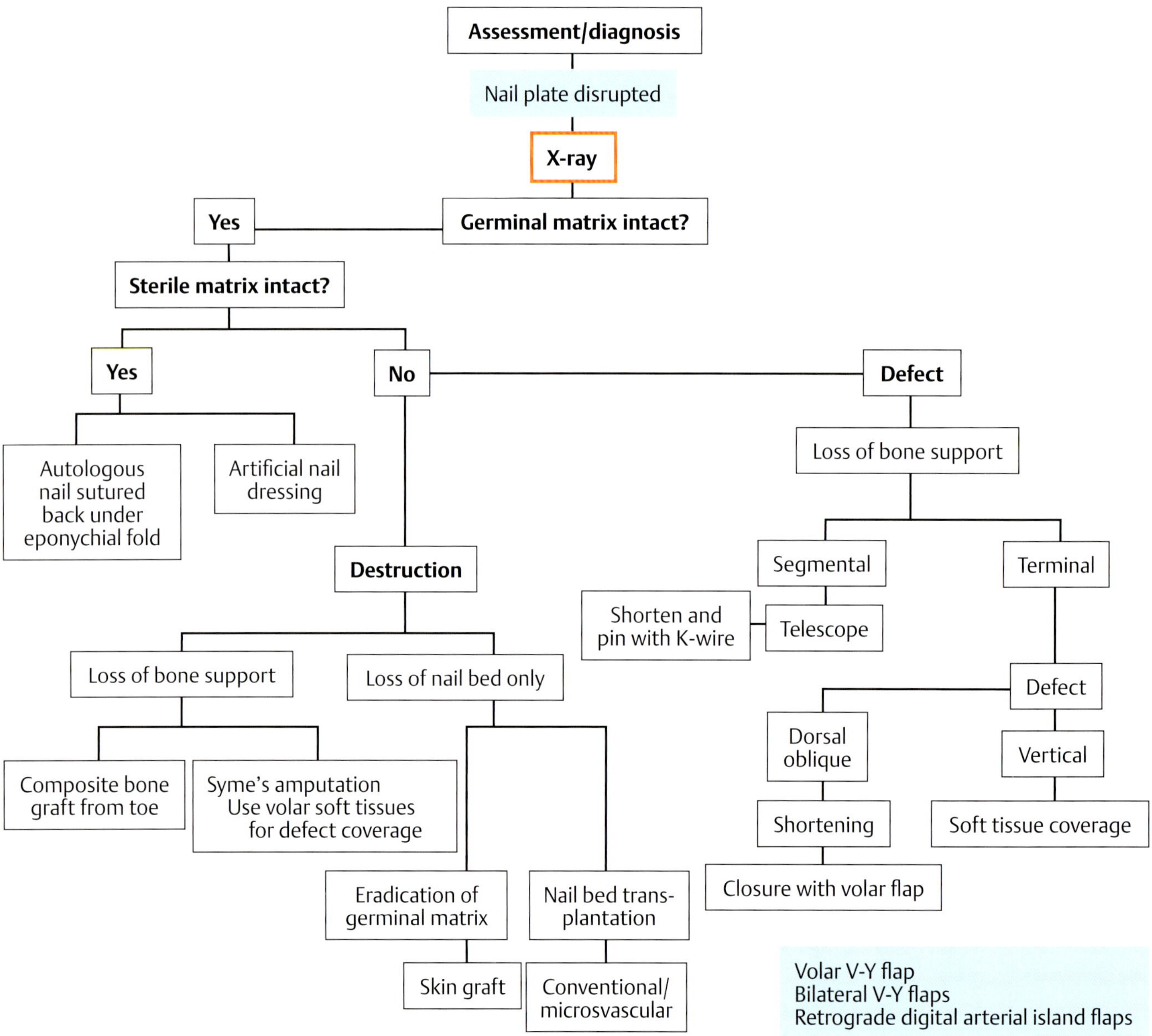

Algorithm 22.1

Parameters in decision-making	Additional options or guidelines	Warnings, precautions, or pitfalls	Emphasis on a particular waypoint

Chapter 23

Dorsal Soft Tissue Injury to Finger and Hand

Case history: 18-year-old man with avulsion injury of the dorsum of the left hand after a fall from a motorcycle.

Abrasion Injury

Assessment/diagnosis

Loss of skin and subcutaneous tissue
Paratenon preserved–thick subcutaneous layer

Soft tissue reconstruction

Groin flap

Advantages
- Favorable donor site
- Reliable tissue cover

Disadvantages
- 3 weeks of immobilization
- Total of 4–5 procedures until treatment goal is achieved!

Free temporal fascial flap
Lateral arm flap
Skin graft from scalp! or from arch of foot to cover free fascial flap (no visible donor site)

Advantages
- Inconspicuous donor site
- Excellent cosmetic result
- "One-stage reconstruction"

Disadvantages
- Complex microsurgical procedure with risk of flap failure

Decision is based on philosophy of the surgeon and the patient's request!

A one-stage reconstruction should be attempted.
Primary skin graft is not recommended in this case, because it leaves a contour and color deformity.
It also prolongs rehabilitation time and increases treatment cost.

Algorithm 23.1

Parameters in decision-making	Additional options or guidelines	Warnings, precautions, or pitfalls	Emphasis on a particular waypoint

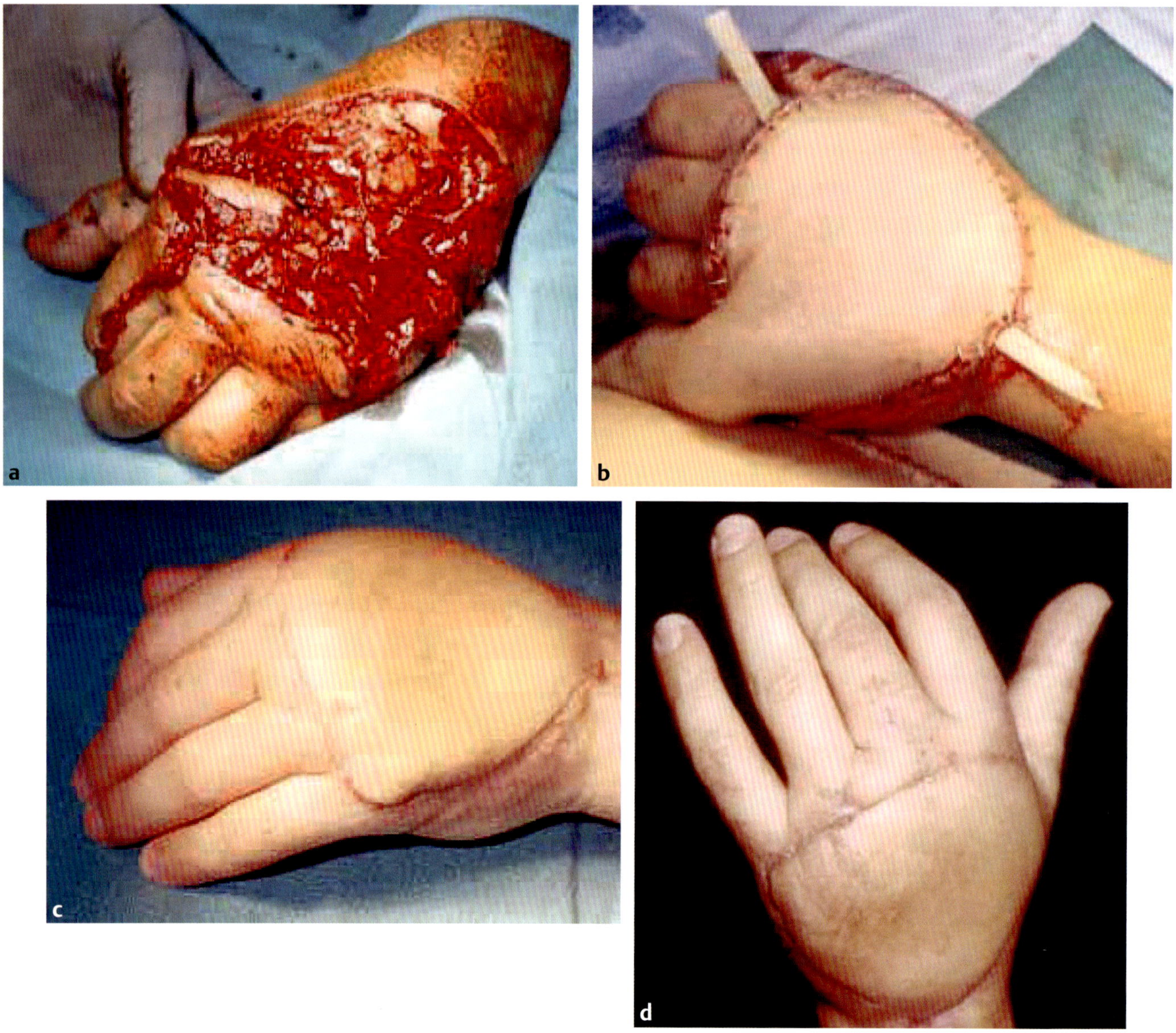

Fig. 23.1 In this case we selected a multiple-stage approach because of the contamination of the wound. **(a)** This patient had a dorsal avulsion injury that involved damage of the skin and the extensor tendons. **(b)** A pedicle flap was grown for dorsal soft tissue coverage. Note the position of the pedicle and the hand position. **(c)** The flap was allowed to heal before second-stage extensor tendon reconstruction was performed with Hunter rods followed by tendon grafts. **(d)** Digital extension is shown after second-stage reconstruction with free tendon grafts.

Chapter 24

Volar Soft Tissue Injury to Finger and Hand/Palm

Case history: A 34-year-old woman injured her palm in an industrial grinder accident. She has loss of functional structures.

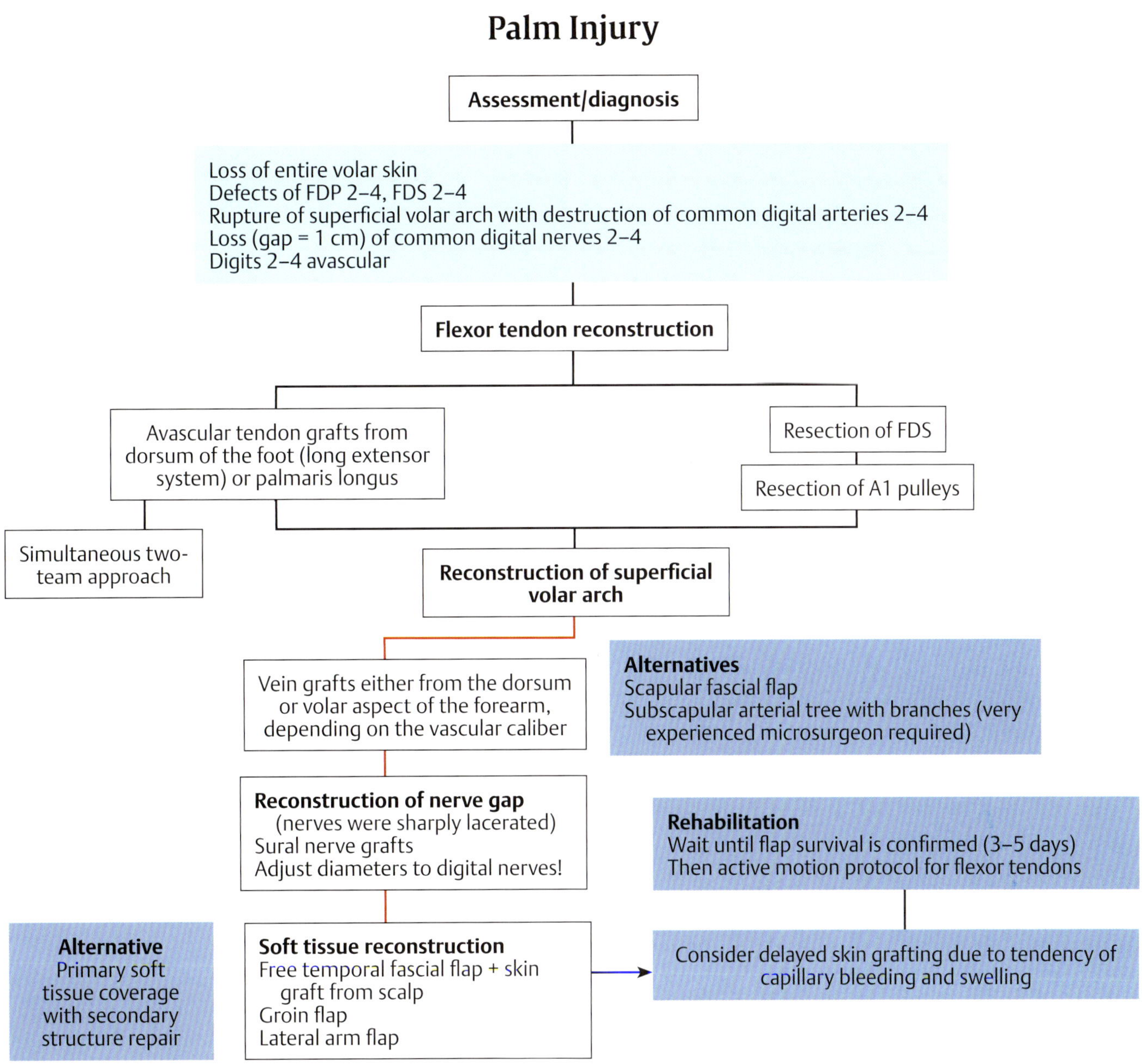

Algorithm 24.1

Parameters in decision-making	Additional options or guidelines	Warnings, precautions, or pitfalls	Emphasis on a particular waypoint

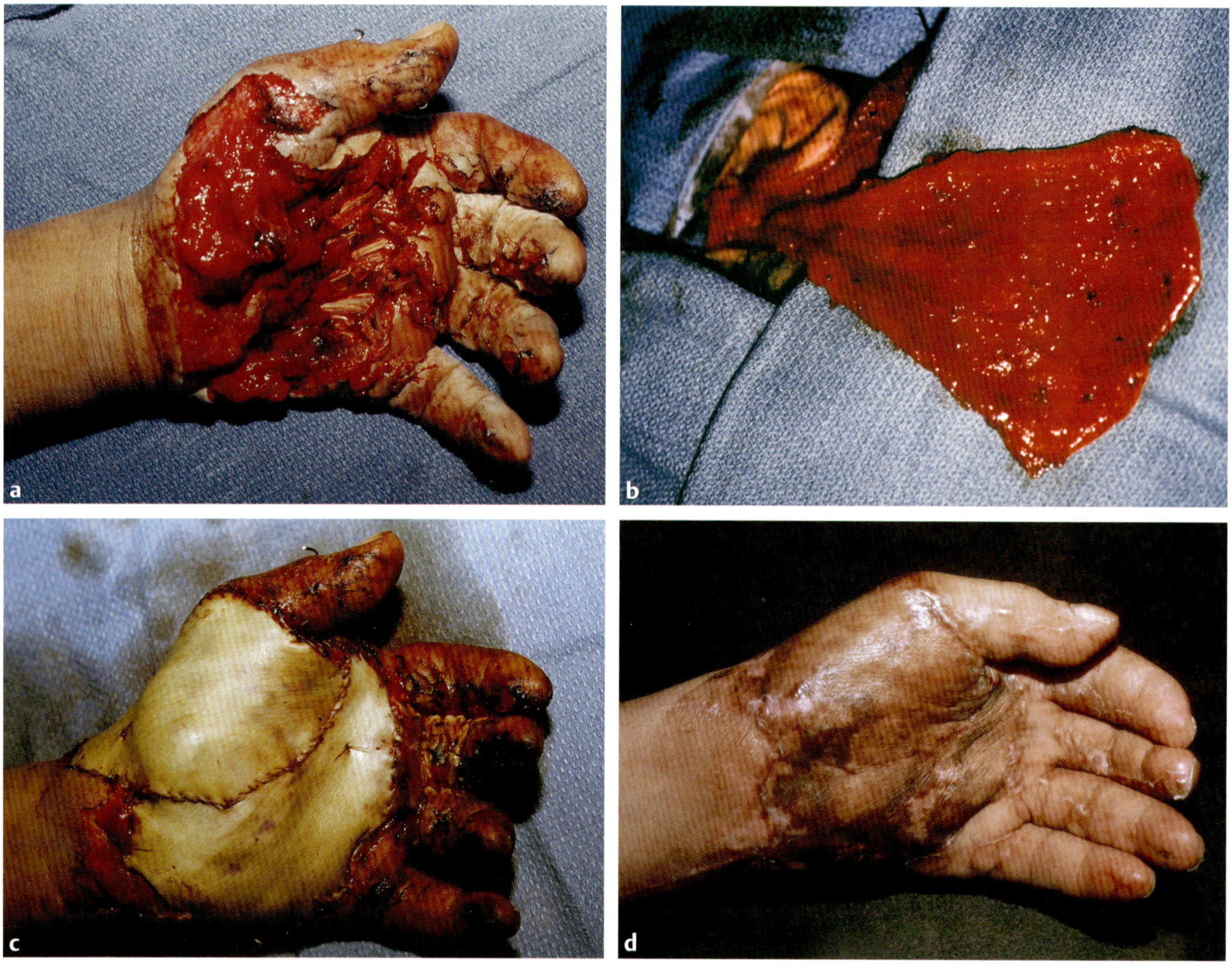

Fig. 24.1 (a) This patient had a volar crush injury caused by an incendiary device. **(b)** A TPF flap was created. **(c)** The transferred flap was covered with an FTSG. **(d)** The patient's hand is shown 3 months after flap transfer.

Chapter 25

Digital Amputation

Case history: 23-year-old man with circular saw injury to the dominant, right long finger.

Circular Saw Injury

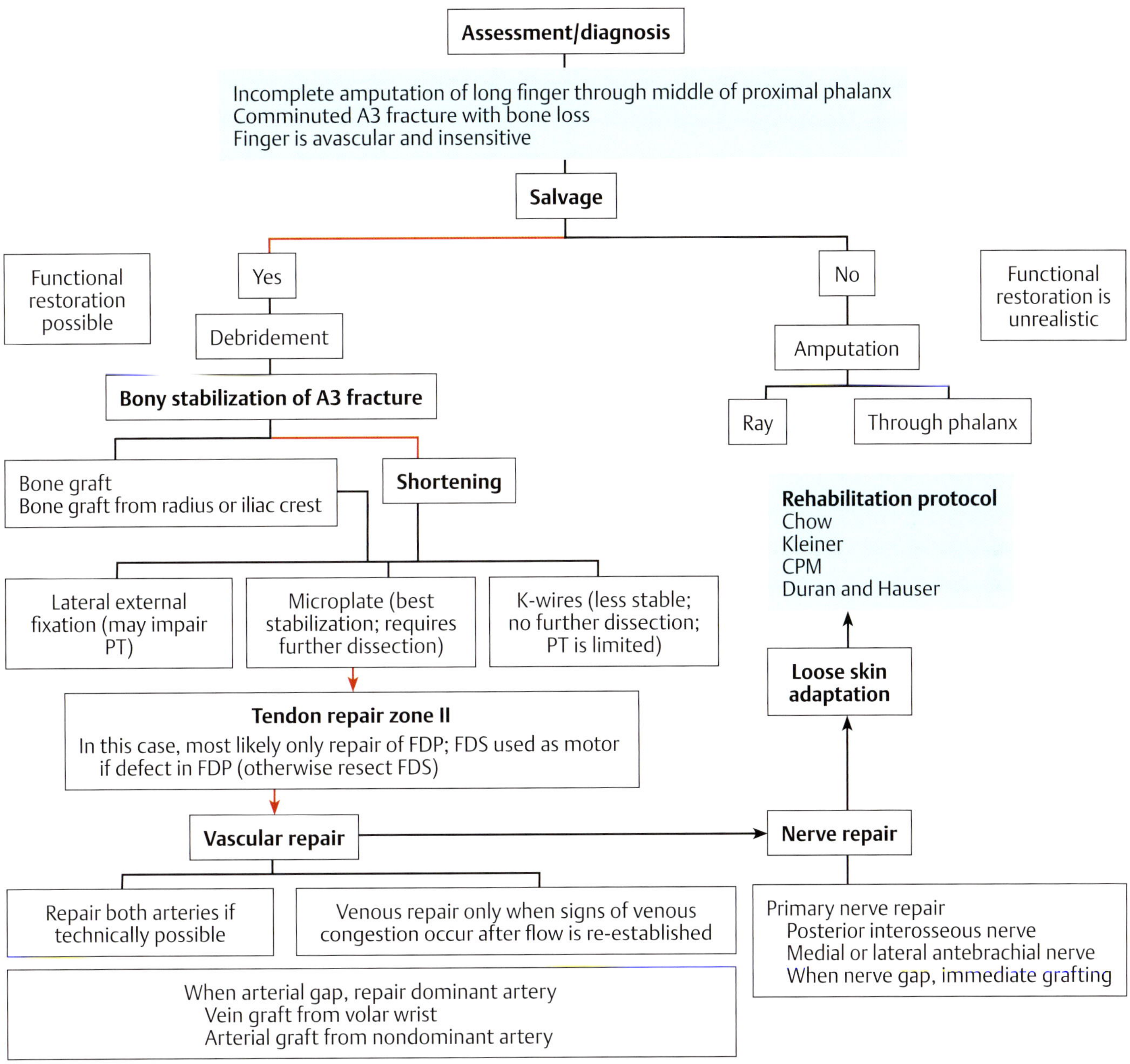

Algorithm 25.1

Parameters in decision-making	Additional options or guidelines	Warnings, precautions, or pitfalls	Emphasis on a particular waypoint

Digital Amputation

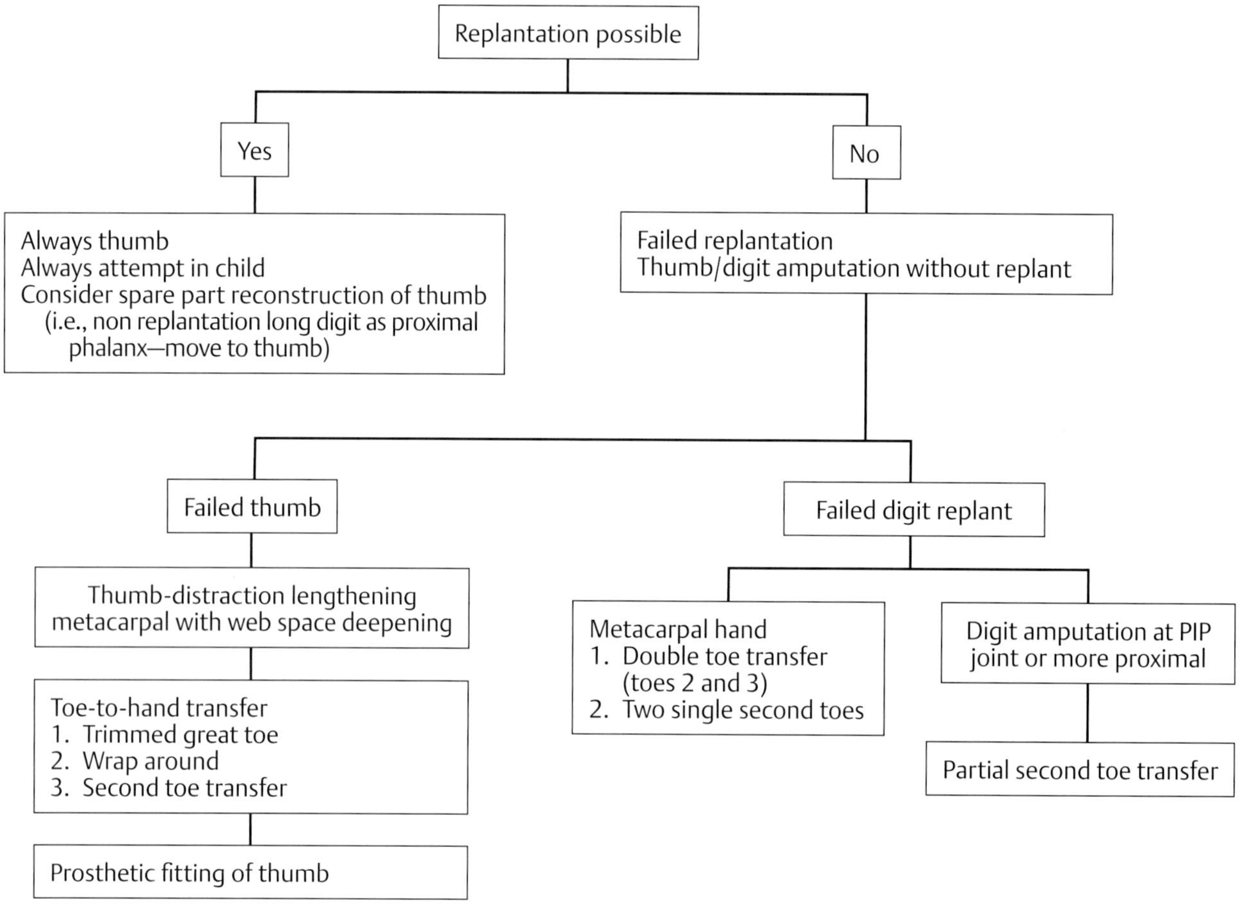

Algorithm 25.2

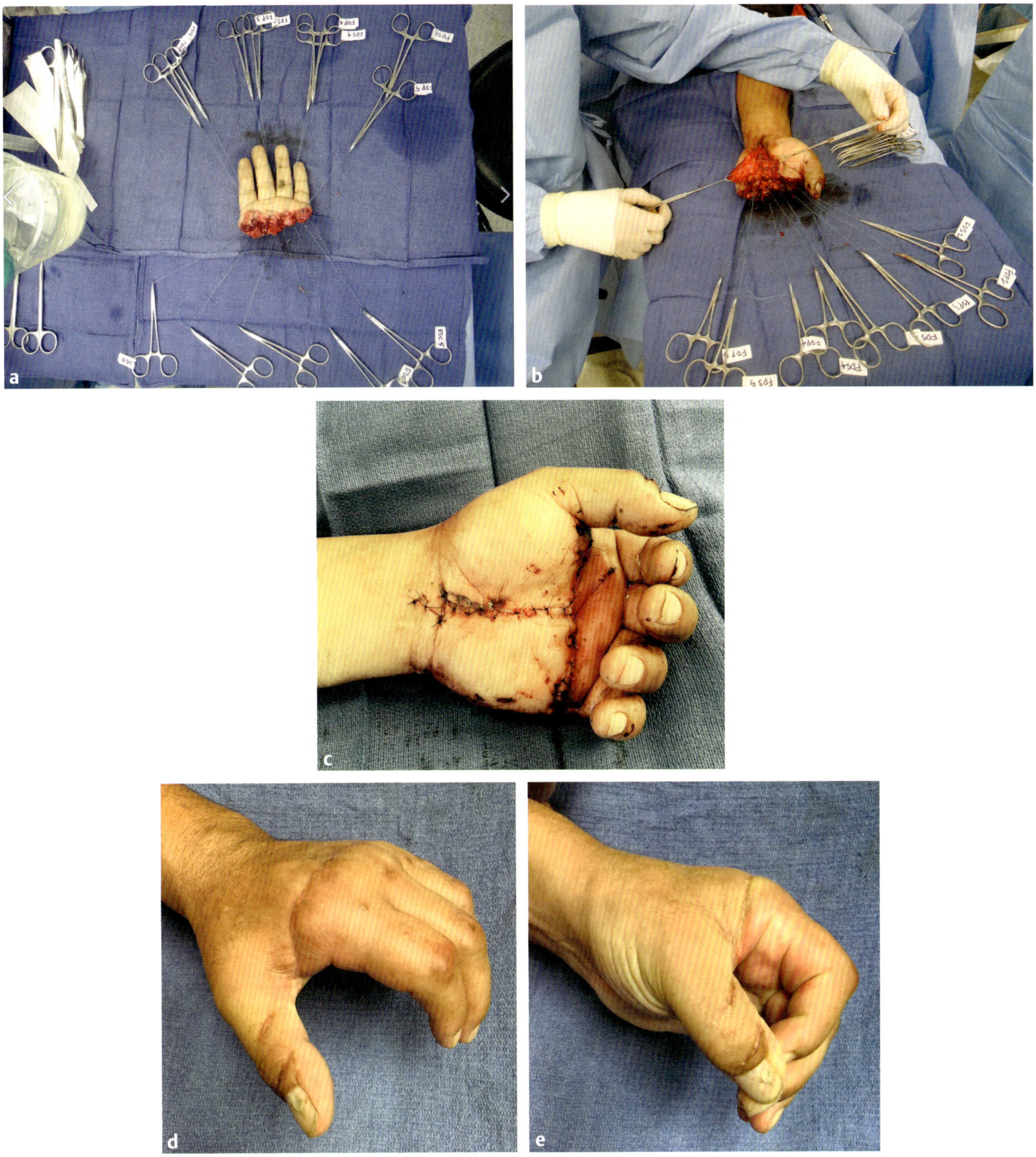

Fig. 25.1 (a) Amputated digits after transmetacarpal amputation. All structures have been tagged to facilitate replantation. **(b)** All structures in the stump have also been tagged and labelled. **(c)** Complete amputation through metacarpals. **(d,e)** The final functional result is shown 1 year after surgery.

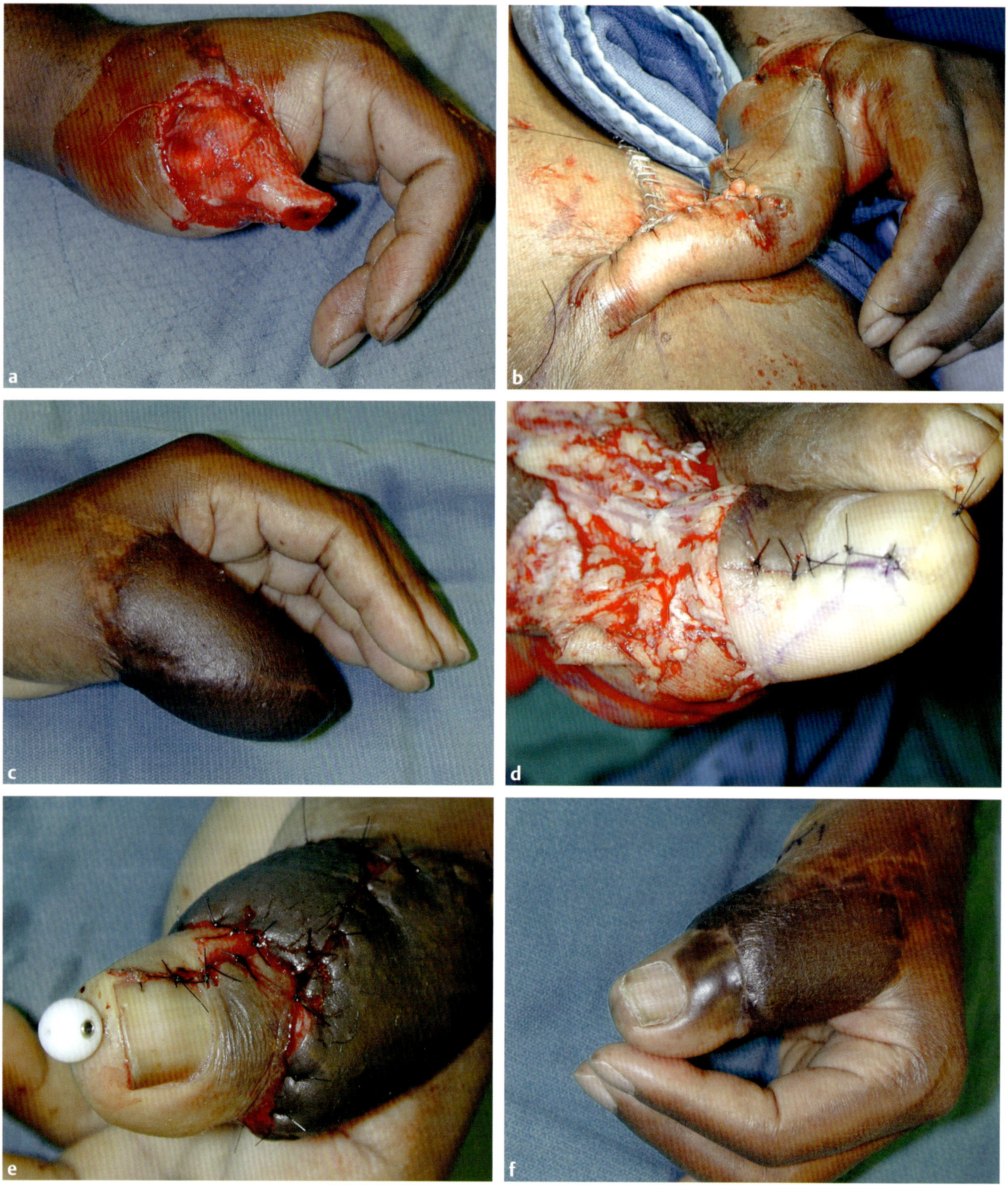

Fig. 25.2 (a) Thumb avulsion injury with nonreplantable thumb part. **(b)** Immediate groin flap for coverage in preparation for trimmed toe transfer. **(c)** Divided and inset groin flap as first stage prior to toe transfer. **(d)** Intraoperative photograph demonstrating reduction of nail plate phalanx and pulp. Toe perfusing in situ prior to transfer to thumb. **(e)** Immediate postoperative appearance with toe transfer. Note the use of the groin flap to limit donor site morbidity from foot. **(f)** Final result at six months with good opposition and sensibility.

Chapter 26

Forearm Trauma

Forearm Trauma

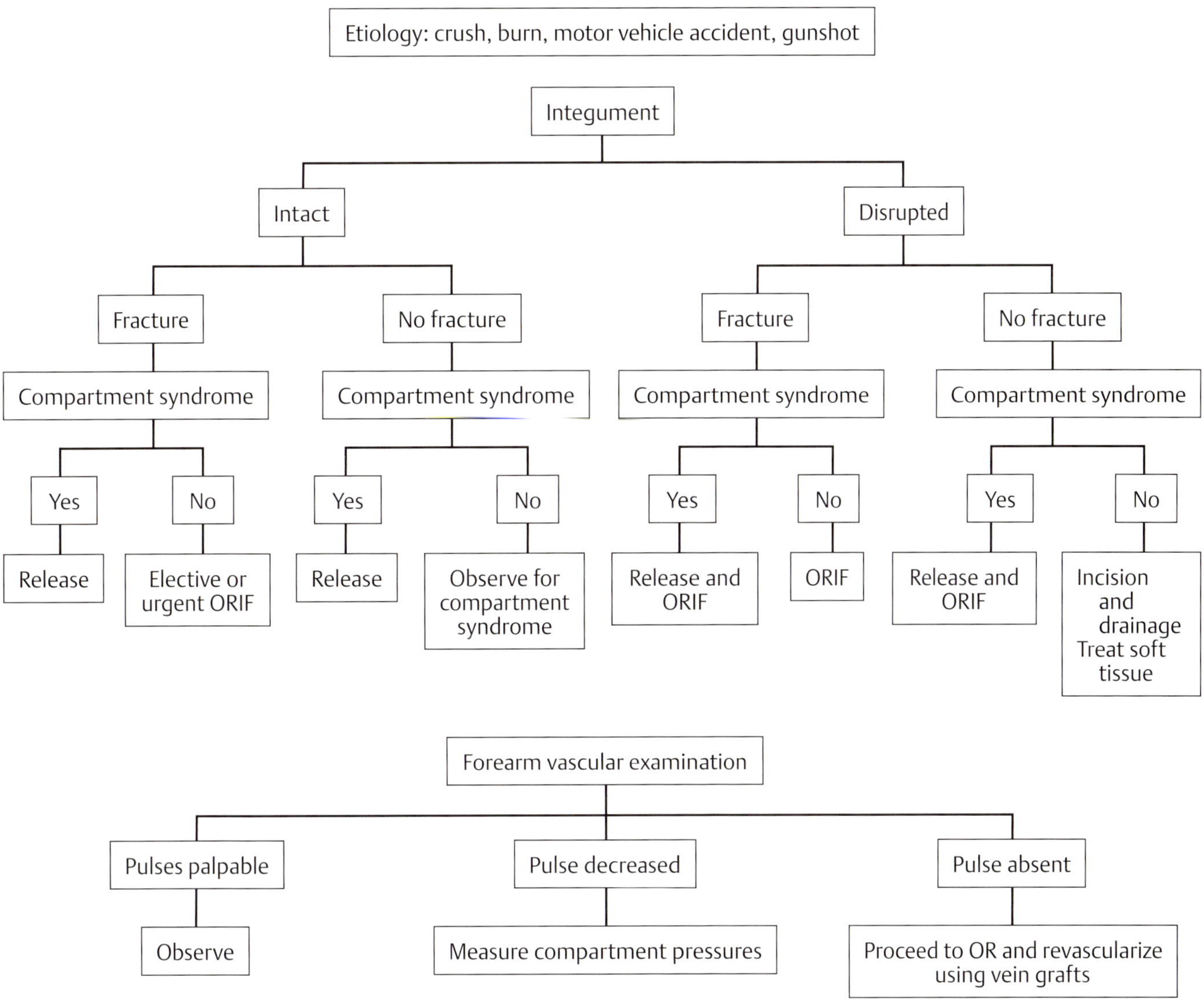

Algorithm 26.1

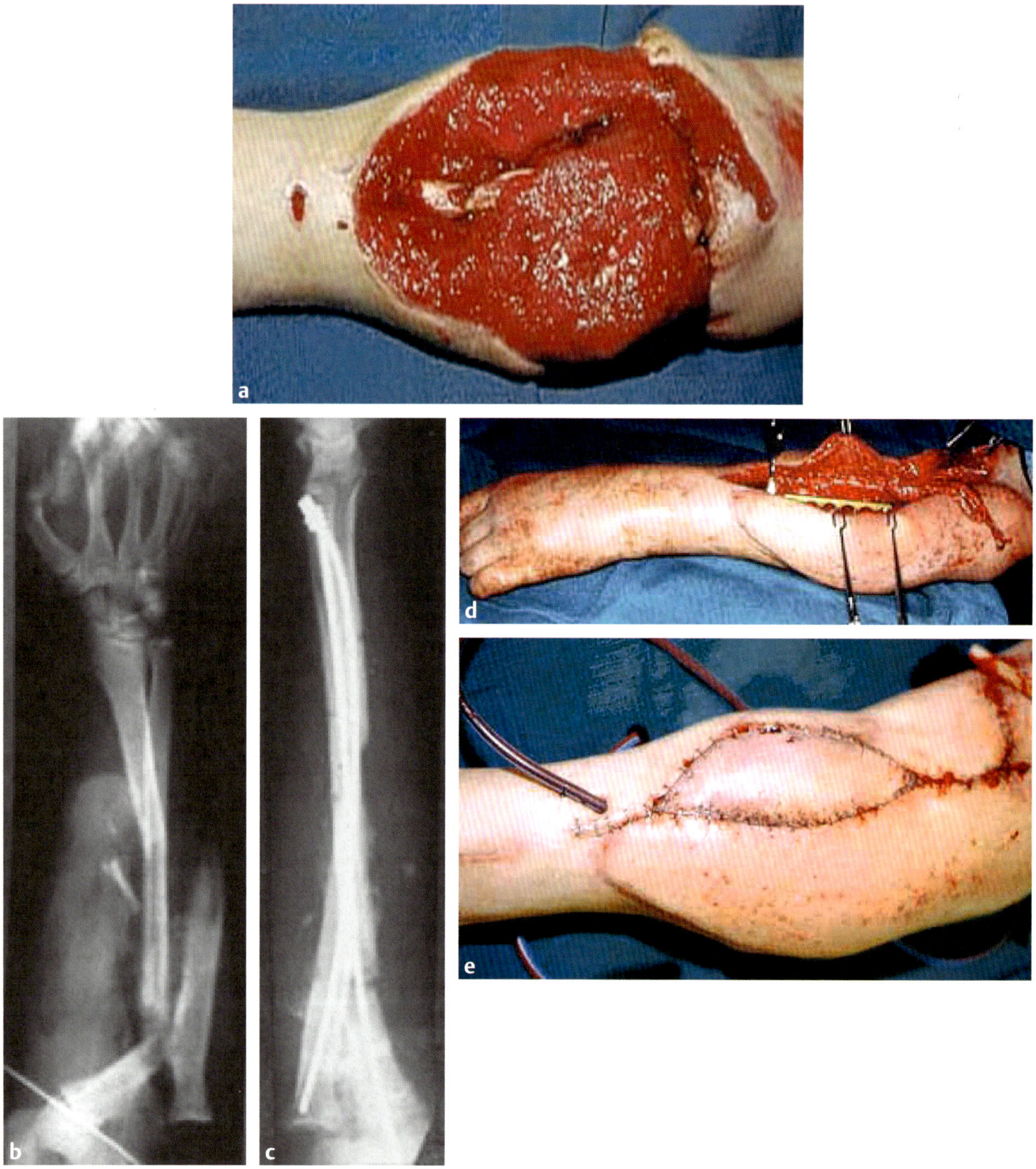

Fig. 26.1 (a) This patient had an infected open forearm fracture that had not received definitive treatment. This photograph was taken 3 weeks after the injury. **(b)** The initial presentation of the bone. **(c)** After revision stabilization with intramedullary locking rods. **(d)** The patient's arm is shown after the application of a free scapular flap for wound coverage and treatment with an approach involving vascularized osteocutaneous fibula for the radius defect. **(e)** After free fibular transfer (*continued*).

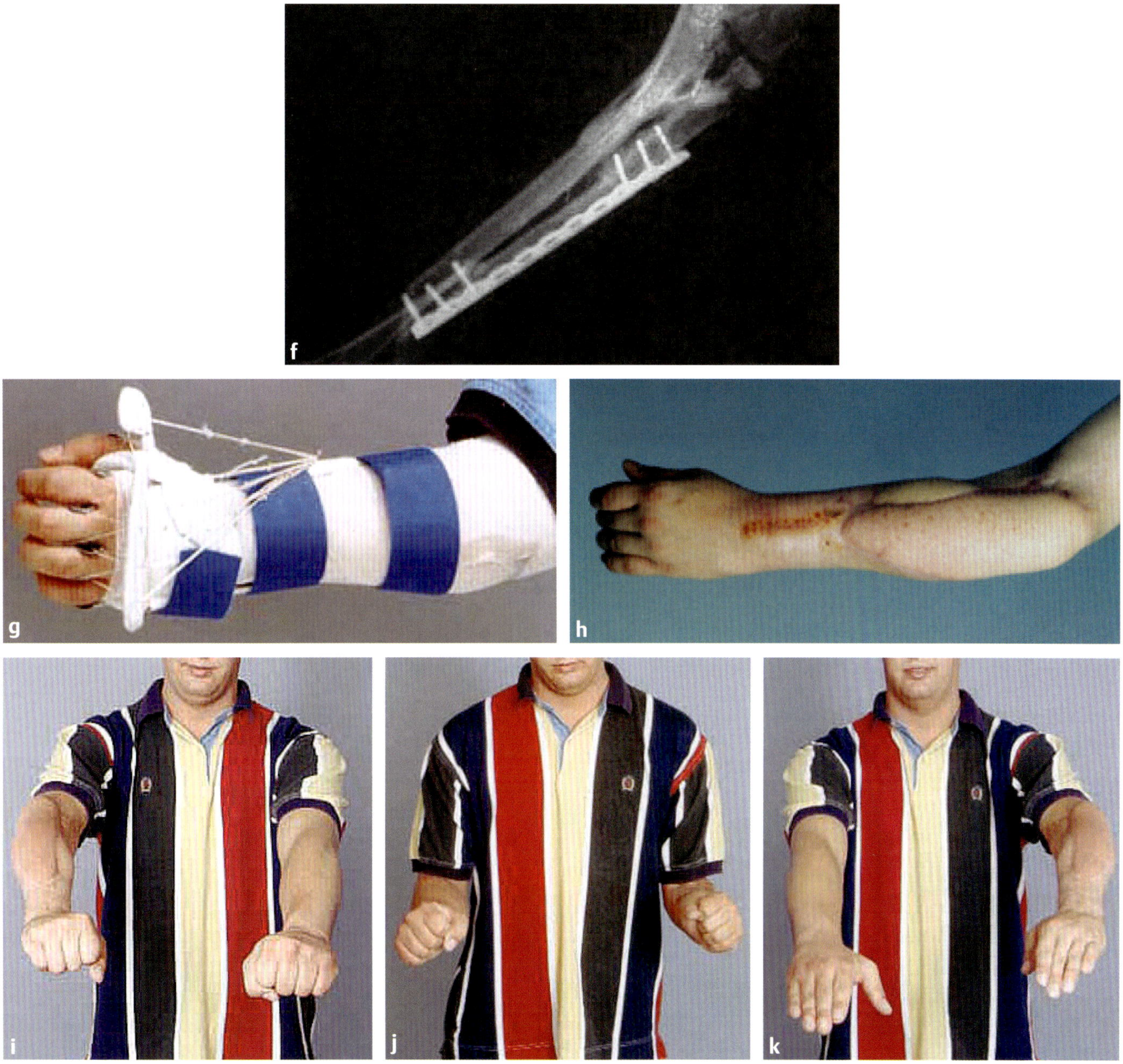

Fig. 26.1 (*continued*) **(f)** The spanning plate and healed radius. **(g)** Radial nerve tendon transfers were performed. **(h)** The healed scapular flap and osteocutaneous fibula flap are shown. **(i–k)** Functional results.

Chapter 27

Compartment Syndrome

Case history: A 10-year-old girl has chronic Volkmann's contracture secondary to compartment syndrome after posterior dislocation of the elbow.

Chronic Volkmann's Contracture

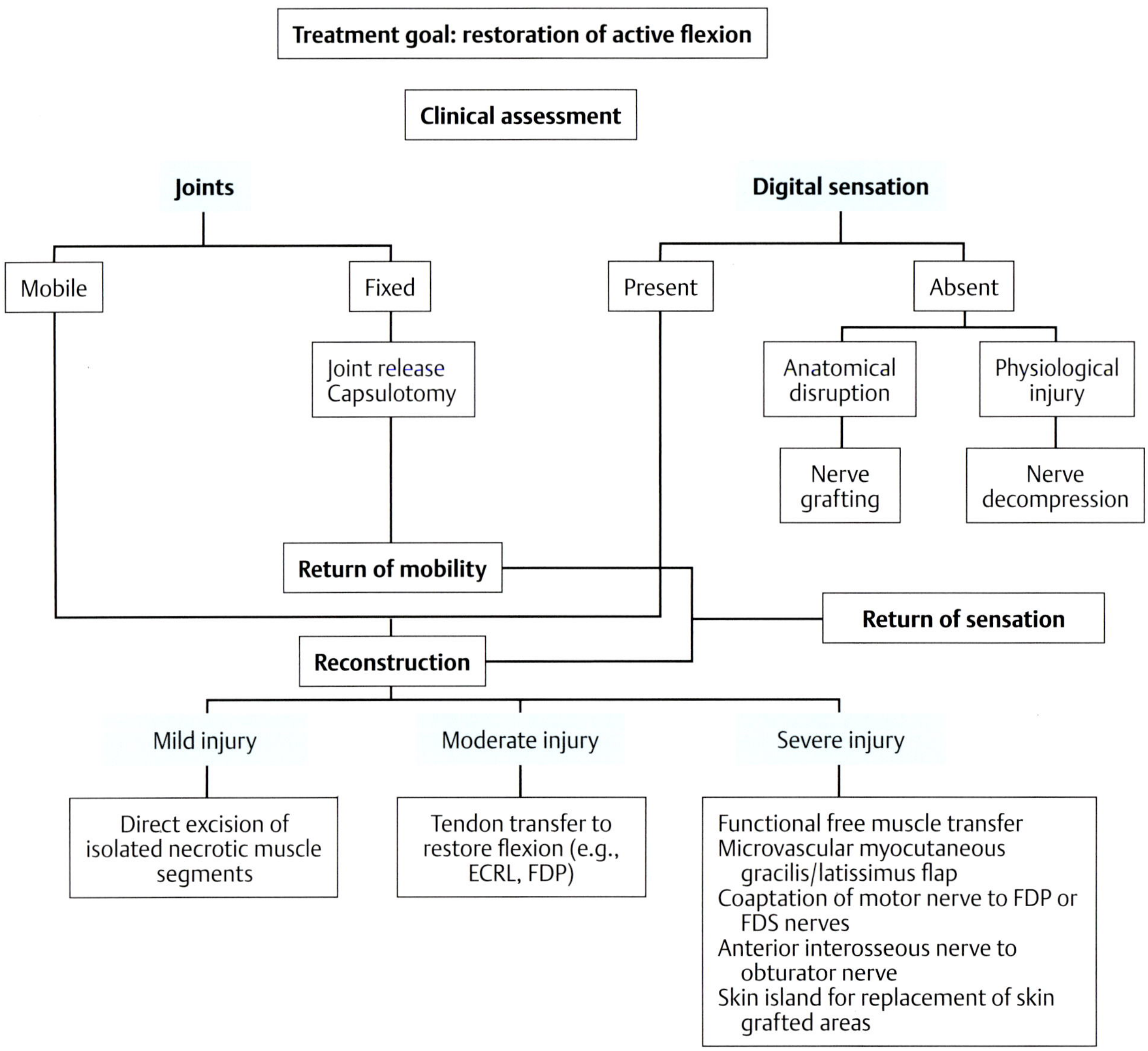

Algorithm 27.1

Parameters in decision-making	Additional options or guidelines	Warnings, precautions, or pitfalls	Emphasis on a particular waypoint

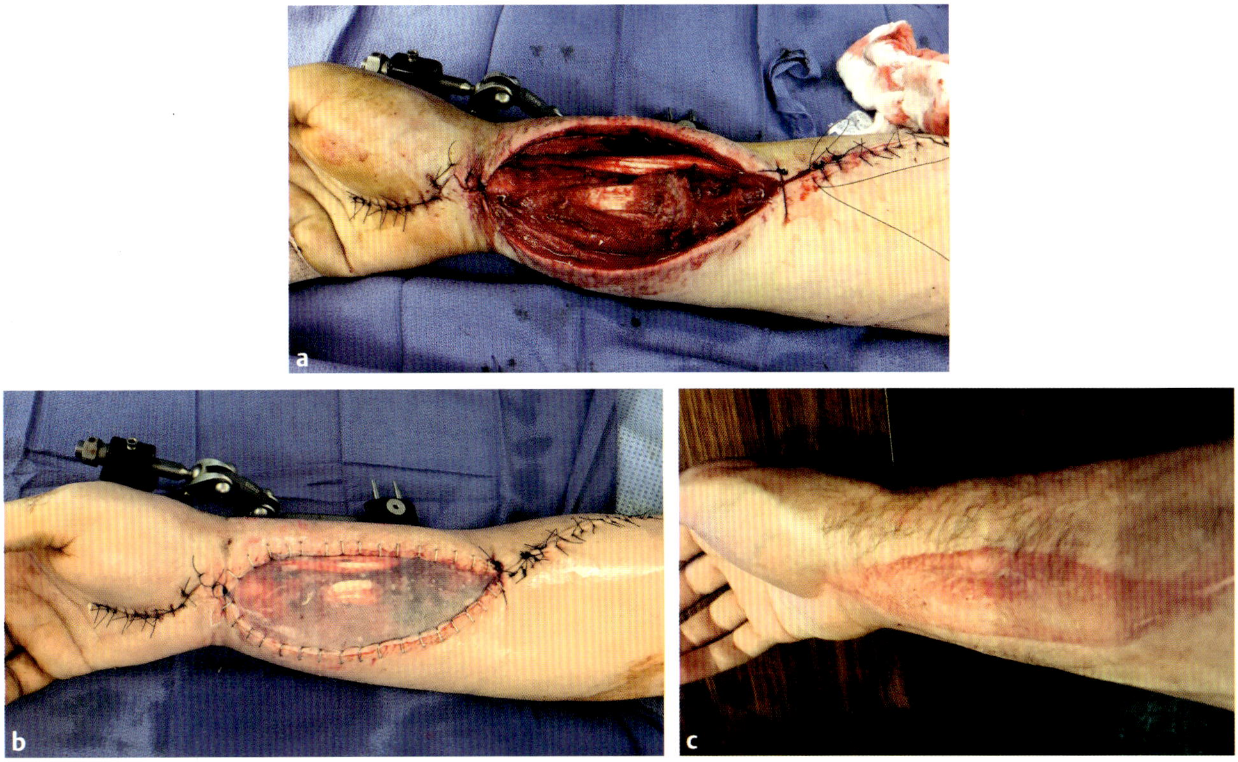

Fig. 27.1 (a) Volar release for the treatment of compartment syndrome, which was diagnosed in this patient 24 hours after an aborted open reduction and internal fixation procedure for a right distal radius fracture. **(b)** A thin STSG was placed on the granulating wound bed 1 week after initial debridement and after several dressing changes with vacuum-assisted closure. **(c)** The graft took well and is shown 8 weeks after decompression. Note the significant decrease in circumferential swelling.

Chapter 28

Tumor

Case history: 55-year-old man with a mass in the triceps muscle.

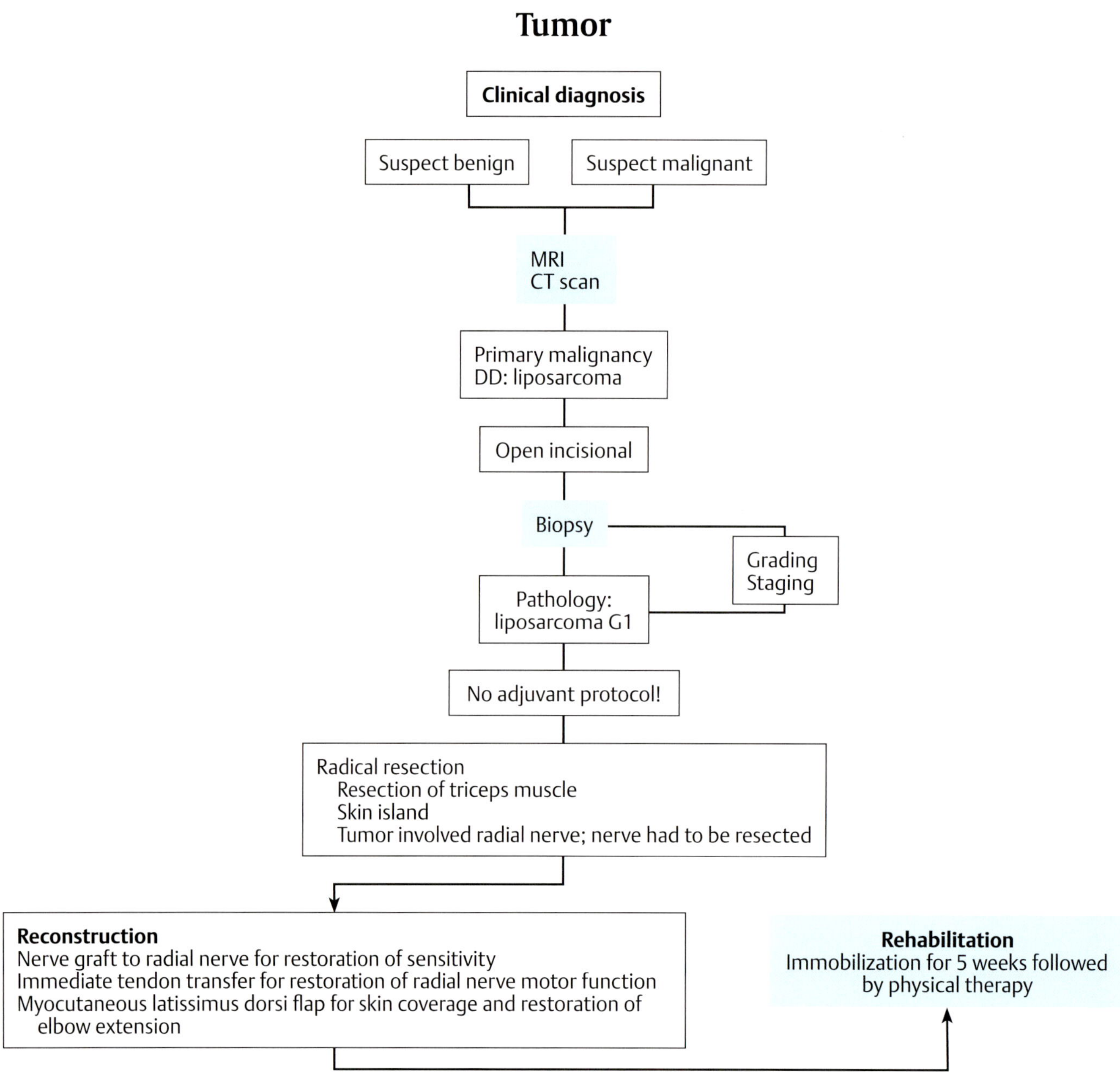

Algorithm 28.1

Parameters in decision-making	Additional options or guidelines	Warnings, precautions, or pitfalls	Emphasis on a particular waypoint

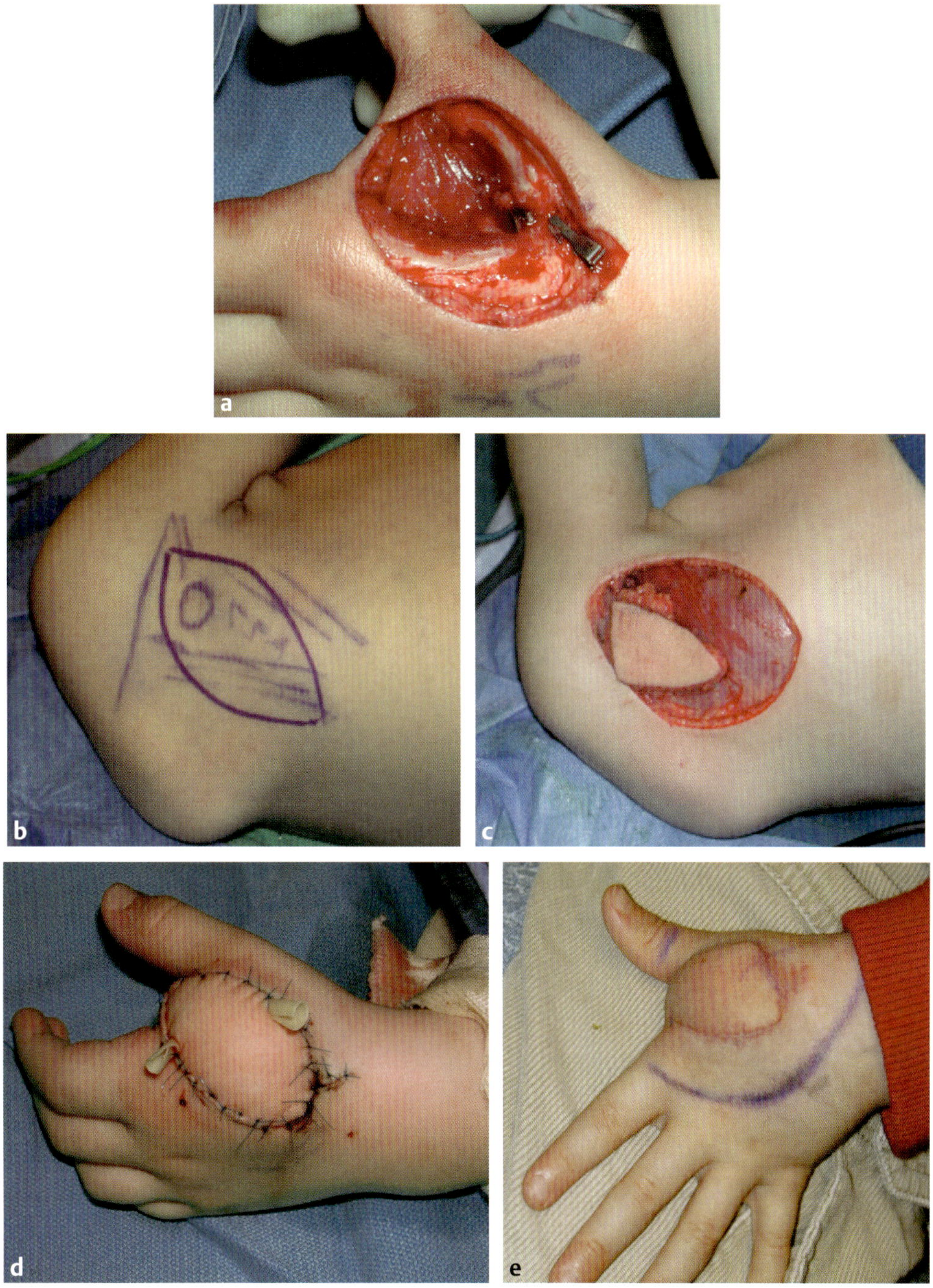

Fig. 28.1 (a) Defect after the treatment of rhabdomyosarcoma in a 4-year-old child. **(b,c)** Outline and elevation of the prescapular flap. **(d)** The appearance of the child's hand immediately after surgery. **(e)** The healed flap and radiation portal.

Part V

Atlas of Flaps—Pearls and Pitfalls

Chapter 29

Cross-Finger Flap

Table 29.1 Cross-finger flap	
Flap	
Tissue	Skin (conventional flap) or adipofascial tissue (reverse flap)
Course of the vessels	Axially in the subcutaneous tissue (no identifiable named vessel)
Dimensions	2.5 × 2 cm for both conventional and reverse flaps
Extensions and combinations	—
Anatomy	
Neurovascular pedicle	No defined pedicle
Artery	—
Veins	—
Length and arc of rotation	—
Diameter	—
Nerve	—
Surgical technique	
Preoperative examination and markings	Preferred donor site: middle phalanx
Flap design	—
Patient position	Arm on arm table to avoid tourniquet-induced ischemia
Dissection	Conventional flap: incise at the dorsolateral border of the digit and raise the flap in the plane above the tendon, with preservation of the paratenon; free the laterovolar vessels as far as possible without violating the neurovascular bundle, then suture the flap into the defect; apply a skin graft to the donor site Reverse flap: incise and raise a thin skin flap, with preservation of the subdermal plexus; raise a flap of adipofascial tissue, with preservation of the paratenon; flip the subcutaneous flap into the defect; cover the donor site with the previously dissected skin flap
Advantages	
Dissection	Simple and reliable
Flap size and shape	Sufficient for most typical defects over the flexor and extensor tendons
Combinations	Refinement in design with axial vessel included (C-ring flap)
Disadvantages	
Flap size	Not optimally suited for a longitudinal oval defect over several joints
Donor site morbidity	Skin graft for the conventional flap may be conspicuous during the postoperative period but improves with time
Pearls and pitfalls	
Dissection	Preservation of the paratenon is of utmost importance for skin graft take; preservation of the subdermal plexus guarantees excellent reconstruction of the donor site with a reverse flap
Extensions and combinations	—
Contouring and correction	Rarely required
Clinical applications	Conventional flap: volar digital defects Reverse flap: dorsal digital defects

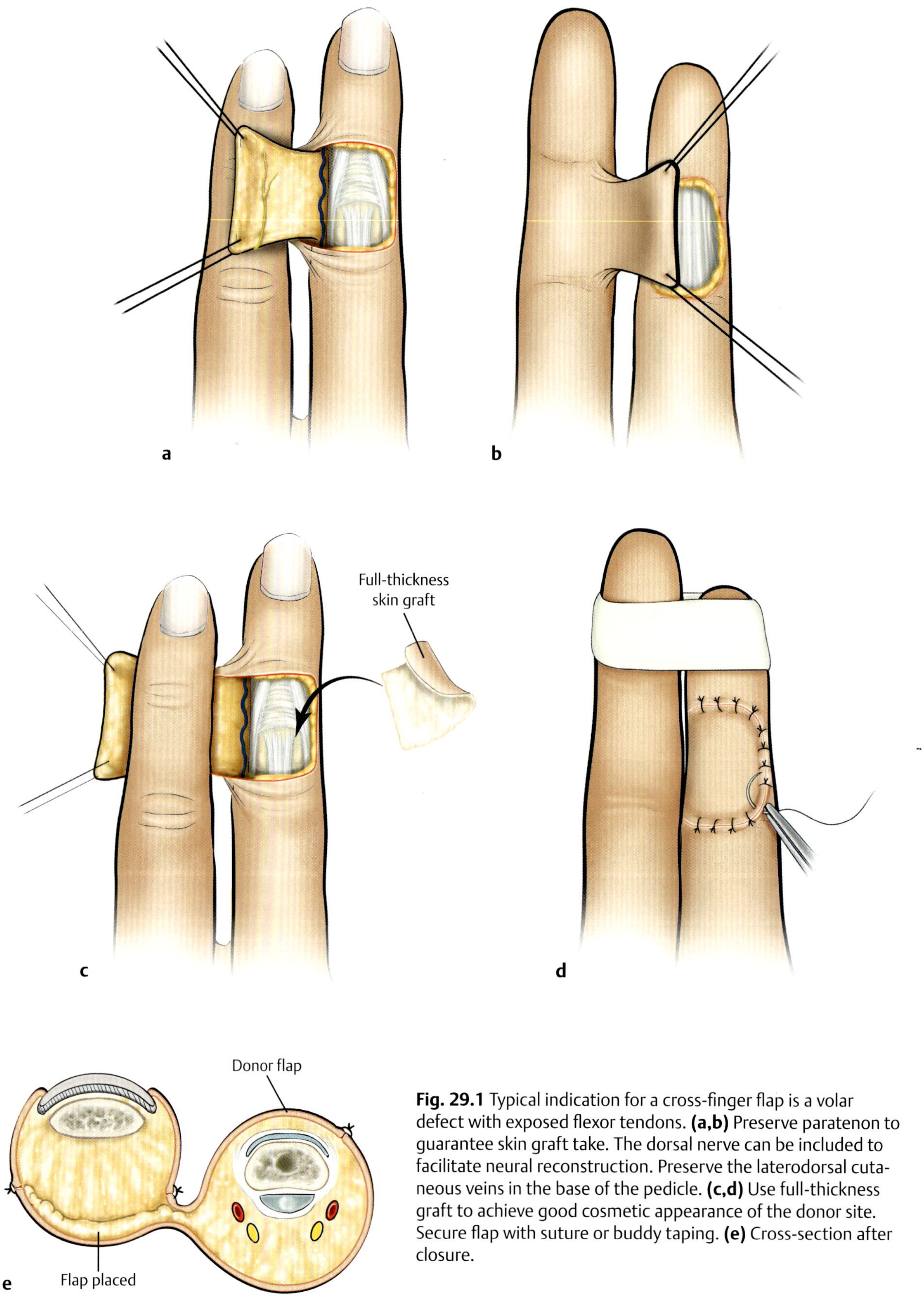

Fig. 29.1 Typical indication for a cross-finger flap is a volar defect with exposed flexor tendons. **(a,b)** Preserve paratenon to guarantee skin graft take. The dorsal nerve can be included to facilitate neural reconstruction. Preserve the laterodorsal cutaneous veins in the base of the pedicle. **(c,d)** Use full-thickness graft to achieve good cosmetic appearance of the donor site. Secure flap with suture or buddy taping. **(e)** Cross-section after closure.

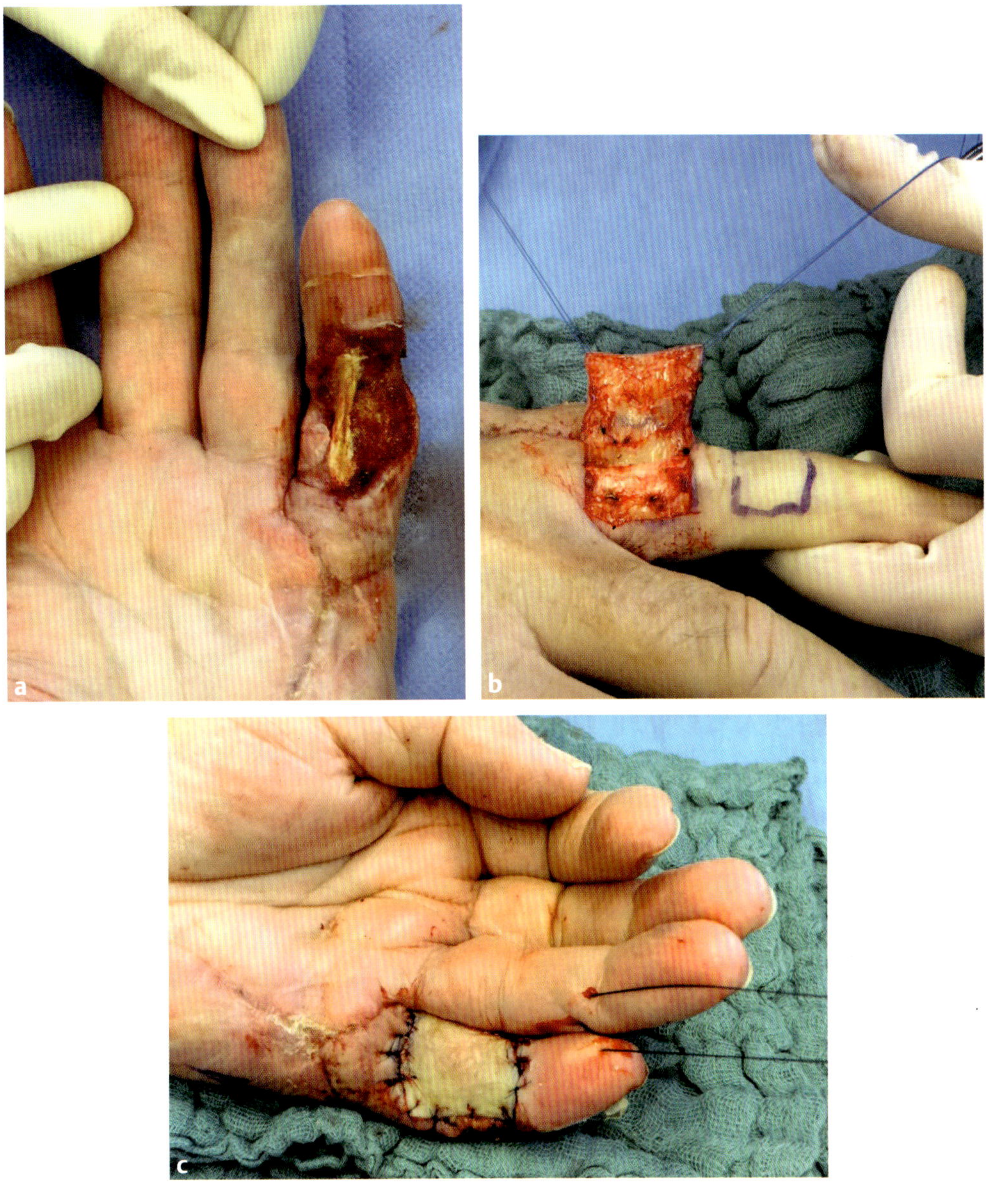

Fig. 29.2 (a) This patient's flexor tendons are exposed as a result of wound-healing problems after surgery for Dupuytren's contracture. **(b)** A cross-finger flap was raised on the ulnar aspect of the dorsum of the ring finger. **(c)** The patient's hand is shown with the flap sutured in place immediately after surgery.

Chapter 30

Reverse Cross-Finger Flap

Table 30.1 Reverse cross-finger flap	
Flap	
Tissue	Adipofascial subcutaneous tissue
Course of the vessels	Fragile subdermal vascular network
Dimensions	1.5 × 1.5 cm
Extensions and combinations	—
Anatomy	No named or identifiable vessel
Neurovascular pedicle	—
Artery	—
Veins	—
Length and arc of rotation	—
Diameter	—
Nerve	—
Surgical technique	
Preoperative examination and markings	Dorsal aspect of the digits; Doppler identification of the vessels and their courses
Flap design	Mark the defect size on the dorsum of the finger
Patient position	Arm on arm table, with the hand pronated
Dissection	Use an “open the book, close the book” technique: raise the skin flap and preserve the subdermal plexus; arm the skin flap with two stay sutures, and then raise the adipofascial areolar tissue from the paratenon of the extensor tendon; fold the flap into the dorsal defect of the adjacent digit; close the donor site by suturing the skin flap back into place; reconstruct the recipient site with a full-thickness graft, preferably from the hypothenar eminence
Advantages	Local flap with reliable blood supply when flap is not lacerated during dissection; easy to dissect, even for novices; thin flap with stable coverage
Disadvantages	Recipient finger and donor finger have to be immobilized together; we prefer to suture through the pulp to allow for conjoint motion after a few days and to prevent the spreading of the fingers, which risks tearing the pedicle; “buddy taping” is frequently not sufficient Pedicle is divided after 12–14 days; physical therapy can be started after 3–4 days
Pearls and pitfalls	
Dissection	Carefully peel off the flap tissue from the paratenon; with this particular flap, a violation of the paratenon is not harmful, because the defect is closed again with a vascularized skin flap
Extensions and combinations	—
Contouring and correction	Secondary contouring is rarely necessary
Clinical applications	Dorsal defects of the digits

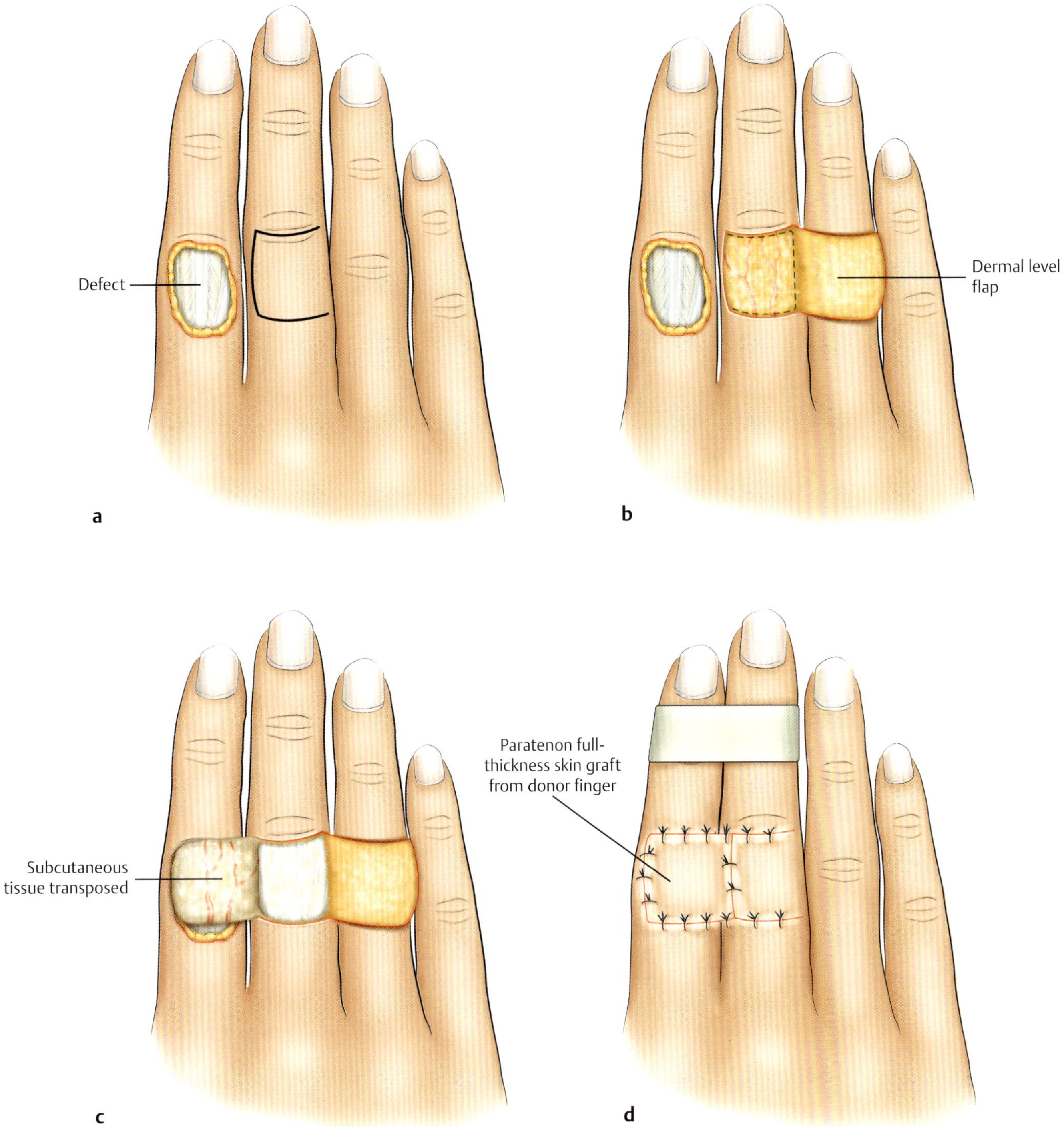

Fig. 30.1 Reverse cross-finger flap. **(a)** Dorsal defect over the PIP joint. A reverse cross-finger flap is designed on the adjacent finger. **(b)** The skin flap is raised, leaving the subcutaneous tissue layer intact. **(c)** The subcutaneous layer is turned over into the defect and fixated with stay sutures. **(d)** A full-thickness skin graft is applied to the reverse cross-finger flap. The donor site is closed with the skin flap from the donor finger (open the book, close the book technique).

Chapter 31

V-Y Flap

Table 31.1 V-Y flap for fingertips

Flap	
Tissue	Volar V-Y (Tranquilli-Leali, Atasoy); lateral V-Y (Geissendörfer, Kutler)
Tissue	Skin
Course of the vessels	In the subcutaneous tissue of the pulp
Dimensions	1 × 1.5 cm
Extensions and combinations	—
Anatomy	
Neurovascular pedicle	No defined pedicle
Artery	—
Veins	—
Length and arc of rotation	—
Diameter	5–10 mm
Nerve	—
Surgical technique	
Preoperative examination and markings	Slightly laterally curved triangular incision
Patient position	Arm on arm table, digital block or plexus anesthesia, tourniquet
Dissection	Volar flap: incise the skin without violating the subcutaneous tissue; release the fibrous septa from the pulp to the periosteum; trim the bone; pull the flap distally with a Gillies hook; divide the remaining septa; fixate the flap in the defect with a needle; no distal suture needed Lateral flap: cover the defect with bilateral triangular flaps; the limbs of the incision should meet at the distal flexor crease; incise the skin without violating the subcutaneous tissue; release the fibrous septa from the periosteum; trim the bone; pull the flap medially with a Gillies hook; release the remaining septa; fixate the flap to the contralateral flap with sutures or use two needles
Advantages	
Dissection	Simple and reliable
Flap size and shape	Small defects of the fingertip can be covered with sensate skin
Donor site	Primary closure with V-Y technique or loose approximation of the skin
Disadvantages	
Flap size	Sometimes too small
Pearls and pitfalls	
Dissection	Do not injure the subcutaneous tissue; do not suture the flap distally, because this will impair the blood supply; the flap is frequently pale after release of the tourniquet, wait and then rinse with warm saline
Extensions and combinations	—
Contouring and correction	Very rarely required
Clinical applications	Small defects of the fingertips

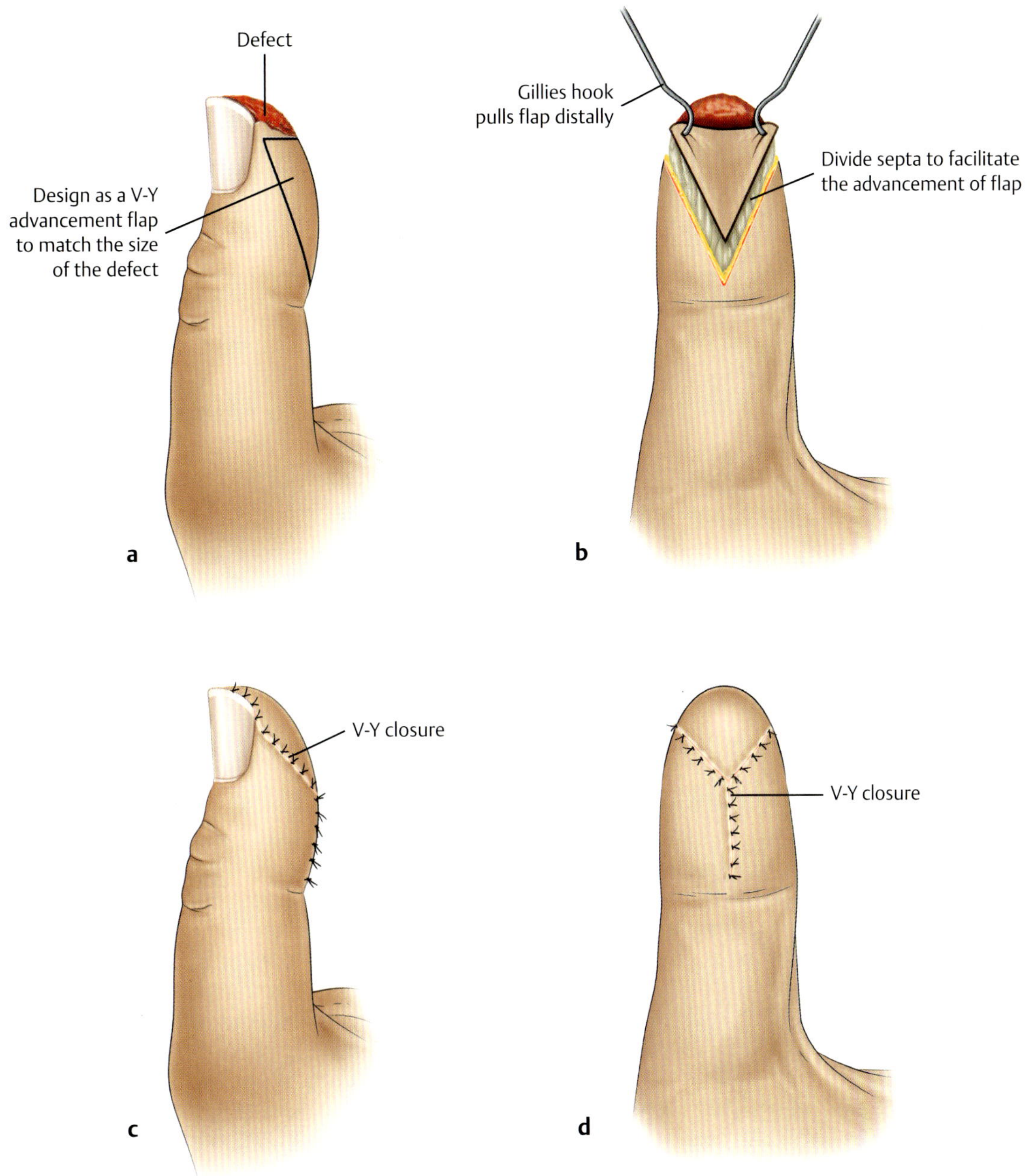

Fig. 31.1 (a) The V-Y advancement flap should be large enough to cover the defect. **(b)** Use Gillies hooks to pull flap gently distally. Divide all septa to facilitate advancement of the flap. **(c,d)** V-Y closure.

Chapter 32

Lateral Digital Advancement Flap

Table 32.1 Lateral digital advancement flap

Flap	
Tissue	Skin and subcutaneous tissue
Course of the vessels	Undersurface of the flap; attached to the flap through a fragile septum and perivascular areolar tissue
Dimensions	2 × 1–1.5 cm
Extensions and combinations	—
Anatomy	Proper digital artery; no identifiable veins; periarterial plexus
Neurovascular pedicle	—
Artery	—
Veins	—
Length and arc of rotation	—
Diameter	—
Nerve	—
Surgical technique	
Preoperative examination and markings	Lateral half of a digit; digital Allen test
Flap design	Mark the defect size; the flap is designed as a large "V" that is centered over the proper digital artery and that extends toward the volar flexor crease of the metacarpophalangeal joint
Patient position	Arm on arm table, with the hand pronated
Dissection	Incise the flap circumferentially in the marked and required dimensions; dissection starts by identifying the neurovascular bundle proximal to tip of the designed flap; the nerve is identified, isolated, and separated from the artery in its entire length; all areolar tissue around the artery, which provides the venous outflow, should be preserved; after complete dissection of the flap, it is mobile enough to be advanced into the defect; closure is performed in a V-Y fashion; if the defect is not too big, the complete neurovascular bundle can be included in the pedicle flap to provide immediate sensibility
Advantages	Local flap with reliable blood supply; immediate restoration of sensibility is possible
Disadvantages	Some cold intolerance has been reported, but this can also be due to the primary injury
Pearls and pitfalls	
Dissection	Decide before pedicle dissection if the defect allows for the inclusion of the nerve in the pedicle
Extensions and combinations	—
Contouring and correction	Secondary contouring is rarely necessary
Clinical applications	Lateromedial defects of the fingertips that require flap coverage

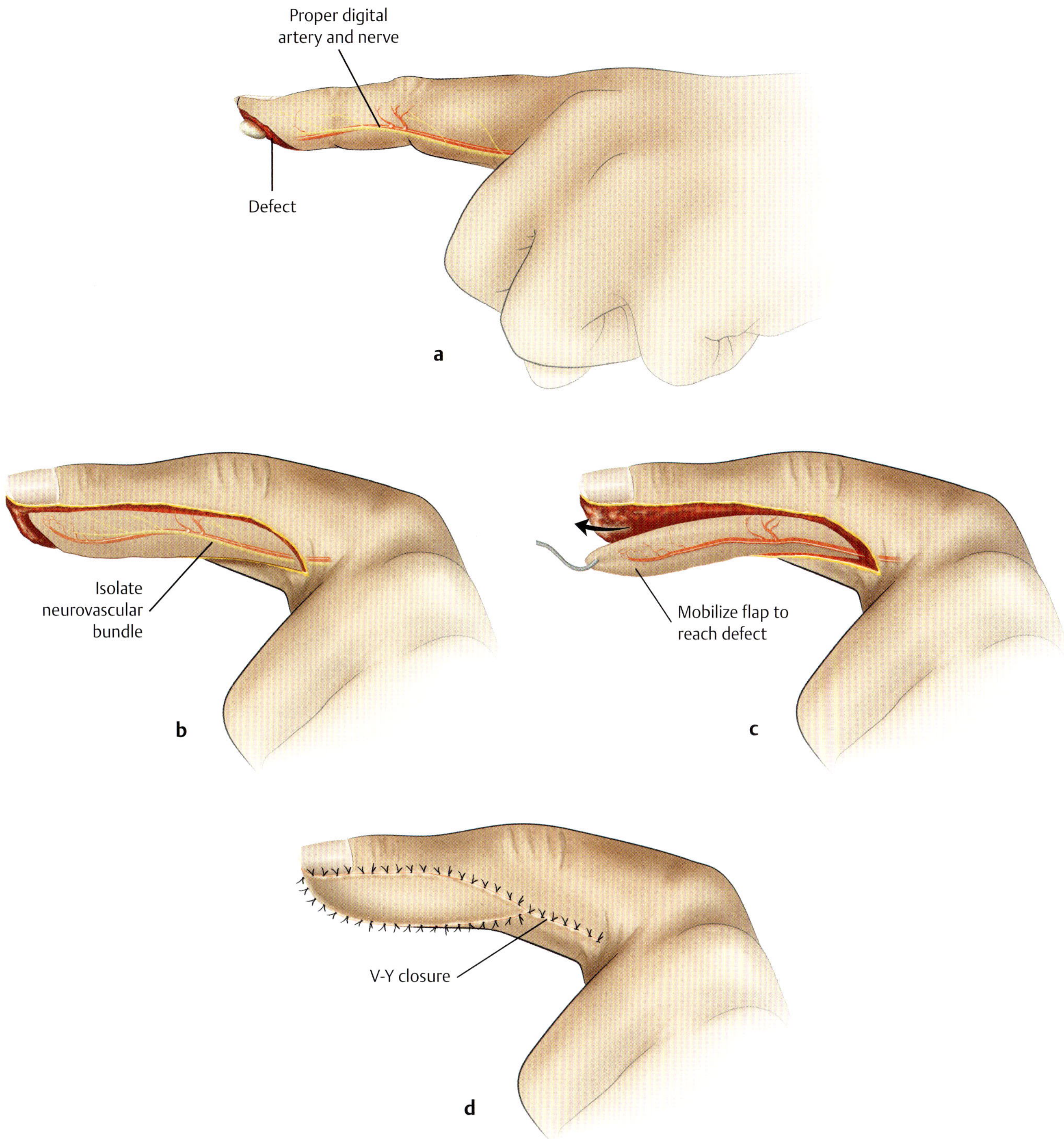

Fig. 32.1 (a) Complex fingertip injury with bone exposed. The patient desired the best possible sensate reconstruction. **(b)** The lateral advancement flap is raised on the ulnar neurovascular bundle. **(c)** Mobilize the flap to reach the defect without tension. Gentle pull with skin hook. **(d)** Flap inset completed and closed with V-Y closure.

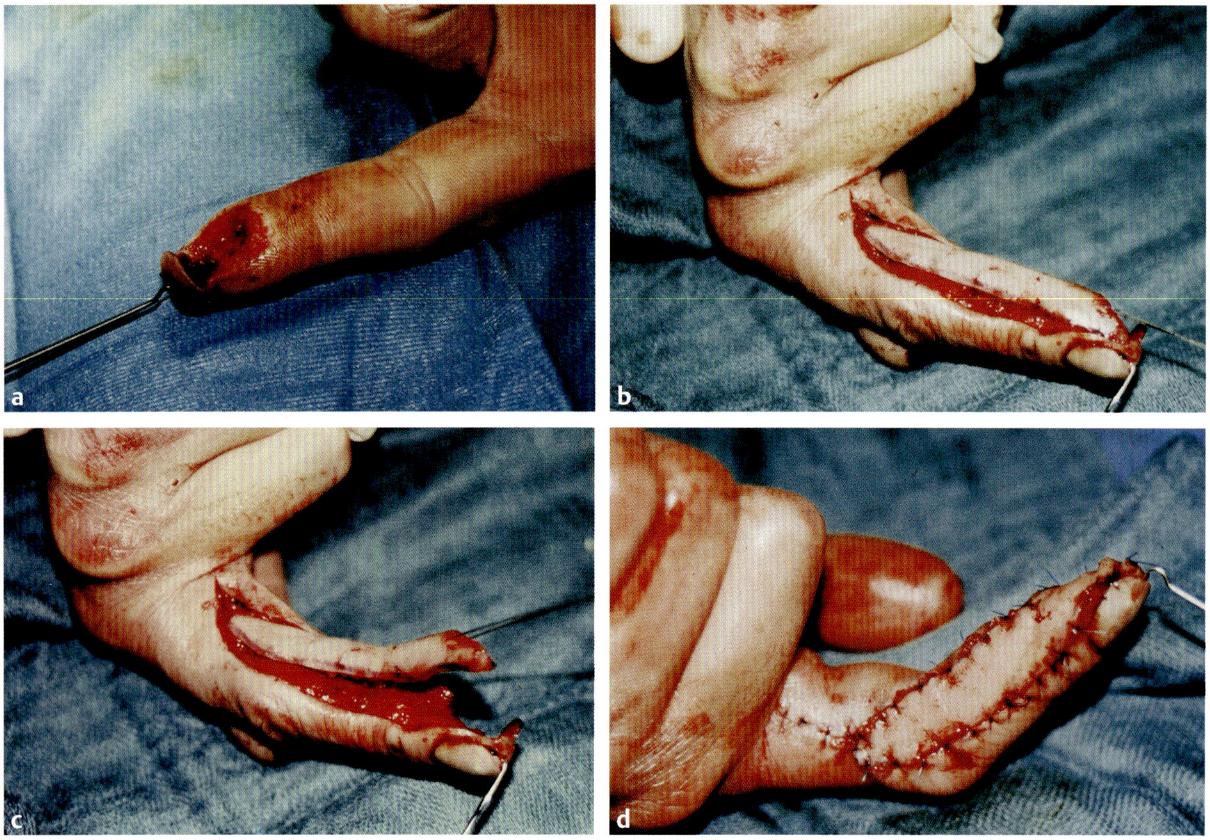

Fig. 32.2 (a) This patient sustained a complex fingertip injury with exposed bone. The patient desired the best possible sensate reconstruction. **(b)** A lateral advancement flap is raised, based on the ulnar neurovascular bundle. **(c)** The flap is further mobilized to reach the defect without tension. **(d)** The flap inset has been completed, with perfect perfusion of the flap.

Chapter 33

Thenar Flap

Table 33.1 Thenar flap

Flap	
Tissue	Volar skin
Course of the vessels	Dermal circulation without a named artery
Dimensions	1.5 × 1.5 cm
Extensions and combinations	—
Anatomy	Relies on the inosculation of the pedicle flap to the wound bed
Neurovascular pedicle	—
Artery	—
Veins	—
Length and arc of rotation	—
Diameter	—
Nerve	—
Surgical technique	The flap is elevated at the subcutaneous plane with a pedicle that is no more than twice the length of the base of the flap; it is oriented to inset into the digital pulp defect of the injured finger
Preoperative examination and markings	—
Patient position	Supine, with the use of a hand table; tourniquet control
Dissection	In the subcutaneous plane, with the preservation of perforating vessels (if seen)
Advantages	Rapid dissection; good color match of skin
Disadvantages	This is a pedicle flap that requires digital flexion and attachment of the digit to the volar flap for 2–3 weeks
Pearls and pitfalls	Risk of proximal IP flexion contracture in elderly patients
Dissection	—
Extensions and combinations	—
Contouring and correction	—
Clinical applications	—

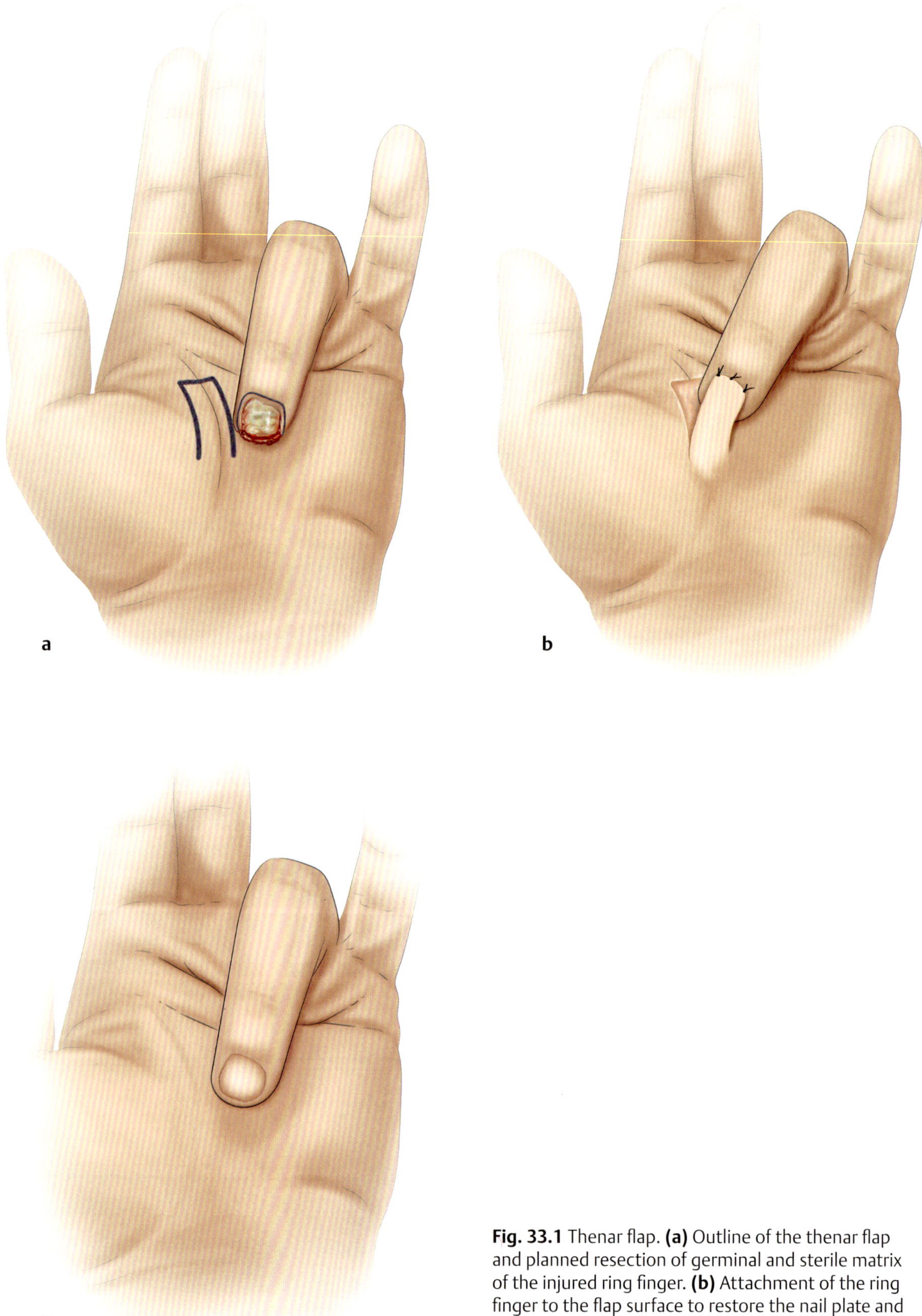

Fig. 33.1 Thenar flap. **(a)** Outline of the thenar flap and planned resection of germinal and sterile matrix of the injured ring finger. **(b)** Attachment of the ring finger to the flap surface to restore the nail plate and to provide a flap that has the appearance of a nail. **(c)** After division and insetting.

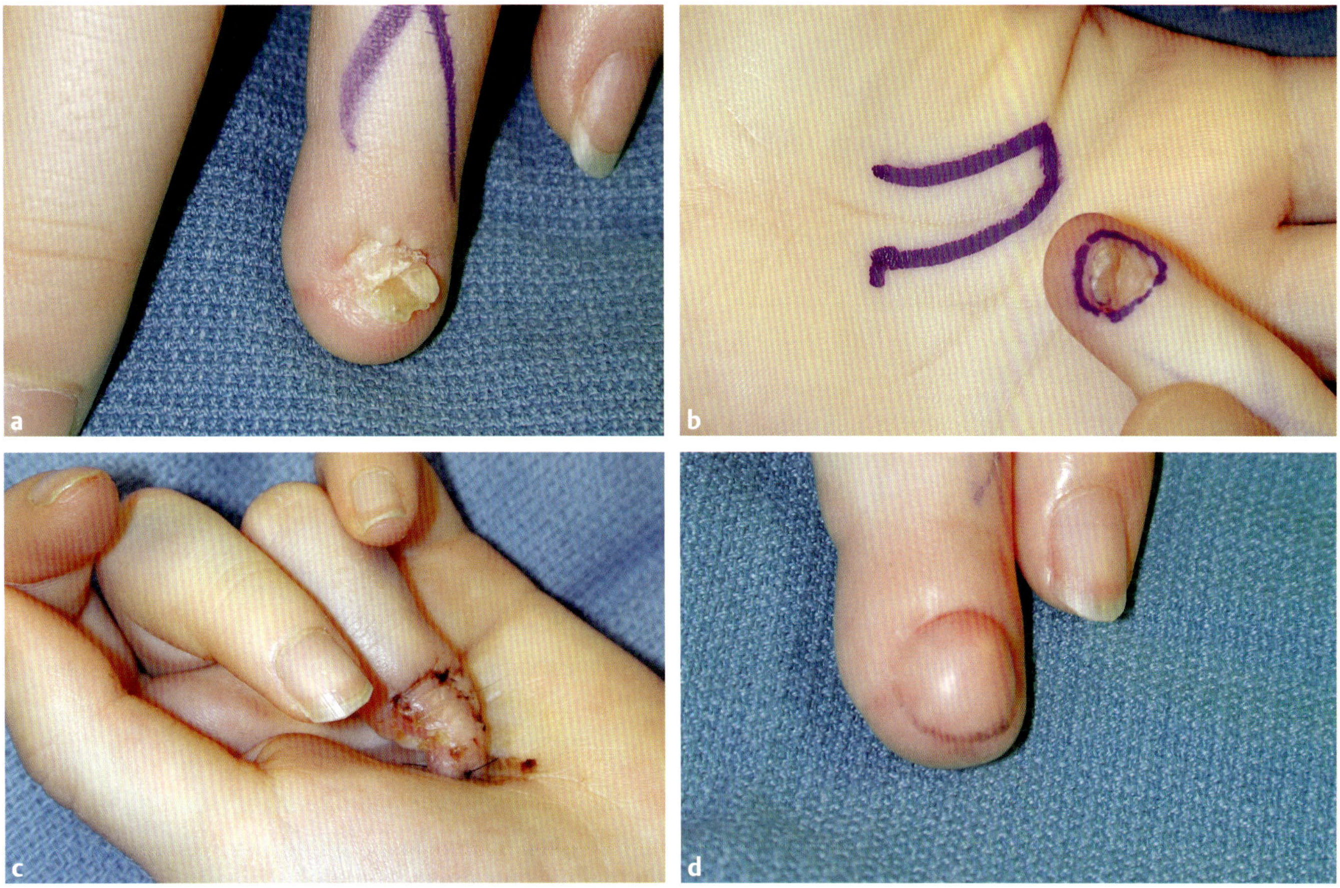

Fig. 33.2 Thenar flap. **(a)** This scarred and mutilated nail bed resulted from a crush injury the patient had as a child. **(b)** The outlines show the thenar flap and the planned resection of the germinal and sterile matrix of the injured ring finger. **(c)** Attachment of the ring finger to the flap, with the intent to restore the surface of the nail plate and to provide a flap that has the appearance of a nail. **(d)** After division and insetting.

Chapter 34

Volar Advancement Flap (Moberg)

Table 34.1 Volar advancement flap (Moberg)	
Flap	Volar advancement flap (Moberg); O'Brien modification
Tissue	Skin
Course of the vessels	Underneath the flap
Dimensions	Can reach the dimension of the entire volar surface of a digit or the thumb
Extensions and combinations	–
Anatomy	
Neurovascular pedicle	–
Artery	Proper digital artery
Veins	Concomitant veins of the digital artery
Length and arc of rotation	Maximal defect size: longitudinal; mobilization: 1.5–2 cm
Diameter	–
Nerve	Proper digital nerves
Surgical technique	
Preoperative examination and markings	Midlateral skin markings; the digital Allen test is recommended
Patient position	Hand on arm table to avoid tourniquet ischemia
Dissection	Moberg: midlateral incision; identification of the neurovascular bundles; unilateral preservation of the dorsal branches; volar advancement; distal flap fixation with a needle; frequently the flexion of the digit is necessary to allow for the closure of the defect O'Brien modification: bilateral dissection of the neurovascular bundles; volar flap advancement; skin graft to the donor site (i.e., the dissection site of the vessels)
Advantages	
Flap	Sensate flap to restore sensibility of the pulp
Dissection	Straightforward and simple
Vascular pedicle	Reliable
Flap size and shape	Pulp defects of 1.5–2 cm
Disadvantages	
Flap	Only small to midsize defects
Donor site morbidity	Flexion contracture may occur if defect is too large and mobilization has not been sufficient
Pearls and pitfalls	
Dissection	Preserve the dorsal collaterals on one side; suture the flap distally only with the needle to avoid further tension and impairment of the distal flap supply; a relaxing incision can be made at the base of the thumb or converted into an O'Brien modification to reduce the risk of flexion contracture, especially in older patients; insert a Z-plasty into a regular Moberg flap to avoid tension at the flap base
Extensions and combinations	–
Contouring and correction	Extremely rare
Clinical applications	Defects of the pulp of the thumb

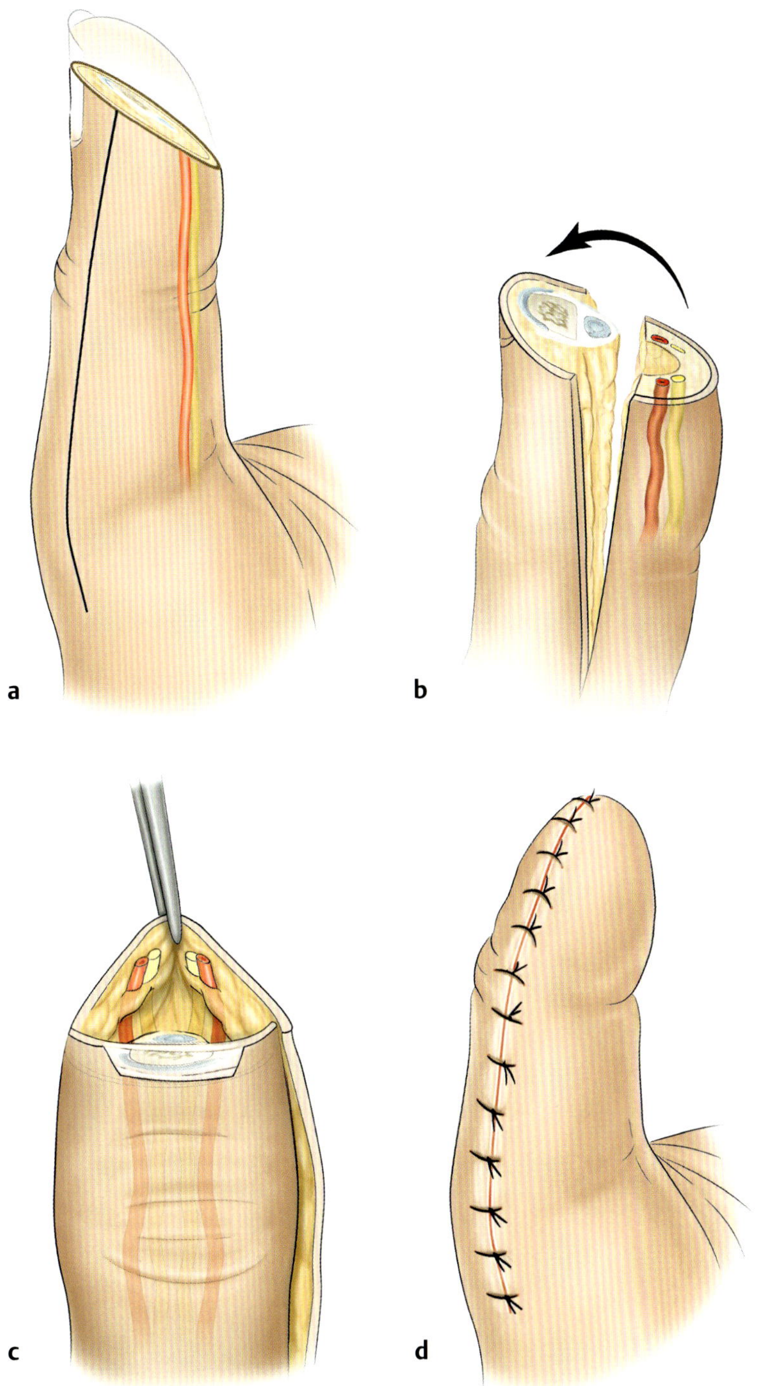

Fig. 34.1 Volar advancement flap (Moberg). **(a)** Midlateral incision to preserve neurovascular bundles. **(b)** Divide all subdermal septa to increase mobility. **(c)** Use forceps to pull flap distally. **(d)** IP joint flexion may be required to achieve closure. If closure can only be achieved with excessive flexion, use other option to prevent flexion contracture.

Chapter 35

Reverse First Dorsal Radial Metacarpal Flap (Moschella)

Table 35.1 Reverse first dorsal radial metacarpal flap (Moschella)

Flap	
Tissue	Skin and subcutaneous tissue
Course of the vessels	On the undersurface of the flap
Dimensions	3 × 1.5 cm
Extensions and combinations	—
Anatomy	Recurrent radial branch of the princeps pollicis artery; no identifiable vein
Neurovascular pedicle	—
Artery	—
Veins	—
Length and arc of rotation	—
Diameter	—
Nerve	—
Surgical technique	
Preoperative examination and markings	Dorsal aspect of the first metacarpal; Doppler identification of the vessels and their course
Flap design	Mark the defect size and include the cutaneous extension distally to facilitate skin closure of the donor site and rotation of the flap into the defect; the flap can be considered a "propeller" flap because it is rotated on an isolated vascular pedicle into an adjacent defect
Patient position	Arm on hand table, with the hand pronated
Dissection	Incise the flap circumferentially in the marked and required dimensions; dissection starts close to the paratenon of the abductor pollicis longus; the vessel that runs along the periosteum of the first metacarpal and has to be "peeled off" of the periosteum; dissect toward the pivot point, where the vessel exits from underneath; rotate the flap into the defect, and then close the skin without tension
Advantages	Local flap with reliable blood supply when the vessel can be identified with a handheld Doppler
Disadvantages	The vessel is very fragile and difficult to dissect
Pearls and pitfalls	
Dissection	It may be necessary to leave a small dog-ear around the pivot point when the perforating vessel is not clearly visible
Extensions and combinations	—
Contouring and correction	Secondary contouring is rarely necessary
Clinical applications	Dorsal defects of the thumb distal to the interphalangeal joint

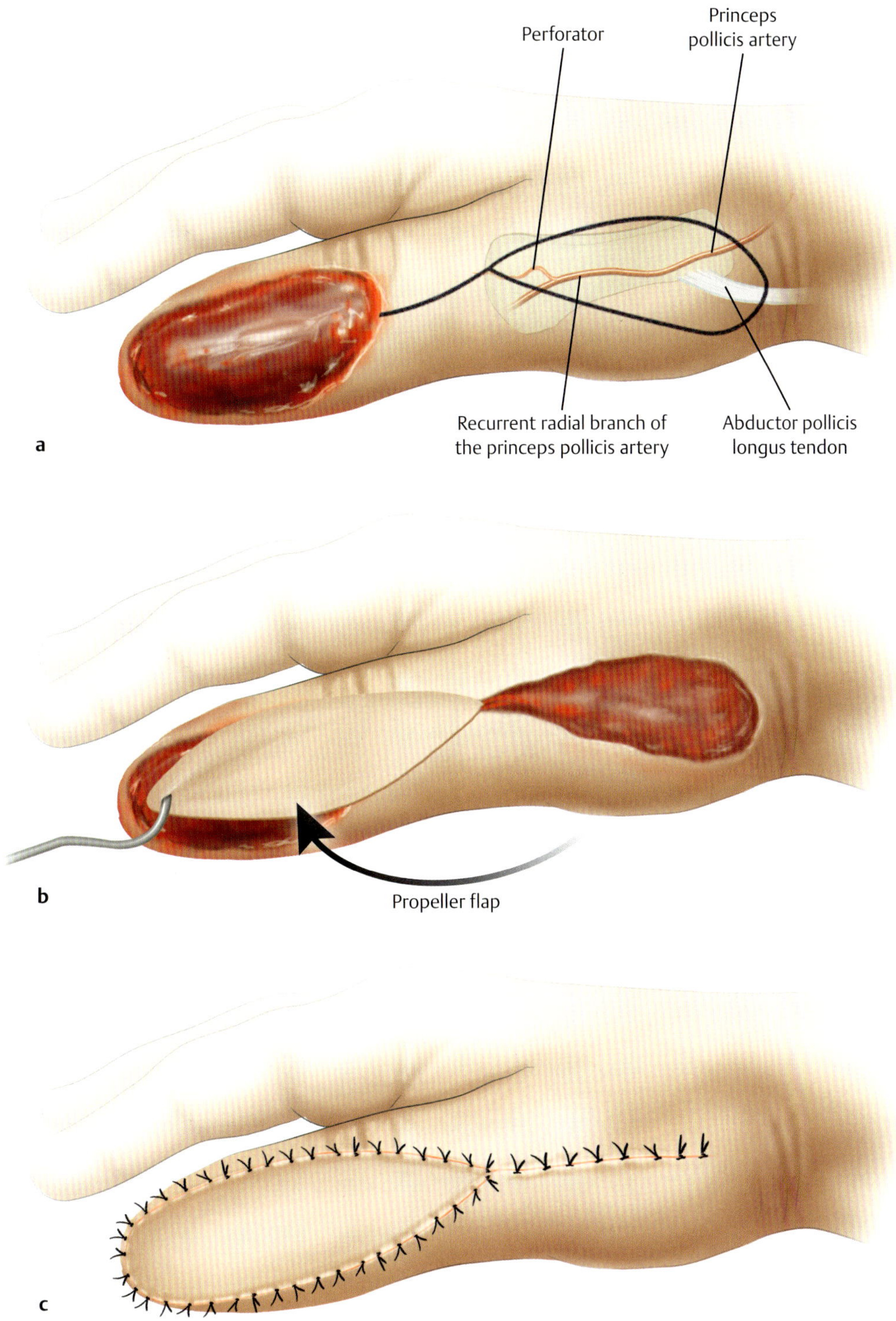

Fig. 35.1 Reverse first dorsal radial metacarpal flap (Moschella). **(a)** Perforator and recurrent radial branch of the princeps pollicis artery. **(b)** Propeller flap. **(c)** Flap inset.

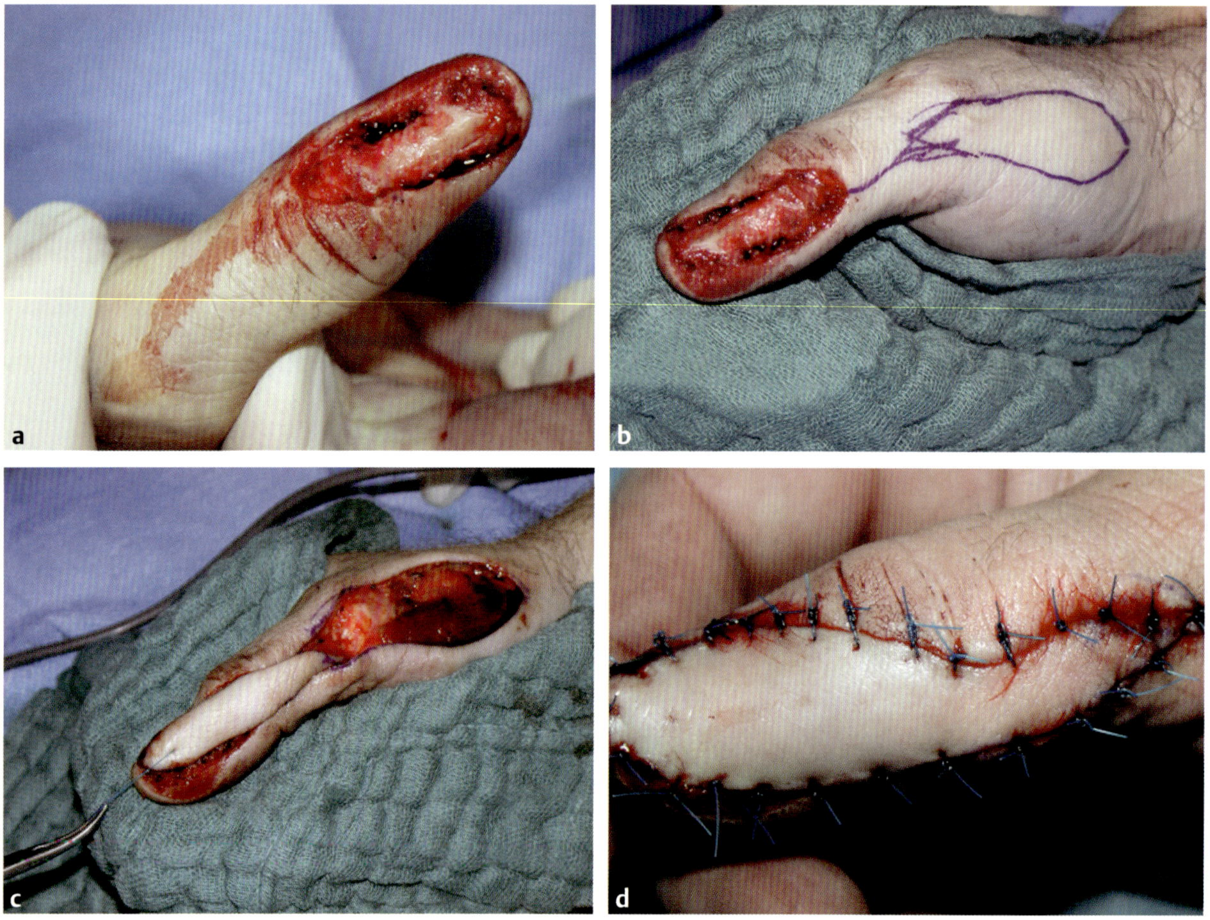

Fig. 35.2 Reverse first dorsal radial metacarpal flap (Moschella). **(a)** This patient sustained a dorsal thumb wound that included the entire nail bed. **(b)** The flap outline is based on a vessel from the princeps pollicis artery. **(c)** The flap has been elevated and transposed. **(d)** The flap after inset. Please note the tiny suture bites on the flap to decrease surface tension and avoid ischemia.

Chapter 36

Reverse First Dorsal Ulnar Perforator Flap (Brunelli)

Table 36.1 Reverse first dorsal ulnar perforator flap (Brunelli)

Flap	
Tissue	Skin and subcutaneous tissue
Course of the vessels	On the undersurface of the flap
Dimensions	3 × 1.5 cm
Extensions and combinations	—
Anatomy	
Neurovascular pedicle	—
Artery	Recurrent ulnar branch of the princeps pollicis artery
Veins	No identifiable vein
Length and arc of rotation	—
Diameter	—
Nerve	—
Surgical technique	
Preoperative examination and markings	Dorsal aspect of the first metacarpal; Doppler identification of the vessels and their courses
Flap design	Mark the defect size and include the cutaneous extension distally to facilitate skin closure of the donor site and rotation of the flap into the defect; the flap can be considered a "propeller" type flap since it is rotated on an isolated vascular pedicle into an adjacent defect
Patient position	Arm on arm table, with the hand pronated
Dissection	Incise the flap circumferentially in the marked and required dimensions; begin the dissection close to the paratenon of the extensor pollicis longus; the vessel that runs along the periosteum of the first metacarpal must be "peeled off" of the periosteum; dissect toward the pivot point, where the vessel exits from underneath; rotate the flap into the defect and then close the skin without tension
Advantages	Local flap with reliable blood supply, when the vessel can be identified with a handheld Doppler
Disadvantages	Not an easy dissection for novices, because the vessel is very fragile
Pearls and pitfalls	
Dissection	It may be necessary to leave a little dog-ear around the pivot point if the perforating vessel is not clearly visible
Extensions and combinations	—
Contouring and correction	Secondary contouring is rarely necessary
Clinical applications	Dorsal defects of the thumb distal from the interphalangeal joint

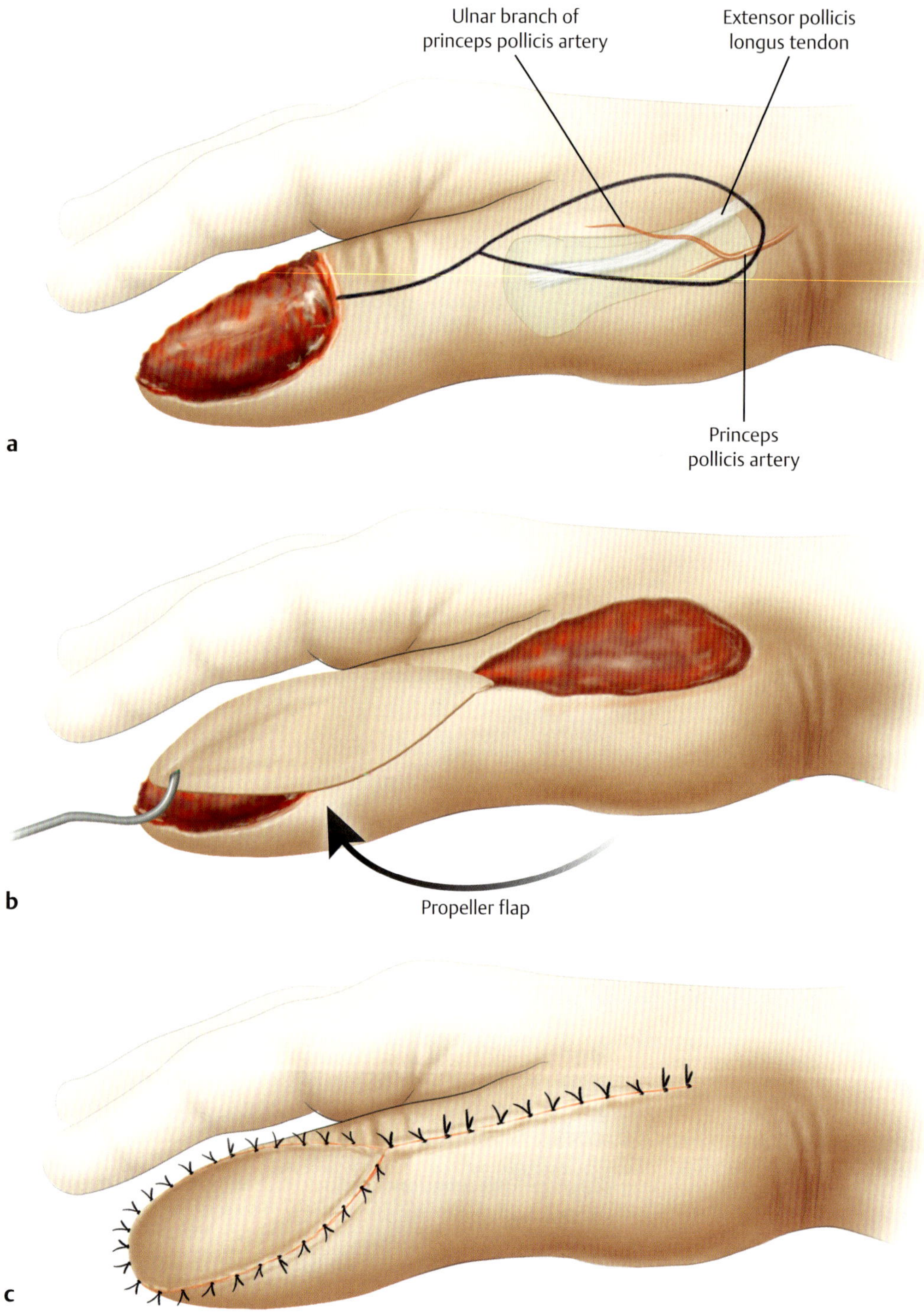

Fig. 36.1 Reverse first dorsal ulnar perforator flap (Brunelli). **(a)** Dorsal ulnar branch of the princeps pollicis artery. **(b)** Propeller flap. **(c)** Flap inset.

Chapter 37

Axial Digital Island Flap

Table 37.1 Axial digital island flap

Flap	
Tissue	Skin and adipofascial subcutaneous tissue
Course of the vessels	On the undersurface of the flap
Dimensions	2 × 1.5 cm
Extensions and combinations	—
Anatomy	
Artery	Proper digital artery
Veins	Periarterial venous plexus
Nerve	Proper digital nerve (if included in flap)
Surgical technique	
Preoperative examination and markings	Midlateral aspect of the digits; Doppler identification of the artery and its course
Flap design	Flap should be centered over the course of the proper digital artery; usually harvested from the middle phalanx
Patient position	Arm on arm table with tourniquet; forearm mobile so that hand can be rotated
Dissection	Starts away from the designed flap, either proximal or distal from the flap ("Go there—where the flap is *not!*"); identify the proper digital artery and nerve; nerve is isolated and armed with a vessel loop; use a vascular clip (not a hemostat) to secure the vessel loop; include all tissue that contains the areolar network around the artery in the flap pedicle so that venous outflow is secured, the nerve is spared, and the flap is centered over the pedicle; the pedicle is dissected in a way that provides a sufficiently wide arc of rotation; the tourniquet is released after a vascular clamp has been placed on the artery distal to the flap; the artery is divided when the flap is well perfused and does not show signs of venous congestion; the flap is rotated into the defect; the donor site can be reconstructed with a full-thickness graft from the hypothenar eminence
Advantages	Local flap with reliable blood supply; microsurgical dissection requiring some expertise; provides stable coverage with a rather inconspicuous donor site
Disadvantages	Proper digital nerve can show some irritation for a few weeks but this usually resolves completely
Pearls and pitfalls	
Dissection	Carefully free the nerve from the vascular structures; the arc of rotation has to be wide enough to avoid kinking and venous congestion
Extensions and combinations	—
Contouring and correction	Secondary contouring is rarely necessary
Clinical applications	Dorsal defects of the digits that are proximal from the flap donor site; defects over the MP joint

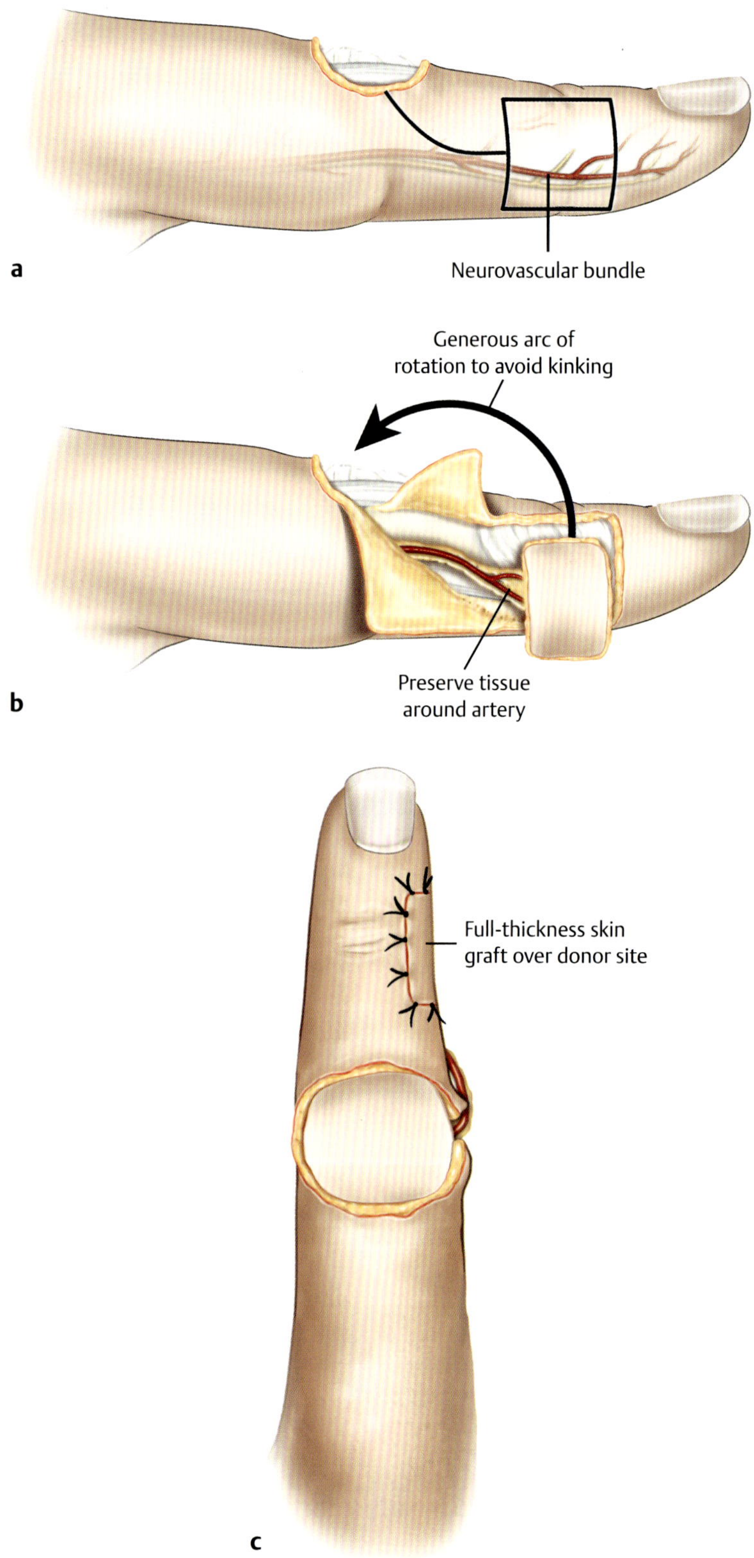

Fig. 37.1 Axial digital island flap. **(a)** Center the flap over the neurovascular bundle. If an innervated flap is required, include the proper digital nerve. If only skin coverage is required, free the nerve carefully from the artery. If an innervated flap is designed (Littler flap), split the common digital nerve intraneurally to increase pedicle length. **(b)** The arc of rotation should be generous to avoid kinking and venous congestion. Preserve areolar tissue around the artery to maintain venous outflow. **(c)** Close the donor site with a full-thickness skin graft.

Chapter 38

Reverse Axial Digital Island Flap

Table 38.1 Reverse axial digital island flap

Flap	
Tissue	Skin and adipofascial subcutaneous tissue
Course of the vessels	On the undersurface of the flap
Dimensions	2 × 1.5 cm
Extensions and combinations	–
Anatomy	
Artery	Proper digital artery
Veins	Periarterial venous plexus
Nerve	Proper digital nerve (if included in flap)
Surgical technique	
Preoperative examination and markings	Midlateral aspect of the digits; Doppler identification of the artery and its course; usually harvested from the proximal phalanx
Flap design	Flap should be centered over the course of the proper digital artery
Patient position	Arm on arm table with tourniquet; forearm mobile so that the hand can be rotated
Dissection	Perform a digital Allen test if there is suspicion of disturbed circulation in the digit; dissection always starts away from the designed flap ("Go there where the flap is *not!*"), and this may be proximal or distal from the flap; identify the proper digital artery and nerve, and isolate and arm the nerve with a vessel loop; do not use a hemostat to secure the vessel loop, because a vascular clip is perfect for this purpose; include all tissue that contains the areolar network around the artery into the flap pedicle so that venous outflow is secured, the nerve is spared, and the flap is centered over the pedicle; dissect the pedicle in a way that provides a sufficiently wide arc of rotation; release the tourniquet after a vascular clamp is placed on the artery proximal to the flap; divide the artery when the flap is well perfused through reverse flow and shows no signs of venous congestion, then rotate the flap into the defect; reconstruct the donor site with a full-thickness graft from the hypothenar eminence
Advantages	Local flap with reliable blood supply; provides stable coverage with an inconspicuous donor site
Disadvantages	The proper digital nerve can be irritated for a few weeks, but this usually resolves completely
Pearls and pitfalls	
Dissection	Carefully free the nerve from the vascular structures; the arc of rotation has to be wide enough to prevent kinking and venous congestion; the flap can be harvested to include the proper digital nerve if sensate fingertip reconstruction is intended; the nerve can be coapted to the distal nerve stump
Extensions and combinations	–
Contouring and correction	Secondary contouring is rarely necessary
Clinical applications	Dorsal defects of the digits proximal to the flap donor site; defects that include the proximal interphalangeal joint; distal defects that include fingertip reconstruction

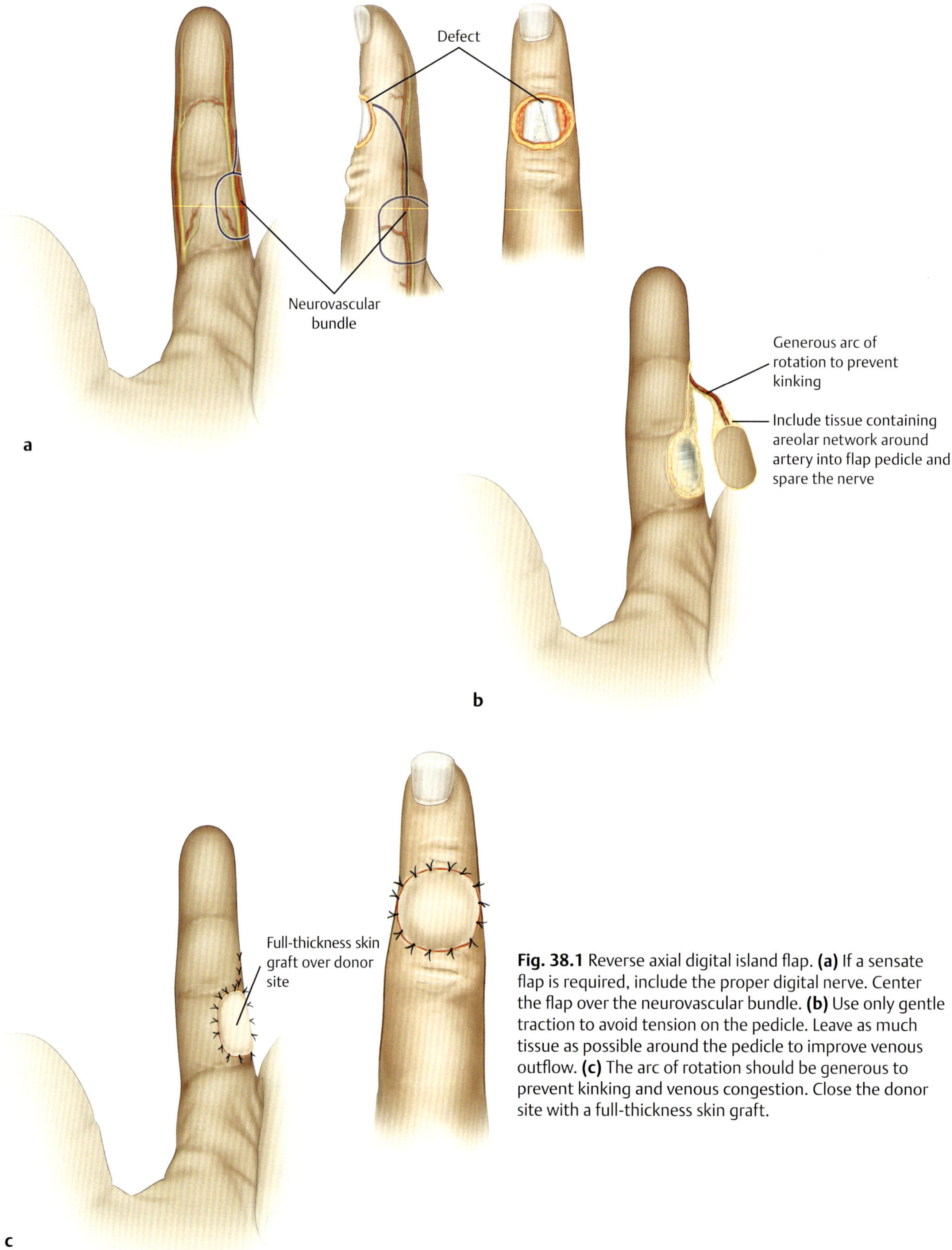

Fig. 38.1 Reverse axial digital island flap. **(a)** If a sensate flap is required, include the proper digital nerve. Center the flap over the neurovascular bundle. **(b)** Use only gentle traction to avoid tension on the pedicle. Leave as much tissue as possible around the pedicle to improve venous outflow. **(c)** The arc of rotation should be generous to prevent kinking and venous congestion. Close the donor site with a full-thickness skin graft.

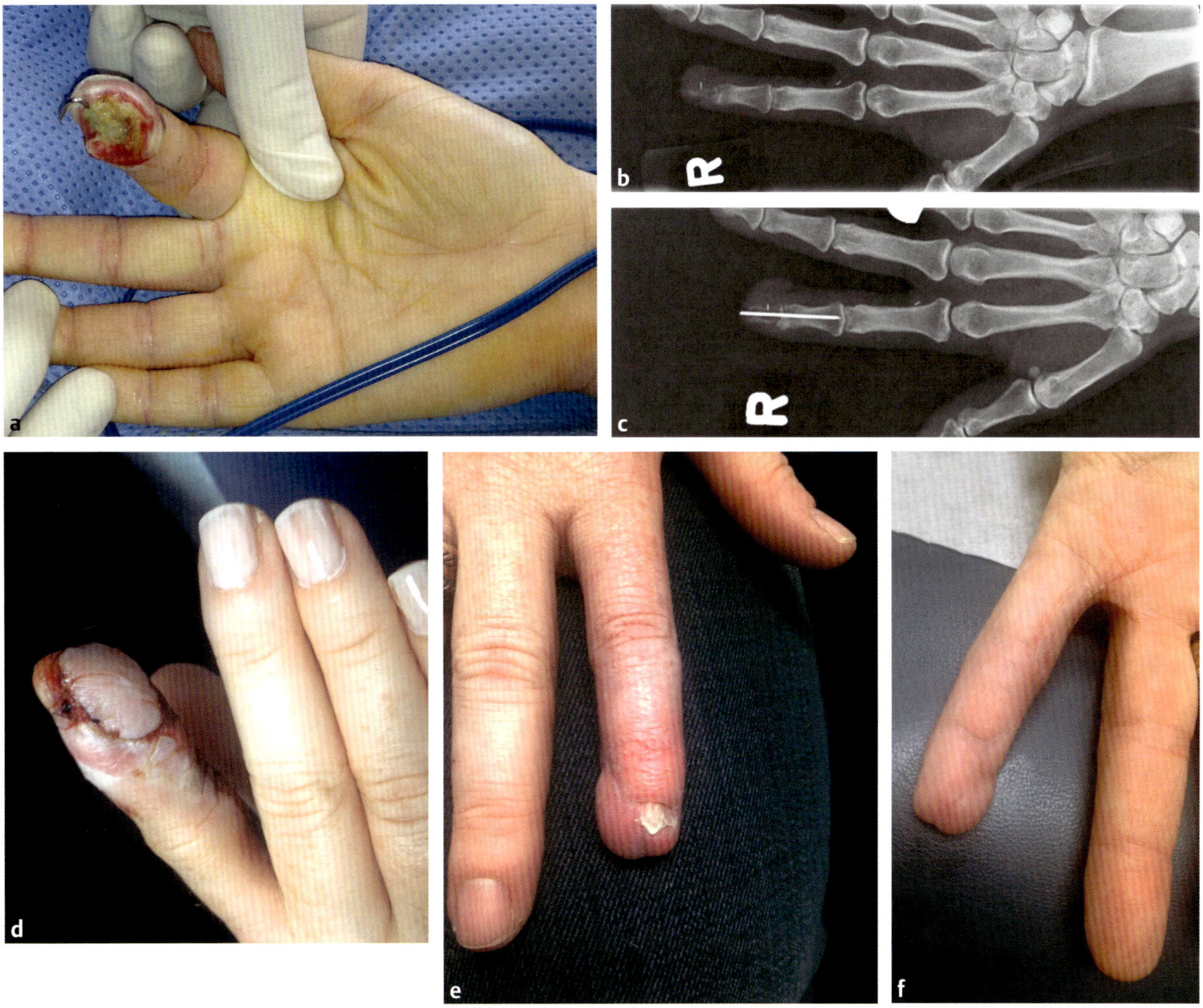

Fig. 38.2 Reverse axial digital island flap. **(a)** This patient sustained a crush injury that resulted in the necrotic pulp shown here. Bony stabilization of the phalangeal remnants is seen **(b)** preoperatively and **(c)** postoperatively. **(d)** An early postoperative view of the flap in place is shown. The repair is shown three months postoperatively in **(e)** dorsal view and **(f)** volar view.

Chapter 39

First Dorsal Metacarpal Artery Flap (Kite Flap)

Table 39.1 First dorsal metacarpal artery flap (neurofascioseptocutaneous flap or kite flap)

Flap	
Tissue	Skin
Course of the vessels	Runs with the fascia of the first dorsal interosseous muscle
Dimensions	2 × 4–6 cm; pedicle or free flap located on the proximal phalanx of the index finger
Extensions and combinations	Rarely tendon strips from the proper extensor indicis; terminal branch from the superficial radial nerve
Anatomy	
Neurovascular pedicle	–
Artery	DMCA nourished from the princeps pollicis artery
Veins	Small venae comitantes; larger subcutaneous vein
Length and arc of rotation	Artery, 3–3.5 cm; vein, 3–6 cm
Diameter	Artery at the level of princeps pollicis, 2–3 mm; vein, 3–5 mm
Nerve	Terminal branch of superficial radial nerve
Surgical technique	
Preoperative examinations and markings	Preoperative Doppler examination for the presence of vessels is mandatory; mark the course of the vessels on the skin, because they are always located more radially than presumed
Patient position	Supine with arm on arm table; tourniquet use during harvest
Dissection	Incise skin along the markings along the second metacarpal; incise the interosseous muscle fascia; preserve the intermuscular septum and raise the fasciocutaneous flap, including the fascia; take care to include the nerve; create a de-epithelialized pedicle; leave approximately 0.5–1 cm of fatty tissue around the artery; preserve the paratenon above the extensor hood; open the tourniquet and check for perfusion; inset the flap at the recipient site; wait for normal perfusion to occur; treat the skin graft donor site with a medium- or full-thickness skin graft; be careful when tunneling

Table 39.1, cont'd

Advantages	
Tissue	Sensate thin and pliable flap
Vascular pedicle	Reliable pedicle with a wide arc of rotation; large-caliber vessel when used as a free flap
Flap size and shape	Can cover large defects without sacrificing a proper digital artery
Combinations	Possible to include a tendon strip of the extensor indicis muscle; a bony segment of the second metacarpal may be a future option
Disadvantages	
Pedicle	Flap is often white during the first few minutes after opening the tourniquet; venous congestion may occur if the flap is passed through a tunnel to the recipient site
Donor site morbidity	Donor site is conspicuous at first but improves significantly over time
Pearls and pitfalls	
Dissection	Do not make arc of rotation too narrow, because venous congestion may occur; preserve the paratenon of the extensor tendons for perfect skin graft take at the donor site; when the tunnel for the flap seems too narrow, create a skin graft pedicle; apply leeches early when venous congestion occurs; avoid any tension on the pedicle; when the flap does not show adequate reperfusion after the opening of the tourniquet, rinse with warm saline; it may take 20 minutes to re-establish flow; include part of the sagittal band across the MP joint to protect the pedicle attached to the skin
Extensions and combinations	Bony segment from the metacarpal may be possible
Contouring and correction	Rarely required; flap shrinks with time
Clinical applications	Pedicle flap: small and medium-sized dorsal defects of the thumb; restoration of sensation of the pulp of the thumb Free flap: small and medium-sized defects wherever local flaps are not possible or appropriate

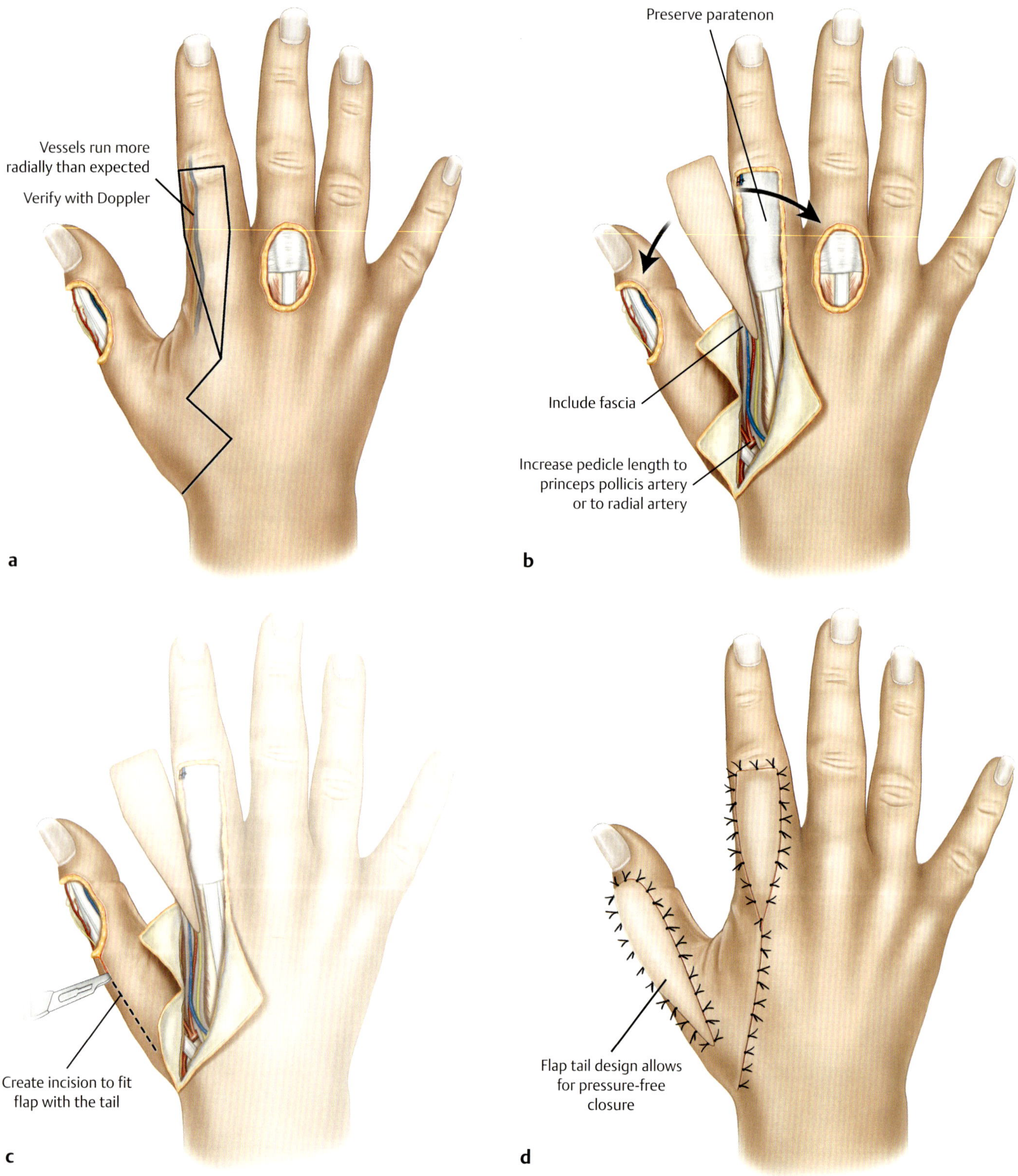

Fig. 39.1 (a) First dorsal metacarpal artery flap design. Vessels always run more radially than usually depicted in illustrations. The vessel's course will be identified by Doppler examination preoperatively. **(b)** Flap dissection. The crucial point of dissection is the area of the extensor hood. Paratenon has to be preserved to guarantee skin graft take. The vessel runs deep in the fascial septum. Include interosseous fascia that contains vessels. The pedicle is traced back to the princeps pollicis artery or radial artery to increase the pedicle length. Try to include a subcutaneous vein for improved outflow. **(c)** Flap movement and placement. Preserve the paratenon over the extensor tendon at the proximal phalanx. To avoid a narrow tunnel or the necessity of skin grafting the pedicle, the "cutaneous tail design" allows for pressure-free closure. Include a branch of the radial nerve to create a neurovascular flap. **(d)** The flap fits perfectly to reconstruct the defect, with no pressure on the pedicle.

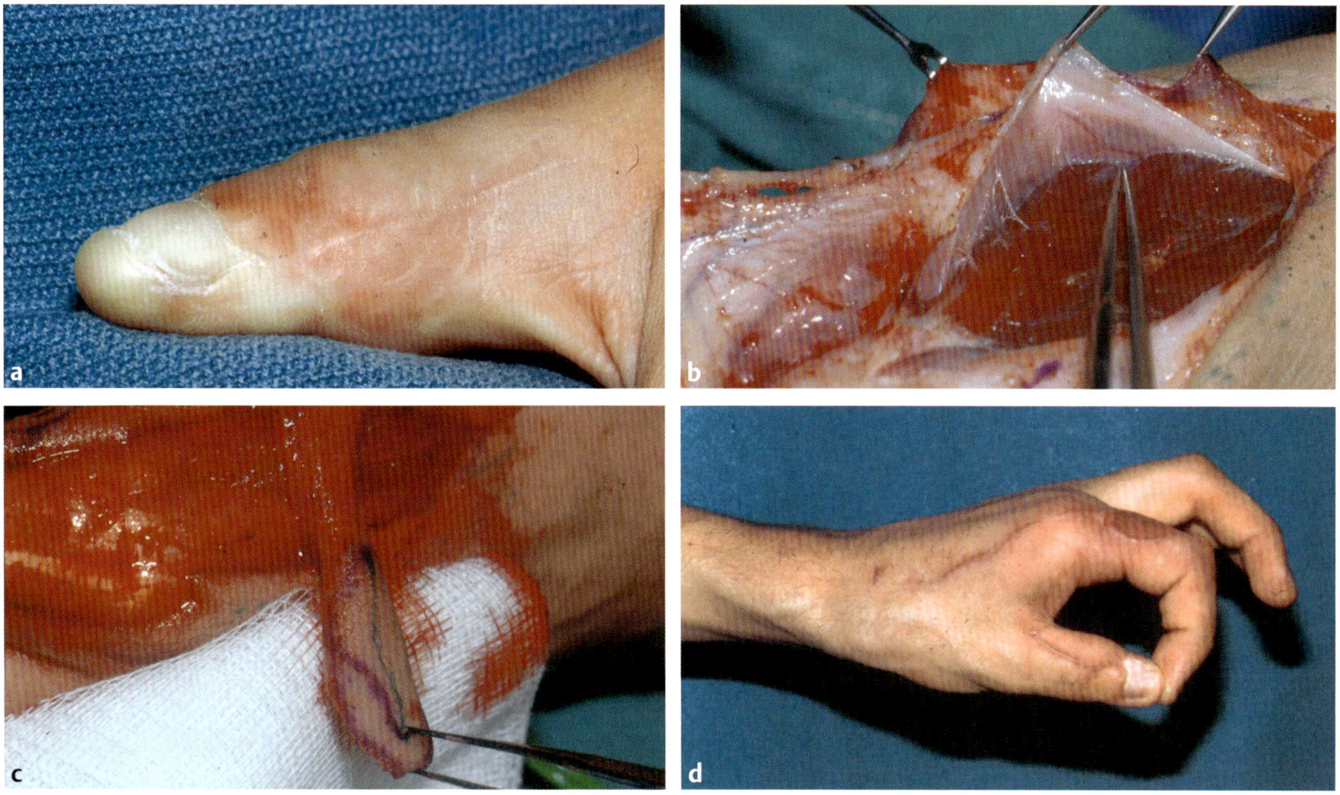

Fig. 39.2 First dorsal metacarpal artery flap (kite flap). **(a)** Insensate deficient soft tissue thumb requiring resurfacing. **(b)** First dorsal interosseous muscle fascia containing first dorsal metacarpal artery. **(c)** Flap elevated and perfusing with tourniquet down. **(d)** Final result with well-healed skin graft over donor site and sensate flap resurfacing ulnar aspect of thumb.

Chapter 40

Dorsal Metacarpal Artery Flap

Table 40.1 Dorsal metacarpal artery flap

Flap	
Tissue	Skin
Course of the vessels	In the intermuscular septum
Dimensions	2 × 4 cm; reverse flap located over the proximal metacarpals; antegrade flap located over the proximal phalanx
Extensions and combinations	Rarely may include tendon strips from the proper extensor indicis or the proper extensor digiti minimi
Anatomy	
Neurovascular pedicle	—
Artery	DMCA nourished from the dorsal arterial arch or through the volar–dorsal perforator from the volar arch
Veins	Small venae comitantes
Length and arc of rotation	Reverse pedicle flap reaches the proximal interphalangeal joint; antegrade flap reaches the proximal wrist extensor crease
Diameter	—
Nerve	—
Surgical technique	
Preoperative examination and markings	Preoperative Doppler examination for the presence of vessels is mandatory; reliability declines from radial to ulnar aspect; the DMCA artery 4 is only present in approximately 80% of patients
Flap design	—
Patient position	Supine with arm on arm table; risk of tourniquet-induced ischemia
Dissection	Antegrade pedicle: incise skin along markings; incise interosseous muscle fascia; preserve intermuscular septum and raise fasciocutaneous flap, including fascia; create de-epithelialized pedicle toward volar–dorsal perforator at the level of the metacarpal head; leave approximately 0.5–1 cm of fatty tissue around the artery; ligate the distal pedicle; open the tourniquet; check for perfusion; inset the flap at the recipient site; wait for normal perfusion Reverse pedicle: incise skin along markings; incise interosseous muscle fascia; preserve intermuscular septum and raise fasciocutaneous flap, including fascia; create de-epithelialized pedicle toward the volar–dorsal perforator at the level of the metacarpal head; leave approximately 0.5–1 cm of fatty tissue around the artery; ligate the proximal pedicle; open the tourniquet; check for perfusion; rotate and inset the flap into the recipient site; wait for normal perfusion

Table 40.1, cont'd

Advantages	
Vascular pedicle	Both are reliable pedicles with wide arcs of rotation
Flap size and shape	Can cover even larger digital defects
Combinations	Can be combined with adjacent DMCA flaps for multidigital injuries
Tissue	Thin and pliable
Disadvantages	
Donor site morbidity	Only donor sites of smaller flaps can be closed primarily; skin grafts on the dorsum of the hand can be conspicuous; contour defects improve with time
Pedicle	Veins cannot be identified in most cases; flaps often appear ischemic during the first few minutes after deflating the tourniquet; venous congestion may occur
Pearls and pitfalls	
Dissection	Do not make the arc of rotation too narrow, because venous congestion may occur; preserve the paratenons of the extensor tendons for perfect skin graft take in the donor site; when the tunnel for the flap seems too narrow, create a skin graft pedicle; apply leeches early when venous congestion occurs; avoid any tension on the pedicle; when the flap does not show adequate reperfusion after the opening of the tourniquet, rinse the area with warm saline; it may take 20 minutes to re-establish blood flow
Extensions and combinations	Bony segment from the metacarpal may be possible
Contouring and correction	Rarely required; flaps shrink with time
Clinical applications	Reserve pedicle flap: small- and medium-sized dorsal digital defects as far as the proximal interphalangeal joint

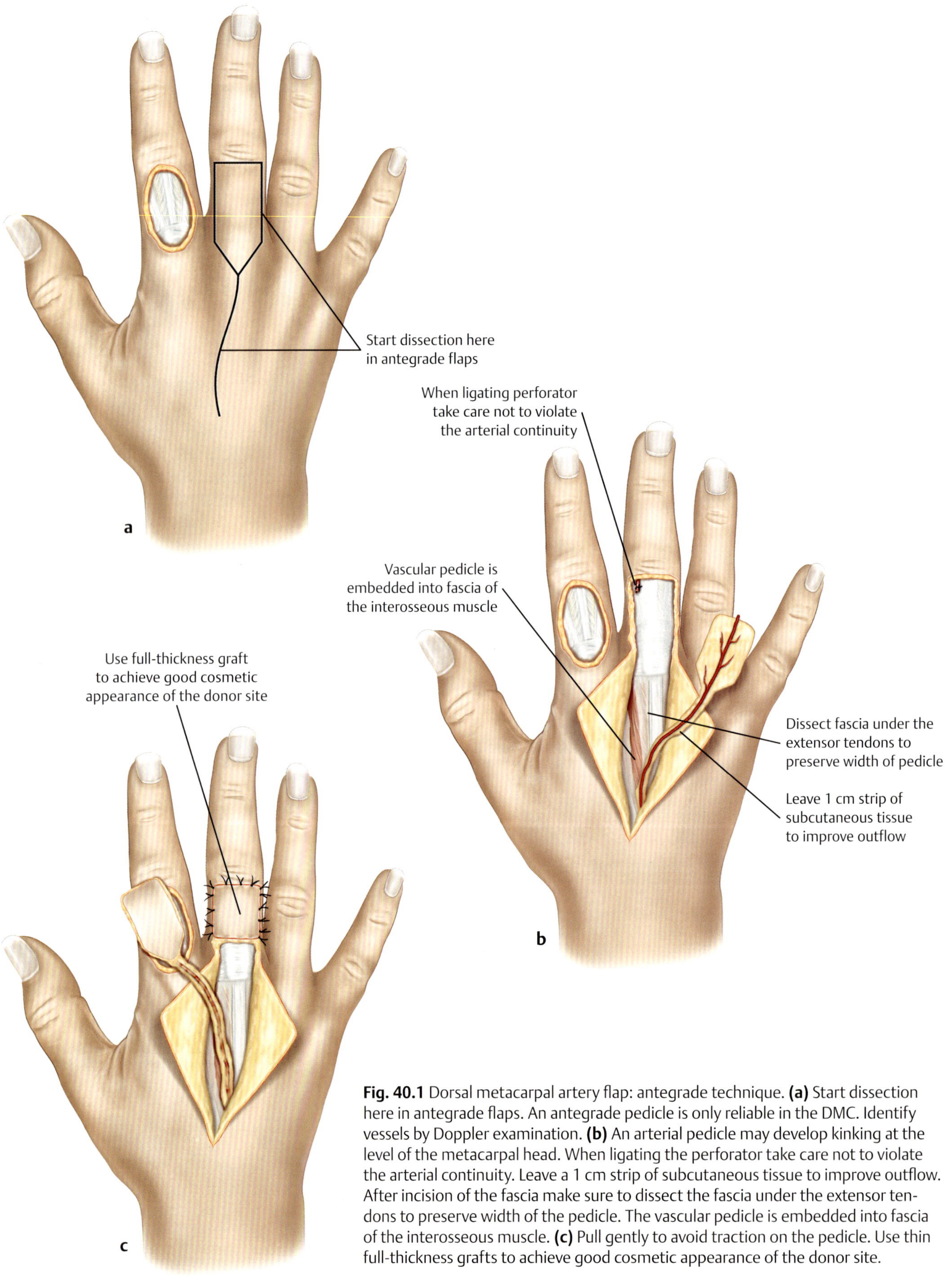

Fig. 40.1 Dorsal metacarpal artery flap: antegrade technique. **(a)** Start dissection here in antegrade flaps. An antegrade pedicle is only reliable in the DMC. Identify vessels by Doppler examination. **(b)** An arterial pedicle may develop kinking at the level of the metacarpal head. When ligating the perforator take care not to violate the arterial continuity. Leave a 1 cm strip of subcutaneous tissue to improve outflow. After incision of the fascia make sure to dissect the fascia under the extensor tendons to preserve width of the pedicle. The vascular pedicle is embedded into fascia of the interosseous muscle. **(c)** Pull gently to avoid traction on the pedicle. Use thin full-thickness grafts to achieve good cosmetic appearance of the donor site.

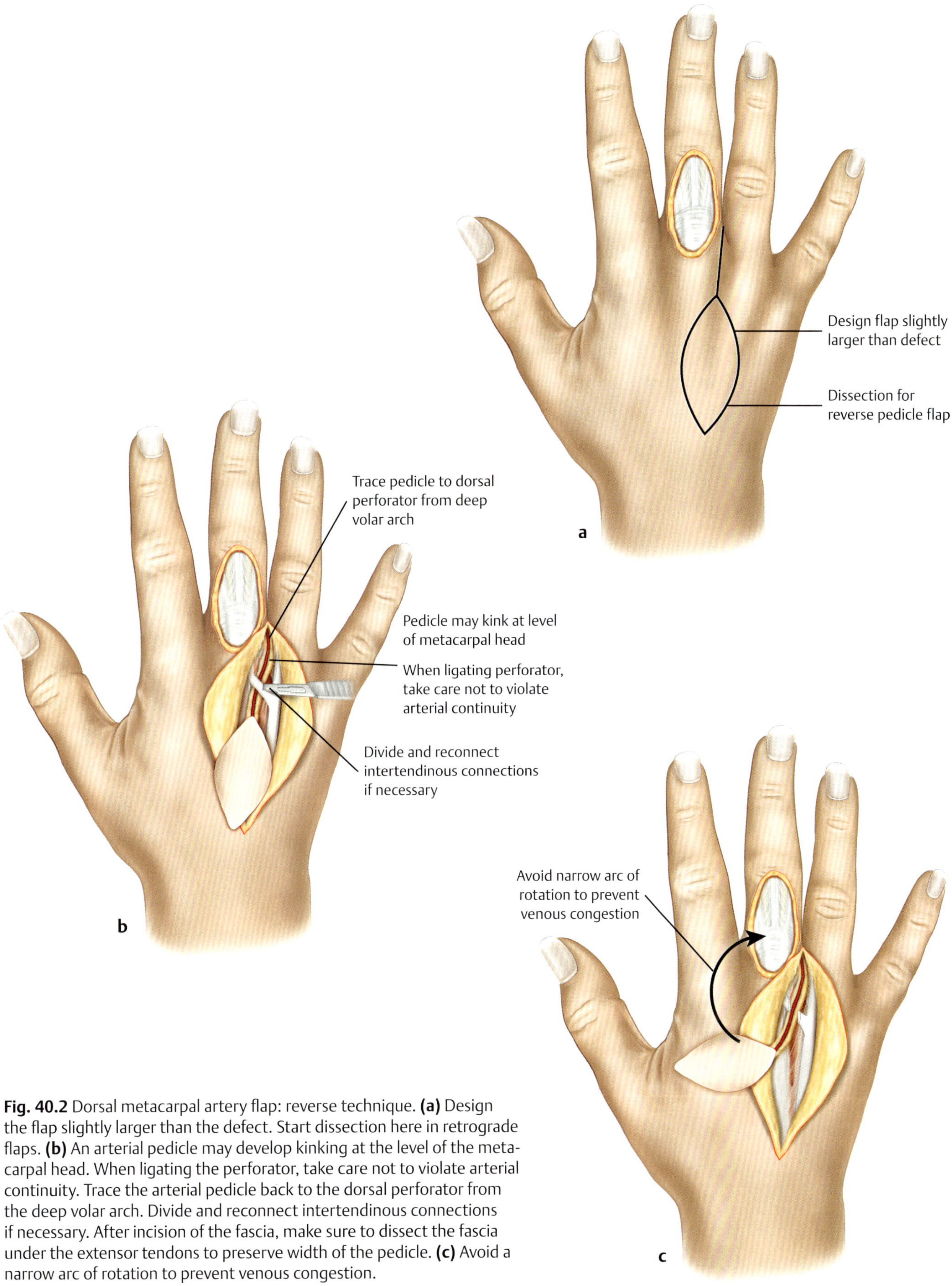

Fig. 40.2 Dorsal metacarpal artery flap: reverse technique. **(a)** Design the flap slightly larger than the defect. Start dissection here in retrograde flaps. **(b)** An arterial pedicle may develop kinking at the level of the metacarpal head. When ligating the perforator, take care not to violate arterial continuity. Trace the arterial pedicle back to the dorsal perforator from the deep volar arch. Divide and reconnect intertendinous connections if necessary. After incision of the fascia, make sure to dissect the fascia under the extensor tendons to preserve width of the pedicle. **(c)** Avoid a narrow arc of rotation to prevent venous congestion.

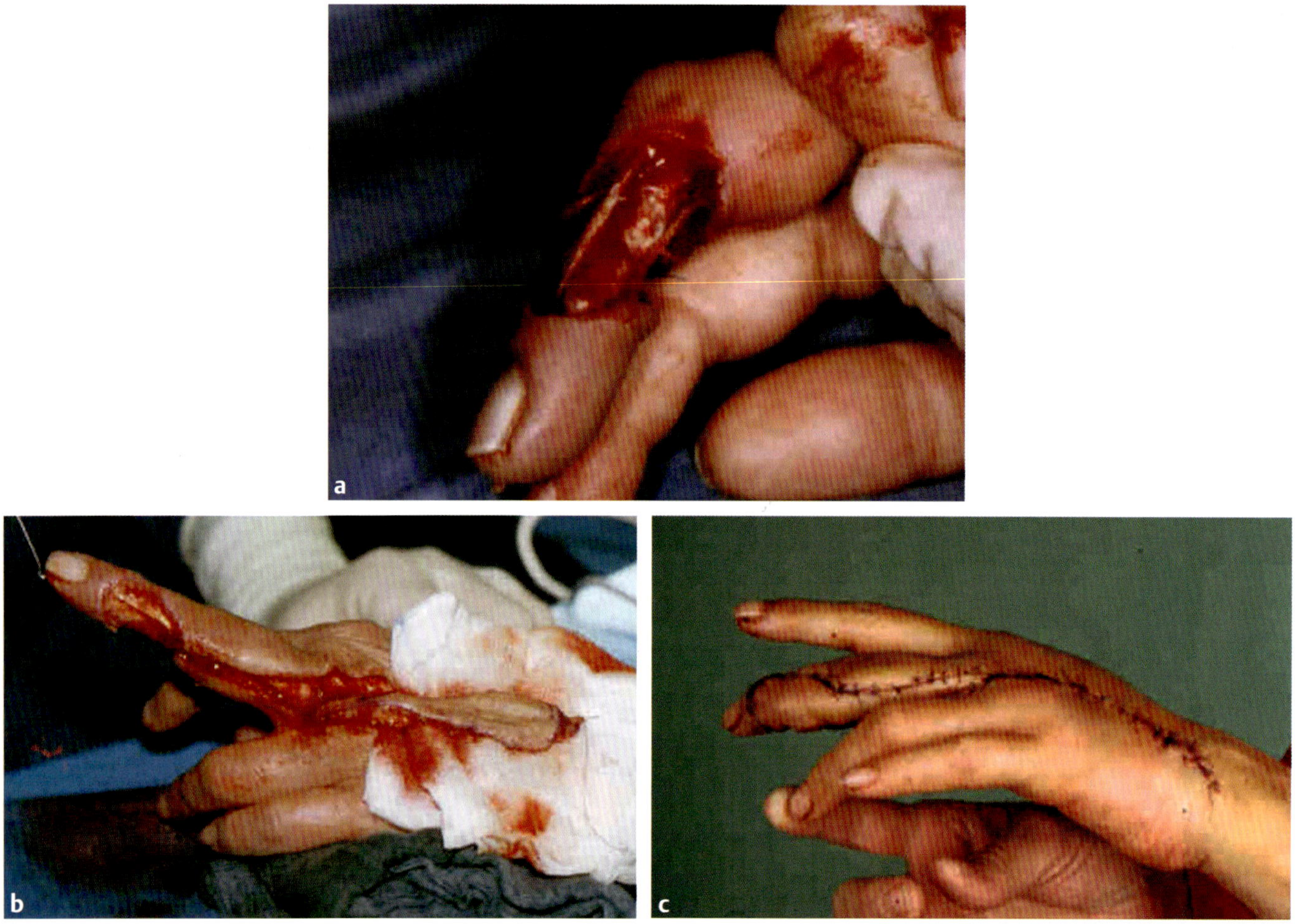

Fig. 40.3 Dorsal metacarpal artery flap. **(a)** The patient's defect is shown after debridement. **(b)** An extended DMCA flap has been created. **(c)** The patient's hand is shown 12 days after surgery.

Chapter 41

Radial Forearm Flap

Table 41.1 Radial forearm flap

Flap	Pedicle or free flap; distal or proximal pedicle
Tissue	Potentially innervated fasciocutaneous flap with little hair; also possible as a fascial flap
Course of the vessels	At the bottom of a fascial septum along the brachioradialis muscle as the leading structure
Dimensions	Maximum 8 × 20 cm
Extensions and combinations	Can be combined with a strip of brachioradialis or palmaris longus tendon, a bony segment of the radius, or a second proximal skin island based on a perforator vessel
Anatomy	
Neurovascular pedicle	—
Artery	Radial artery
Veins	Two concomitant veins or the cephalic system
Length and arc of rotation	Depends on flap location on the forearm; up to 15 cm
Diameter	Artery, 3–4 mm; veins, 3–5 mm (in the case of a free flap)
Nerve	Lateral antebrachial cutaneous nerve
Surgical technique	
Preoperative examination and markings	Identify the course of the radial artery by Doppler examination; Allen test
Patient position	Supine position with arm on arm board
Dissection	Mark the flap centered over the course of the vessel; incise the skin and make a subfascial dissection cuff toward the vessel; stay under the vessels and isolate the pedicle distally; include a cuff of subcutaneous fat and a subcutaneous vein if the flap is raised as a distal pedicle flap
	For experienced surgeons, create a suprafascial dissection and a possible pedicle flap: raise flap from distal to proximal; isolate the vessels proximally; put a vessel clamp on the proximal pedicle; check for perfusion or signs of venous congestion; wait for 15 minutes; leave a subcutaneous vein long; ligate the proximal vessels and rotate the flap to the distal site; check again for perfusion and venous congestion; if the area is congested, connect the vein to a forearm vein (turbocharging)
	Proximal pedicle: put a vessel clamp on the distal pedicle after isolating the flap; check perfusion; ligate the distal vessels

Continued

Table 41.1, cont'd

Advantages	
Vascular pedicle	A long, reliable pedicle with large-caliber vessels; atherosclerosis is rare; can be used as a "flow-through" flap when used as a free flap
Flap size and shape	Large flap; can be raised as a multi-island flap with strips of de-epithelialized subcutaneous tissue and fascia between the skin islands; many shapes possible; usually thin and pliable, even in obese patients
Combinations	Can be combined with extensions or second skin islands based on perforators, strips of tendons, and bony segments of the radius
Dissection	Donor and recipient sites can be dissected simultaneously
Disadvantages	
Donor site morbidity	Very conspicuous donor site with potential impairment of tendon function; indication has to be carefully weighed, especially in women; graft take can be impaired distally
Pedicle	Sacrifice of a major forearm artery
Pearls and pitfalls	
Dissection	Avoid separating the fascial septum from the vessels
Extensions and combinations	Maintain connections to bone and tendons when combined flaps are raised
Contouring and correction	Flap has only a little tendency to sag; contour corrections are rarely required
Clinical applications	Defects where flat, thin, and supple flaps are indicated; forearm, dorsum of the hand, and donor site appearance can be improved with suprafascial dissection

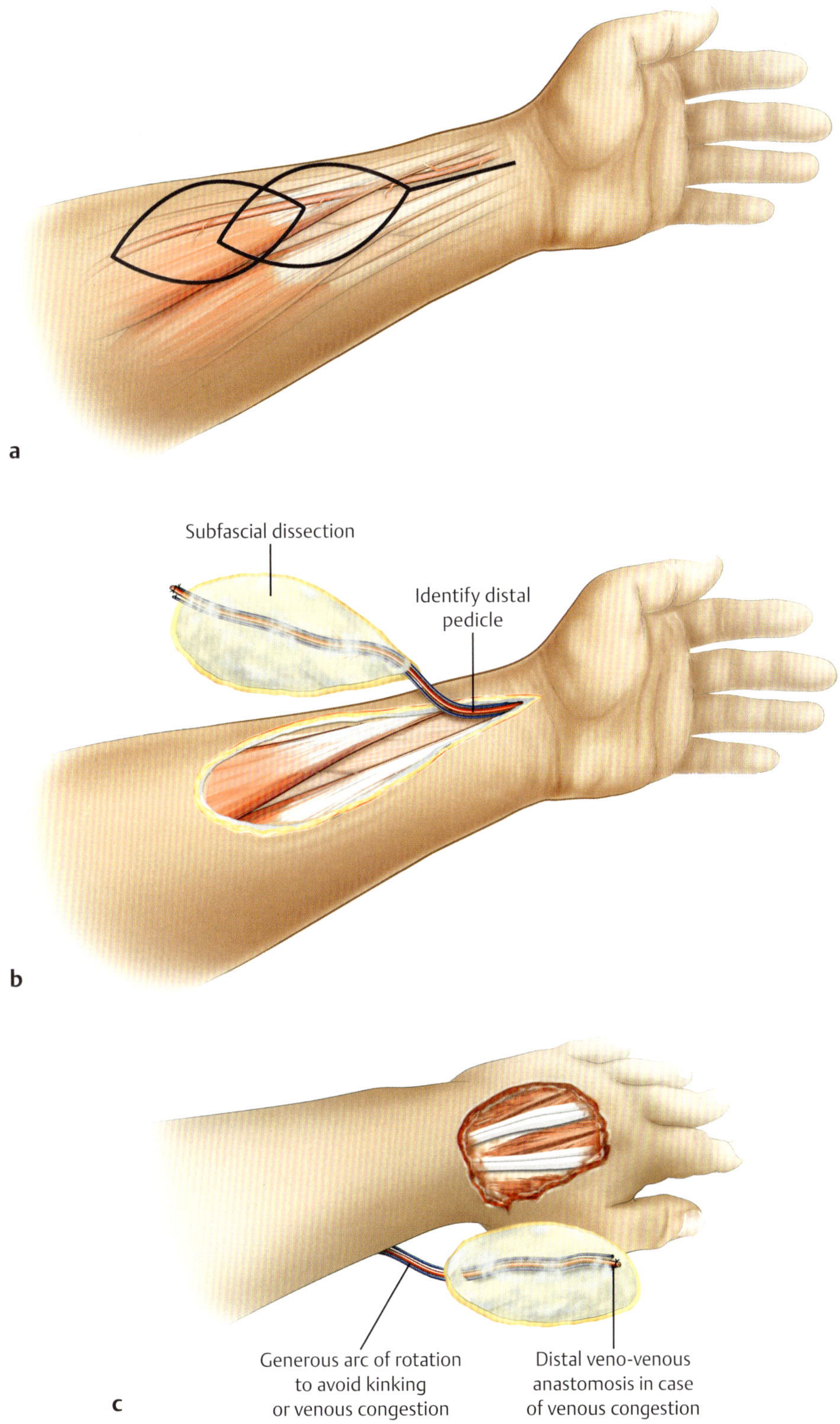

Fig. 41.1 Radial forearm flap. **(a)** Perform a preoperative Allen test. Identify and mark the vessel course preoperatively. **(b)** Dissection is usually subfascial, but epifascial dissection is possible, including only a narrow strip of fascia around the pedicle. Start dissection with identification of the distal pedicle. Start dissection at the ulnar aspect. Try to place the skin island as proximal as possible in reverse pedicle flaps. **(c)** The arc of rotation has to be generous to avoid kinking or venous congestion. Maintain the option of a distal veno-venous anastomosis in case of venous congestion.

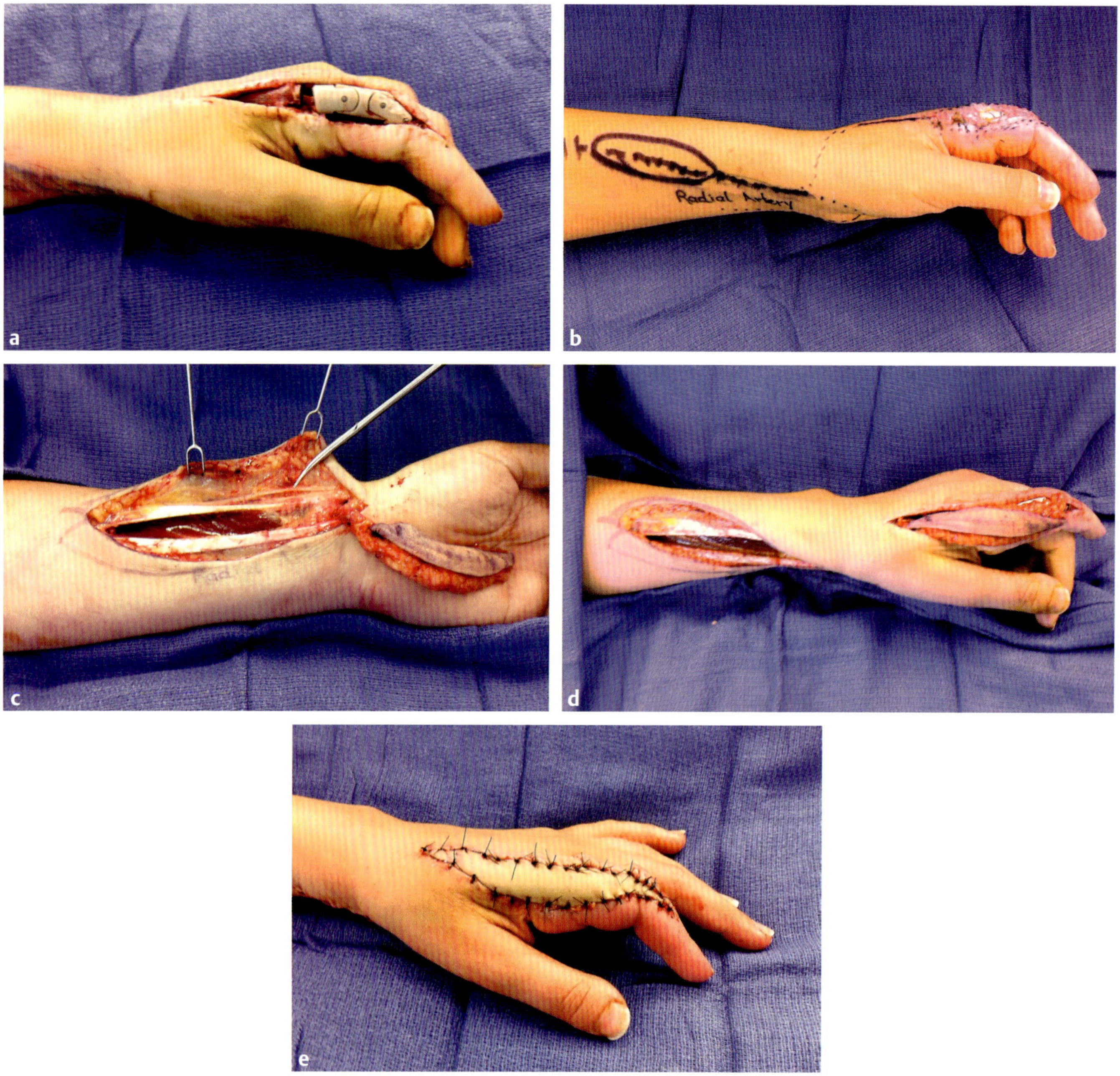

Fig. 41.2 Radial forearm flap. **(a)** An exposed multiarticulated phalangeal prosthesis after successful resection and postoperative irradiation of an osteosarcoma. **(b)** A reverse radial forearm flap was designed for primary donor site closure. **(c)** The flap was raised and islandized with preservation of the superficial branch of the radial nerve. **(d)** The prosthesis was removed and an antibiotic spacer placed. The flap was tunneled and positioned to cover the recipient site defect. **(e)** Radial forearm flap inset.

Chapter 42

Pedicled Vascularized Bone Grafts from the Wrist

Pedicled Bone Grafts for Carpal Pathology

Volar-based

Donor bone from:

Radius
Pronator quadratus
Volar carpal artery

Ulna
Osteoperiosteal branch of ulnar artery

Other
Pisiform
  Dorsal branch of ulnar artery
Thumb metacarpal
  First dorsal metacarpal artery

Dorsal-based

Donor bone from:

Radius
First, second intercompartmental supraretinacular artery
Second extensor compartment branch
Second, third intercompartmental supraretinacular artery
Fourth extracompartmental artery
Fifth extracompartmental artery
Fourth and fifth extracompartmental arteries combined

Ulna
Third and fourth dorsal metacarpal arteries

Other
Thumb metacarpal
Index metacarpal

Algorithm 42.1

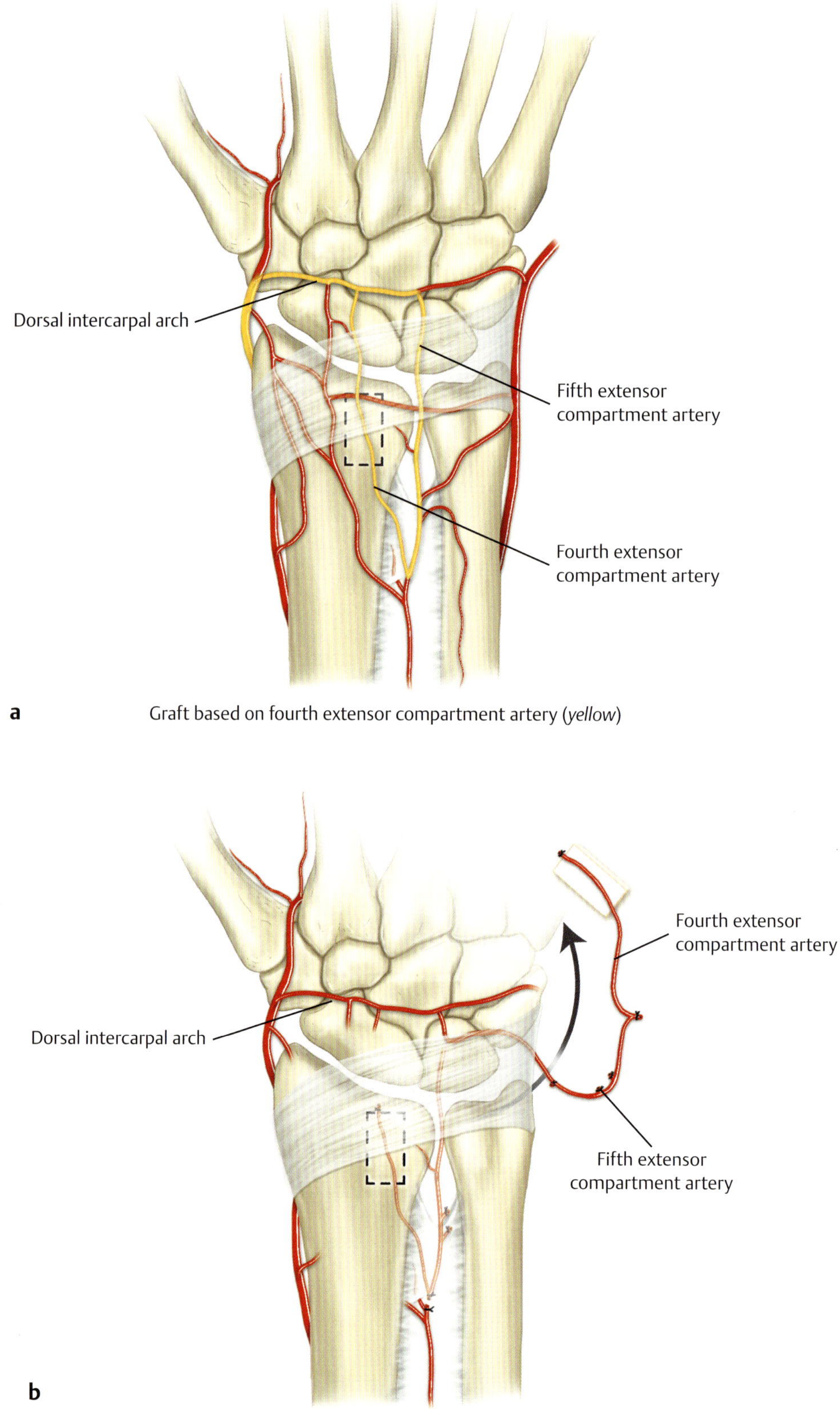

Fig. 42.1 Pedicled vascularized bone grafts from the wrist. **(a)** Graft based on fourth extensor compartment artery (*yellow*). **(b)** Arc of rotation of flap.

Chapter 43

Posterior Interosseous Flap

Table 43.1 Posterior interosseous flap (reverse pedicled flap)

Flap	
Tissue	Skin and fascia
Course of the vessels	Deep to flap surface in a fascial septum; antegrade vessels in the free flap, retrograde vessels in the pedicle flap
Dimensions	8 × 15 cm; donor sites of flaps < 4 cm wide can be closed primarily
Extensions and combinations	Tendon strip from the extensor carpi ulnaris; bony segments from the radius are not reliable
Anatomy	
Neurovascular pedicle	—
Artery	Posterior interosseous artery; recurrent vessels via tenuous anastomoses with anterior interosseous artery through interosseous membrane
Veins	Venae comitantes
Length and arc of rotation	—
Diameter	Artery, 1–1.5 mm; vein, 1 mm
Nerve	Ulnar cutaneous antebrachial branch not reliable for the sensory needs of the innervated flap
Surgical technique	
Preoperative examination and markings	Draw a line from the lateral epicondyle to the dorsal center of the wrist; perform a Doppler examination of the two main perforators at the proximal third of the forearm; outline the flap and center it over this line
Patient position	Supine with arm on arm table
Dissection	Incise laterally along the marking; incise the muscle fascia; perform a subfascial dissection until the fascial septum between the extensor digiti quinti and the extensor carpi ulnaris can be identified; create a medial incision; perform a subfascial dissection until the septum is identified from the other side; free the septum from the periosteum in a distal to proximal direction; raise the flap until the pedicle can be traced to the radial artery; apply a micro-clamp to the proximal pedicle; watch out for nerve branches supplying wrist extensors; open the tourniquet; check for adequate perfusion; rotate the flap after ligation of the pedicle and then inset the flap in the recipient site

Continued

Table 43.1, cont'd

Advantages	
Flap size and shape	Subcutaneous fat can provide excellent gliding tissue for tendon reconstructions
Combinations	Inclusion of tendon strip and bone segments enhances versatility
Disadvantages	
Pedicle	Pedicle can contain very small concomitant veins; a tendency for venous congestion has been reported; nerve transection may be required if motor branches cross between main perforators
Bulkiness	Can be bulky in patients with fleshy forearms
Donor site morbidity	Donor site can be very conspicuous; this flap should not be the first choice for younger patients and females
Pearls and pitfalls	
Dissection	Try to spare the motor nerve; avoid a too narrow arc of rotation, because the flap has a tendency for venous congestion; include a proximal subcutaneous vein for emergency turbocharging; include a wide segment of dorsal fascia with the pedicle; identify the arterial anastomosis to the anterior interosseous artery first (5% of all patients do not have this anastomosis)
Extensions and combinations	Include a tendon strip in the subfascial dissection; stay very close to the periosteum to avoid injury to the pedicle
Contouring and correction	Secondary corrections may be required in many cases
Clinical applications	Dorsal defects of the hand; defects of the first web space; defects around the wrist

Table 43.2 Posterior interosseous flap (free flap and antegrade pedicled flap)

Flap	
Tissue	Skin and fascia
Course of the vessels	Deep to the flap surface in a fascial septum; antegrade vessels in the free flap
Dimensions	8 × 15 cm; donor sites of flaps < 4 cm wide can be closed primarily
Extensions and combinations	Tendon strip from the extensor carpi ulnaris; bony segments from the radius
Anatomy	
Neurovascular pedicle	—
Artery	Posterior interosseous artery; antegrade vessel from the radial artery
Veins	Venae comitantes
Length and arc of rotation	Pedicle length, 3–4 cm
Diameter	Artery, 2–3 mm; vein, 2.5–3.5 mm
Nerve	Ulnar cutaneous antebrachial branch
Surgical technique	
Preoperative examination and markings	Draw a line from the lateral epicondyle to the dorsal center of the wrist; perform a Doppler examination of the two main perforators at the proximal third of the forearm; outline the flap and center it over this line
Patient position	Supine with arm on arm table
Dissection	Incise laterally along the marking; incise the muscle fascia; perform a subfascial dissection until the fascial septum between the extensor digiti quinti and the extensor carpi ulnaris can be identified; create a medial incision; perform a subfascial dissection until the septum is identified from the other side; free the septum from the periosteum in a distally cephalad direction; ligate the pedicle distally; raise the flap until the pedicle branches off toward the radial artery; watch out for nerve branches supplying wrist extensors; open the tourniquet; check for adequate perfusion; rotate the flap or ligate the pedicle and then inset the flap in the recipient site
Advantages	
Vascular pedicle	Adequate caliber
Flap size and shape	Donor sites of flaps < 4 cm wide can be closed primarily; subcutaneous fat can provide excellent gliding tissue for tendon reconstructions
Combinations	Inclusion of tendon strip and bone segments enhances versatility
Disadvantages	
Pedicle	Pedicle is short; nerve transection may be required if motor branches cross between main perforators
Bulkiness	Can be bulky in strong patients with fleshy forearms
Donor site morbidity	Donor site can be very conspicuous; this flap should not be the first choice for younger patients and females
Pearls and pitfalls	
Dissection	Try to spare the motor nerve; avoid a too narrow arc of rotation, because the flap has a tendency for venous congestion; include a proximal subcutaneous vein for emergency turbocharging; include a wide segment of dorsal fascia with the pedicle; identify the arterial anastomosis to the anterior interosseous artery first (5% of all patients do not have this anastomosis)
Extensions and combinations	Include a tendon strip in the subfascial dissection; stay very close to the periosteum to avoid injury to the pedicle
Contouring and correction	Secondary corrections may be required in many cases
Clinical applications	Forearm defects; dorsal hand defects; complex reconstructions with free nonvascularized tendon grafts; defects around the elbow when used as proximal pedicle flaps

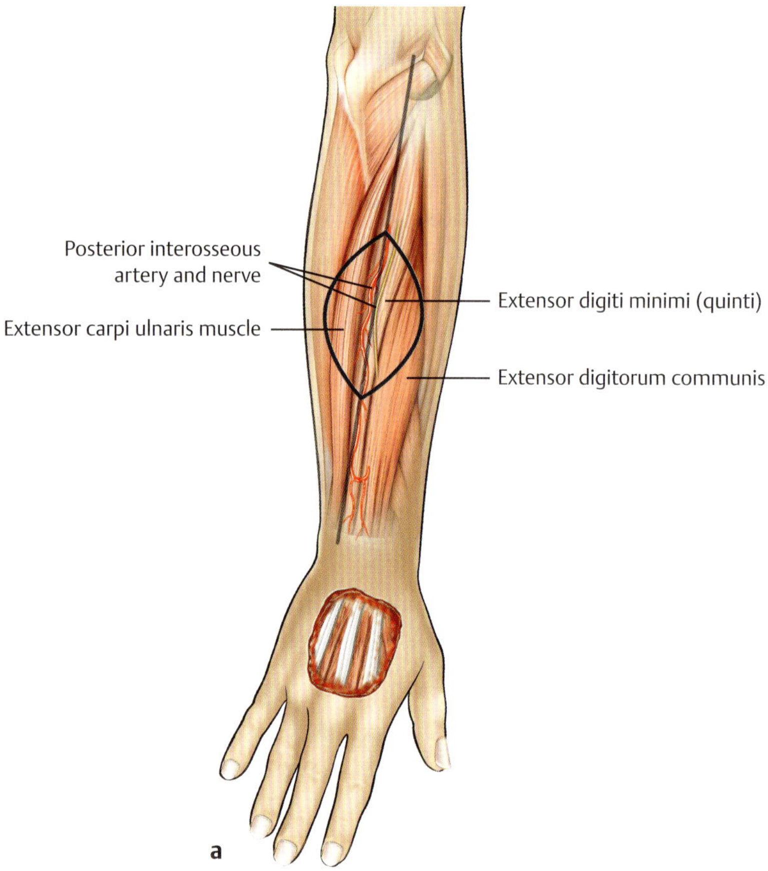

a

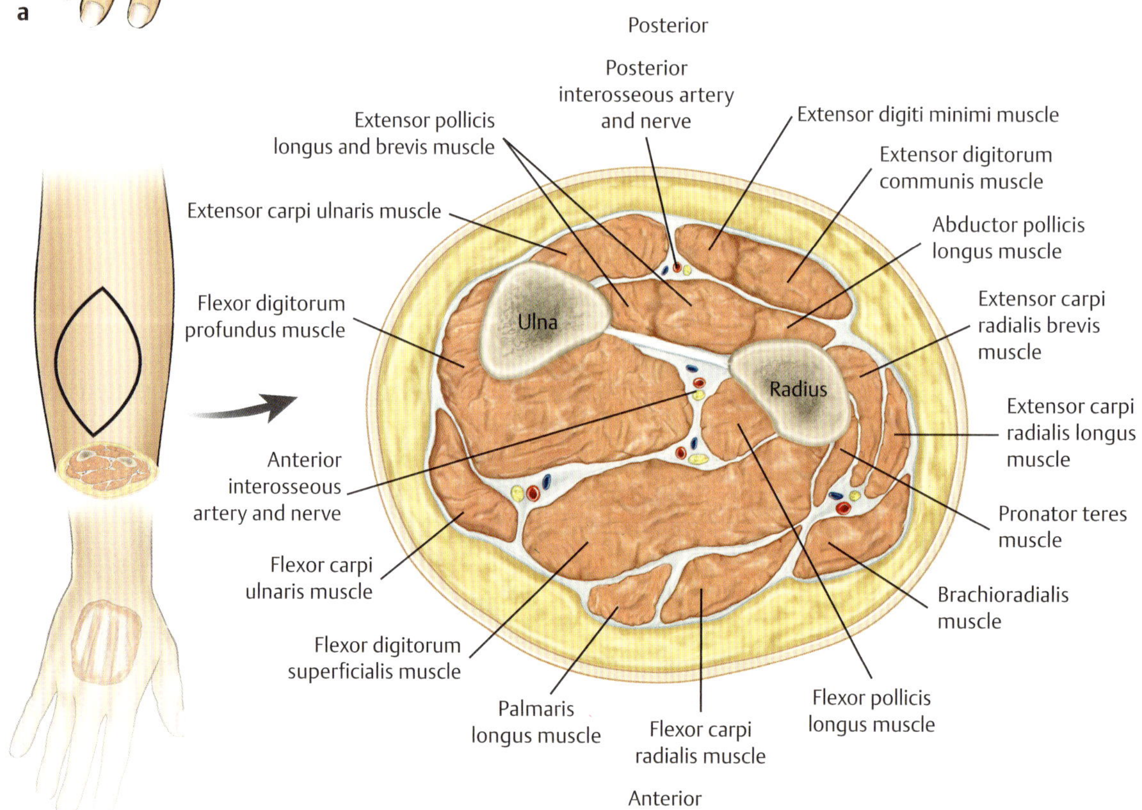

b

Fig. 43.1 Posterior interosseous flap. **(a)** Identify vessel course with Doppler. Identify proximal perforators prior to planning. **(b)** Start dissection here. Try to spare motor nerve to extensor carpi ulnaris (*continued*).

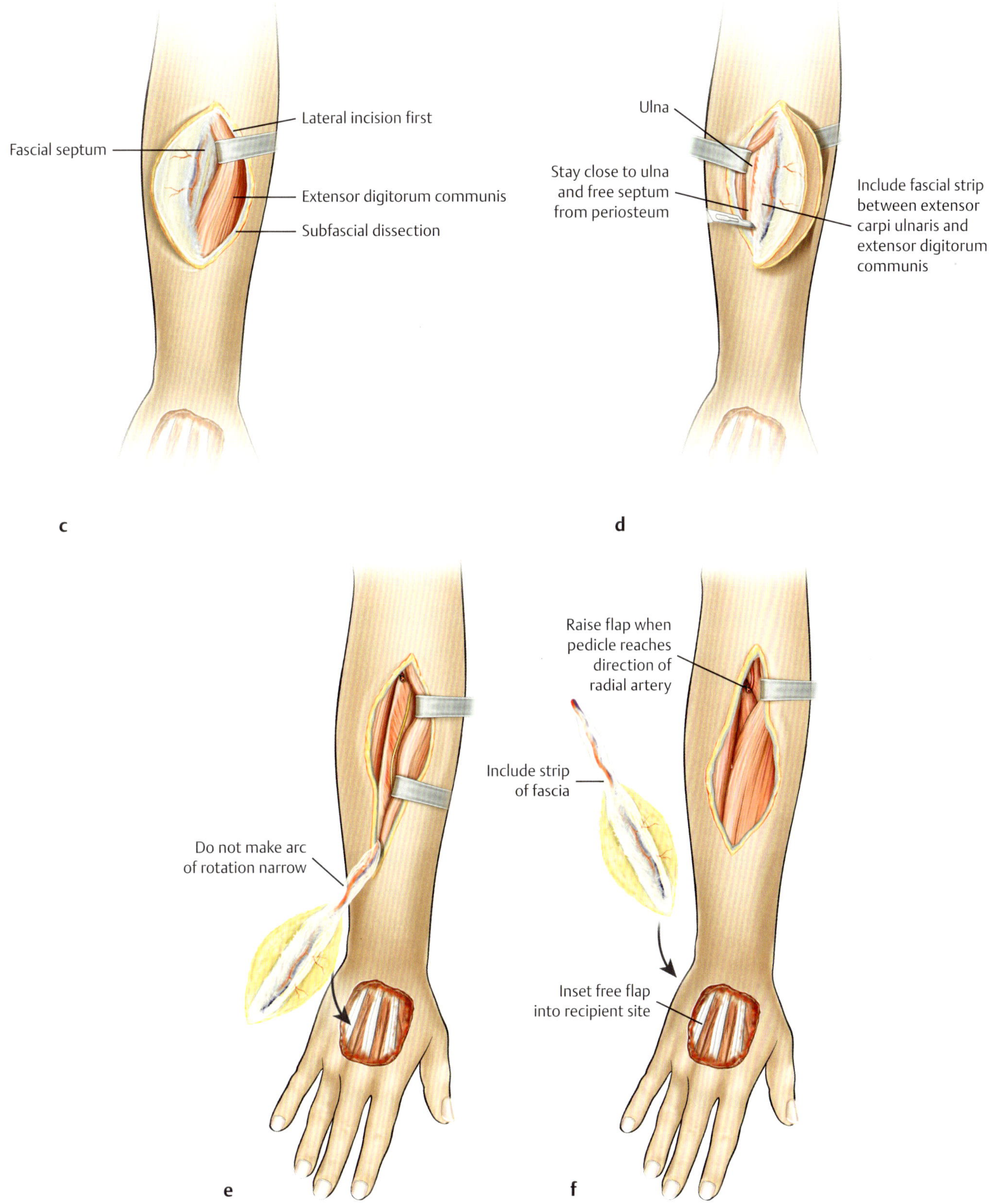

Fig. 43.1 *(continued)* **(c)** Stay close to the ulna to avoid violation of the pedicle. Preserve subcutaneous vein for distal veno-venous anastomosis in case of venous congestion. Do not make arc of rotation too narrow. Include fascial strip between the extensor carpi ulnaris and extensor digiti quinti containing the pedicle vessels. **(d)** Isolation of pedicle. **(e)** Flap elevated as pedicle flap. **(f)** Flap harvested as free flap.

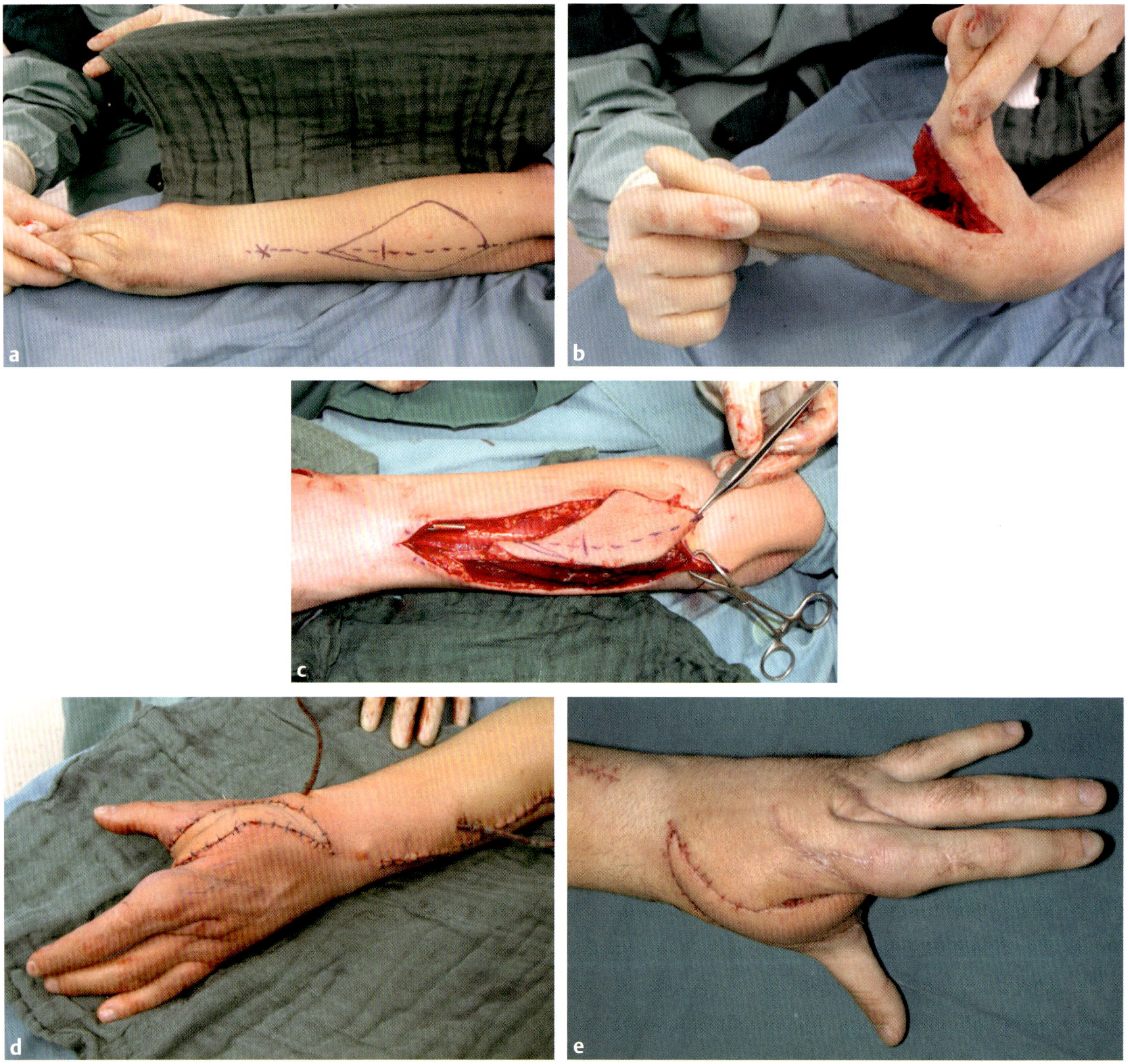

Fig. 43.2 Posterior interosseous flap. **(a)** The patient's flap design is shown. Flap access is from the lateral epicondyle to the distal radial ulnar joint. The midpoint is the location of the posterior interosseous artery. **(b)** Web space release. **(c)** Flap elevation. **(d)** Primary donor site closure and flap insetting. **(e)** The patient's final result, with increased finger-thumb web space, is shown.

Chapter 44

Reverse Ulnar Perforator Forearm Flap

Table 44.1 Reverse ulnar perforator forearm flap

Flap	
Tissue	Skin or fascia
Course of the vessels	Underneath the flap in Scarpa's fascia; passes laterally under the flexor carpi ulnaris
Dimensions	4 × 15 cm at the ulnar aspect of the forearm
Extensions and combinations	—
Anatomy	
Neurovascular pedicle	—
Artery	Distal perforator (4 cm from wrist) of the ulnar artery
Veins	Venae comitantes
Length and arc of rotation	Flap reaches the proximal palm of the wrist joint
Diameter	—
Nerve	—
Surgical technique	
Preoperative examination and markings	Doppler identification of perforator vessel; flap centered over the lateral ulnar aspect of the forearm
Patient position	Supine with arm on arm table to avoid tourniquet ischemia
Dissection	Incise the skin along the markings; perform a subfascial dissection with sparing of ulnar artery and nerve; preserve the extensor paratenon; identify the distal perforator; create a distal skin incision when taking it as an island flap, otherwise leave the distal skin bridge intact; open the tourniquet; check the flap for perfusion; rotate the flap into the defect
Advantages	
Vascular pedicle	Reliable and easy to identify
Flap size and shape	Large flap possible
Combinations	Inclusion of tendon strip possible (flexor carpi ulnaris)
Dissection	Easy and straightforward
Disadvantages	
Flap	Flap leaves dog-ear at pivot point that frequently requires secondary correction; donor site has to be skin grafted in most cases
Bulkiness	Flap may be bulky
Donor site morbidity	Skin grafted area may be conspicuous; impairment of tendon gliding rarely encountered; major risk is injury or division of the ulnar nerve
Pearls and pitfalls	
Dissection	Do not violate the paratenon; identify the perforator before dissection; frequently check the integrity of the perforator when proceeding distally with the dissection
Extensions and combinations	Inclusion of tendon strip (flexor carpi ulnaris)
Contouring and correction	Contouring after 6 months; frequently, smaller dog-ears will appear and can be smoothed out
Clinical applications	Long narrow defects around the wrist

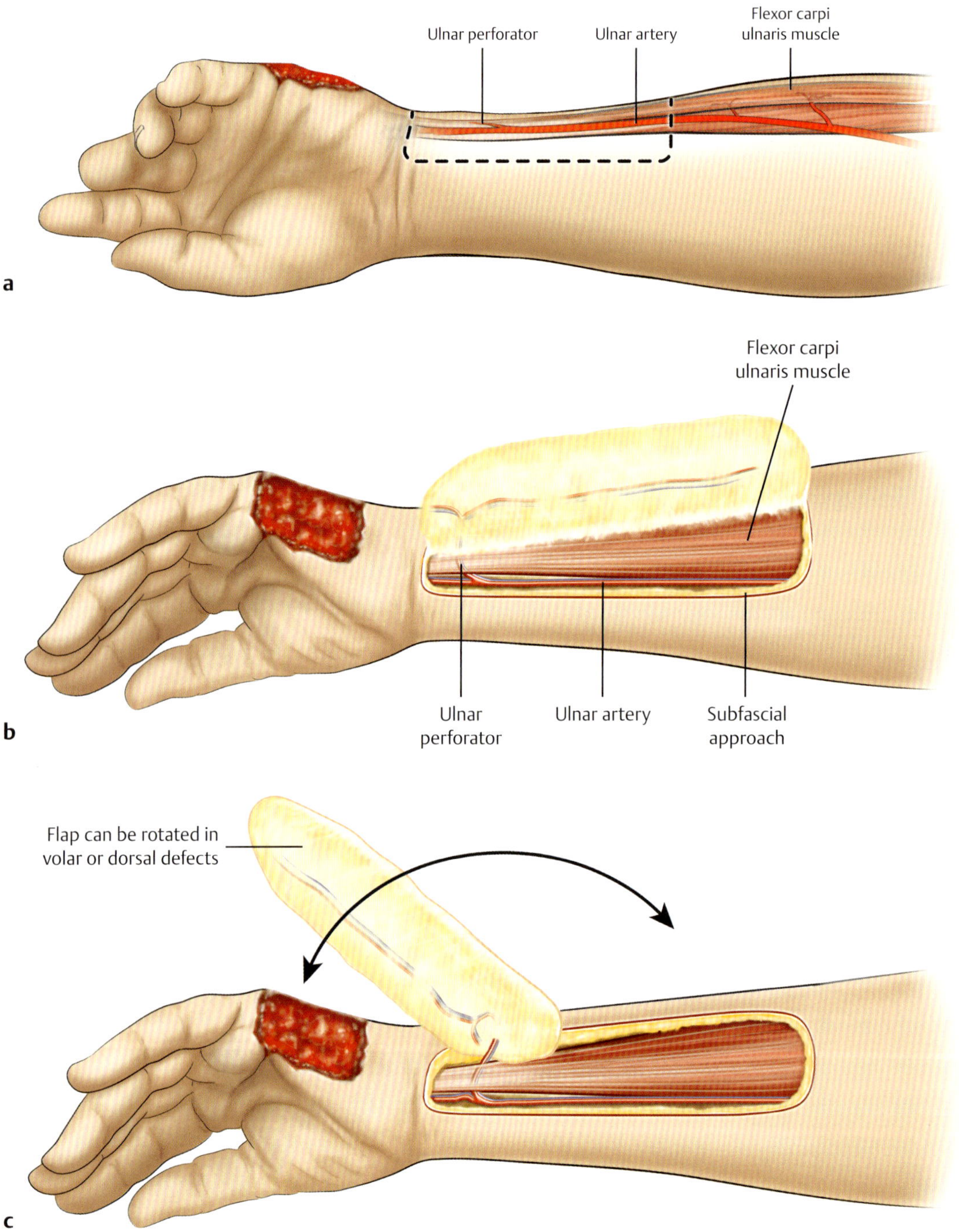

Fig. 44.1 Reverse ulnar perforator forearm flap. **(a)** Center the flap over the course of the ulnar artery. Use Doppler device to identify pedicle approximately 3–4 cm proximal to the wrist crease. **(b)** Start the dissection proximally and proceed distally. Approach pedicle location carefully. Stay subfascial during the dissection. The pedicle passes underneath the flexor carpi ulnaris tendon laterally. **(c)** The flap can be rotated in volar or dorsal defects. When the flap is raised it can be transformed into a true island flap by dividing the distal skin bridge. Preserve the distal skin bridge until perfusion of the flap is confirmed after elevation.

Chapter 45

Lateral Arm Flap

Table 45.1 Lateral arm flap

Flap	Pedicle or free flap, antegrade or reverse pedicle
Tissue	Innervated cutaneous flap, frequently from a non–hair-bearing area; also may be de-epithelialized if a subcutaneous fascial flap
Course of the vessels	In a fascial plane, deep along the humerus; perforators enter the flap via a delicate septum from the undersurface
Dimensions	Up to 15 × 8 cm (primary closure only possible for flaps ≤ 6 × 12 cm)
Extensions and combinations	Can be harvested as an osteocutaneous flap with a segment from the humerus; can include a fasciocutaneous forearm extension
Anatomy	
Neurovascular pedicle	–
Artery	Posterior radial collateral artery (branch of the profunda brachii artery); distal flow from a recurrent radial collateral artery from the articular network around the elbow
Veins	Two concomitant veins and cephalic system
Length and arc of rotation	≤ 8 cm
Diameter	Arteries, 1.5–2 mm; veins, 2–2.5 mm
Nerve	Posterior cutaneous forearm nerve from the radial nerve
Surgical technique	
Preoperative examinations and markings	Doppler identification of vessel course recommended; mark the insertion of the deltoid muscle and the lateral condyle; outline the flap dimensions centered over this line
Patient position	Supine; arm draped to allow for free movement; arm on an arm table or fixed across the chest; tourniquet recommended (but sometimes hard to hold in place)
Dissection	Free flap and antegrade pedicle flap: start with a posterior incision down to the muscle fascia; raise the flap subfascially and tack the fascia to the skin to prevent shearing; continue to the anterior border of the triceps muscle, where the fascia dives deep and inserts into the humerus; perforators are seen in the septum; incise anteriorly down to the fascia; subfascial dissection should include the fascia of the flexor muscles; pursue the fascia down to the humerus; ligate the distal continuation of the posterior radial collateral artery; separate the fascial septum as close as possible to the periosteum; follow the pedicle proximally under the triceps muscle into the spiral groove; separate the lower cutaneous nerve from the radial nerve Reverse pedicle flap: proceed with dissection as described for the free flap dissection; ligate the proximal inflow; pursue the distal pedicle toward the elbow Fasciocutaneous forearm extension: extend the flap 5 cm distal to the elbow, with width that is similar to the lateral arm flap; raise the extension subfascially; include the recurrent pedicle as long as possible

Continued

Table 45.1, cont'd

Advantages	
Dissection	Flap dissection is rapid for experienced surgeons; a simultaneous two-team approach is possible
Vascular pedicle	Reliable and constant pedicle with moderate diameter
Flap size and shape	Thin flap that can be made in various shapes; oval is the optimal shape
Combinations	Very versatile due to optional combinations with bone, tendon strip from the triceps, forearm fascia extension, and/or nerve for both innervation and vascularized flow through the nerve graft
Disadvantages	
Flap	Depending on the patient, the flap can be bulky due to the subcutaneous layer
Donor site morbidity	Scar is conspicuous; only donor sites ≤ 6 cm wide can be closed primarily, or else skin graft is required; no functional loss except numbness on the lateral forearm
Pedicle	Pedicle is short; vascular diameter can be small, especially in women
Pearls and pitfalls	
Dissection	Do not confuse the nerve branches; stay extremely close to the periosteum of the humerus to preserve the delicate septum; tack the fascia to the skin to prevent shearing forces; repair the tendon donor site in the triceps muscle
Extensions and combinations	Try to center a perforator over the strip of periosteum taken with the bony segment; the posterior cutaneous nerve can be harvested as a vascularized nerve graft
Contouring and correction	Flap tends to sag; contour corrections are frequently needed
Clinical applications	Defects of the dorsum of the hand and the first web space; defects around the elbow and the shoulder region when used as a distal or proximal pedicle flap

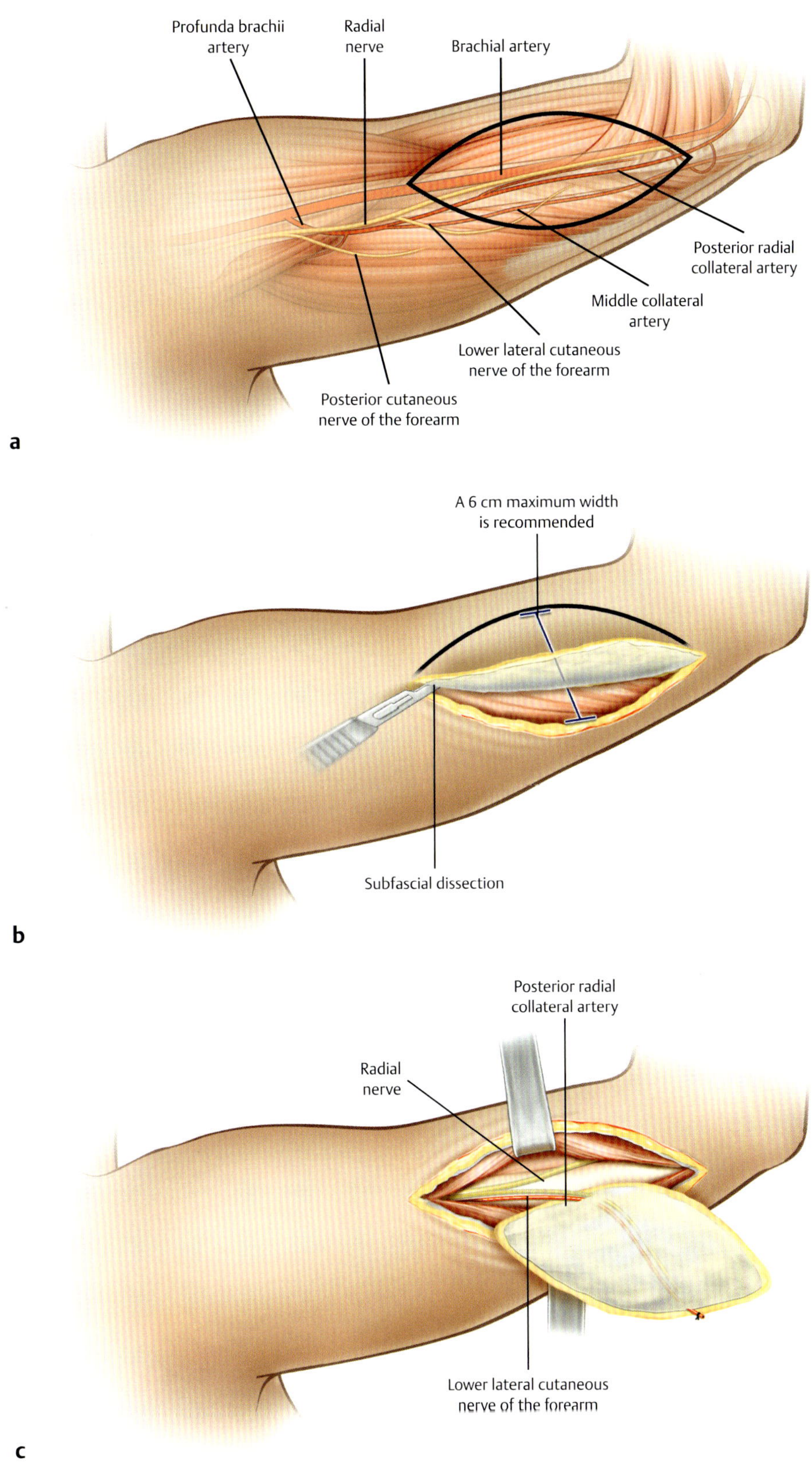

Fig. 45.1 Lateral arm flap. **(a)** Location of the skin island varies with the origin of the vascular pedicle. Proximal skin island is usually only used in distally based pedicle flaps. Incision follows the line between insertion of the deltoid muscle to the lateral epicondyle of the humerus. Distal extension may include proximal fifth of the forearm. **(b)** Stay carefully beneath fascia. **(c)** Identify radial nerve and lower lateral cutaneous nerve. Distal end of posterior radial collateral artery may be used as a flow-through conduit. Flap can be transplanted including a 10 cm nerve segment. Identify posterior radial collateral artery from posterior.

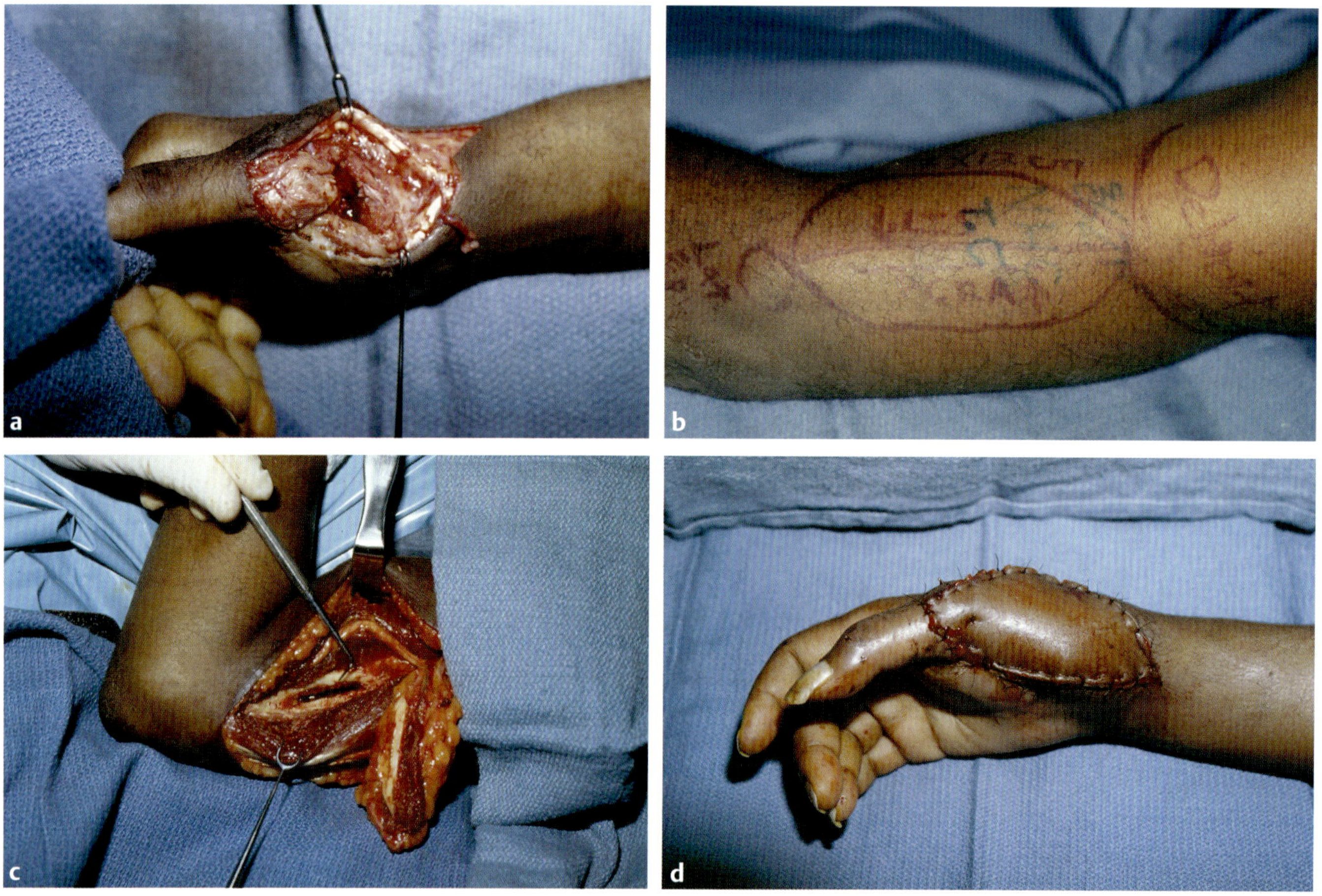

Fig. 45.2 Lateral arm flap. **(a)** This patient sustained a first metacarpal composite injury secondary to a gunshot wound. **(b)** Lateral arm flap. **(c)** Osteocutaneous flap isolated on a pedicle. **(d)** The flap is shown after inset.

Chapter 46

Parascapular and Scapular Flaps

Table 46.1 Parascapular and scapular flap

Flap	
Tissue	Fasciocutaneous/osteocutaneous flap, non–hair-bearing, can also be de-epithelialized as a pedicle or free subcutaneous fascial flap
Course of the vessels	Parallel to the skin above the deep fascia
Dimensions	Parascapular flap, 8–10 × 20–25 cm; scapular flap, 10–15 × 12–25 cm
Extensions and combinations	Fascial extensions; any combination with other flaps from the subscapular system
Anatomy	
Neurovascular pedicle	—
Artery	Constant branch of the circumflex scapular artery; vertical branch for parascapular flap; horizontal branch for scapular flap
Veins	Two concomitant veins
Length and arc of rotation	6–10 cm
Diameter	Artery, 1.5–3 mm; veins, 2–4 mm
Nerve	No sensory nerve
Surgical technique	
Preoperative examination and markings	Doppler identification of vessels (horizontal and descending branch), identification and marking of triangular space (defined by teres major, teres minor, and long head of the triceps), tip of the scapula, scapular spine, spine, and border of latissimus dorsi muscle
Patient position	Midlateral or oblique prone position
Dissection	Parascapular flap: start with a low medial incision (retrograde elevation); identify the epifascial plane; proceed cranially to the area of the triangular space; complete the skin incision; identify the fatty tissue around the pedicle; carefully retract the flap medially; ligate or clip the muscle and bone branches very carefully; follow the pedicle into the triangular space; identify the thoracodorsal or subscapular artery; check for flap perfusion; perform pedicle transection or flap transfer; some authors favor the identification of the vascular pedicle as the first step of the dissection
	Scapular flap: employ the same strategy of dissection as for the parascapular flap, then dissect medially and proceed toward the triangular space; as with the parascapular flap, the vascular pedicle can also be identified first during the course of the dissection

Continued

Table 46.1, cont'd

Advantages	
Vascular pedicle	Long; reliable; large caliber; arc of rotation as a pedicle flap reaches the axillary fold and the dorsal brachium
Flap size and shape	Large flaps possible with medial and lateral extensions and scapular fascial extension; uniform thickness of flap; can also be used as a "buried flap" when de-epithelialized
Combinations	Possible with all flaps from the subscapular system; very valuable: combination with bone parts for segmental forearm defects; bone segments can be harvested medially and laterally
Further options	Preserves most of the other flaps from the subscapular system
Disadvantages	
Bulkiness	Thickness depends on the patient's body habitus; sometimes it is too bulky
Donor site morbidity	No functional loss; conspicuous scarring when scar widens; only donor sites 8–12 cm wide can be closed primarily
Pearls and pitfalls	
Dissection	Watch out for fatty tissue around the pedicle; put some stay sutures in for careful flap retraction; do not sever the large bony/muscular branch, which comes very soon after the pedicle dives deep; have the patient deeply relaxed during the pedicle dissection, which facilitates dissection into the axilla; use long blade retractors to open the triangular space
Extensions and combinations	Most combined flaps can be raised without altering patient position; do not violate the bony/muscular branch when taking a bone segment; include a muscle cuff; an axillary incision is only required when the flap is combined with other flaps from the subscapular system; in the case of combined flaps, do not transect the pedicle before anatomical variations have been excluded
Contouring and correction	May be necessary, as the flap tends to sag; debulking may be required; liposuction can be difficult due to the structure of the dorsal fatty tissue
Clinical applications	Resurfacing of forearm and dorsum of the hand; provision of skin coverage and gliding tissue for flexor and extensor tendons, when the fascial extension is included; perfect for segmental defects of the forearm; defects of the shoulder area and the dorsal brachium when used as a pedicle flap

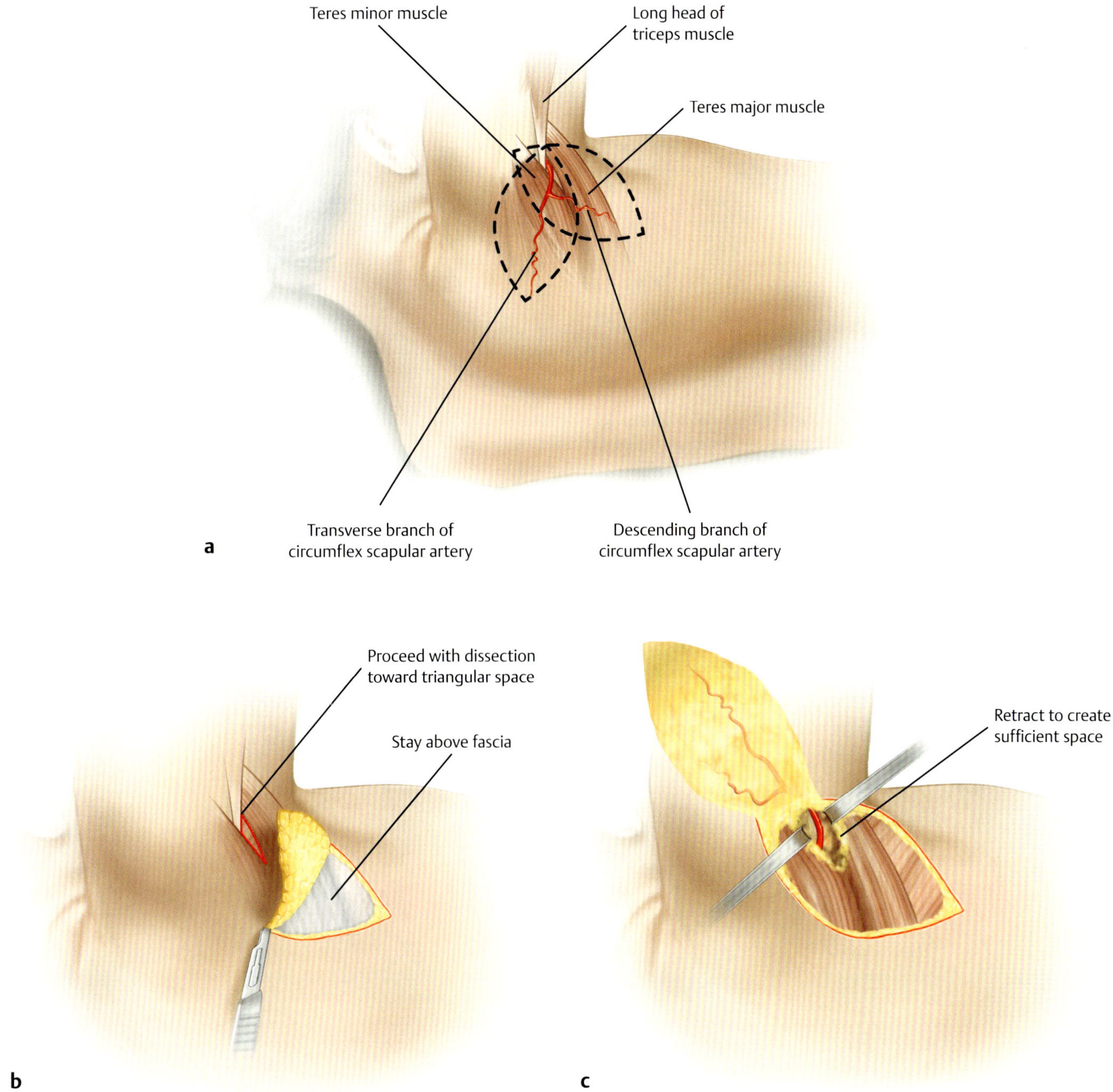

Fig. 46.1 Creation of the parascapular and scapular flaps. **(a)** The rule of "2" should be used when designing the flap: the pedicle is located 2 cm inferior to the scapular spine and 2 cm lateral to the midaxial line. **(b)** Identify the entrance of the pedicle into triangular space preoperatively by Doppler examination. Start the dissection at inferior edge of the flap and proceed toward the triangular space. Stay above the fascia. **(c)** When fatty layers are encountered, use caution near the pedicle and use long blade retractors to create sufficient room within the triangular space. Carefully ligate or clip all branches of the circumflex scapular artery to the lateral border of the scapula and the adjacent muscles. A bony segment can be taken from lateral or medial border.

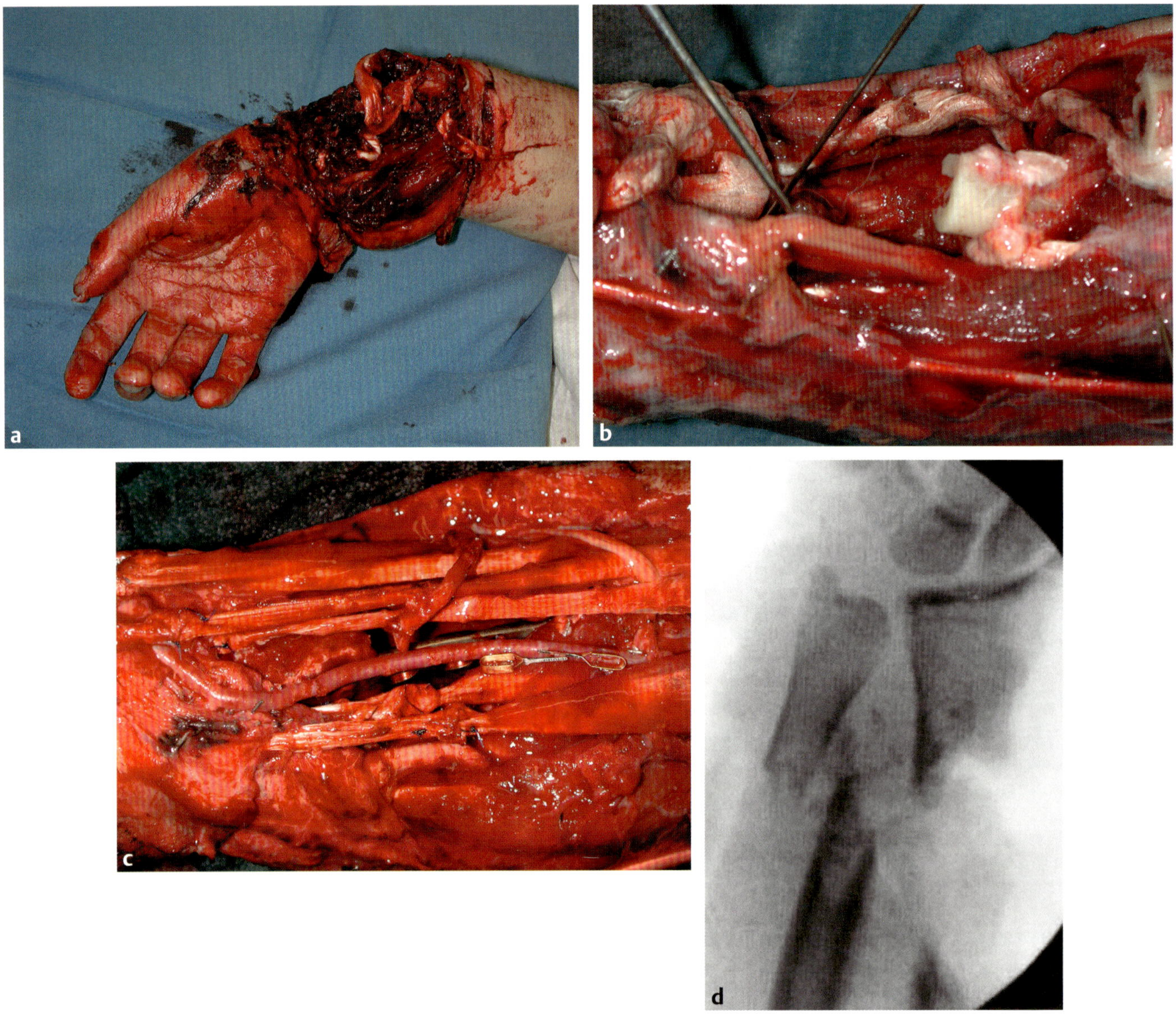

Fig. 46.2 Parascapular and scapular flap. **(a)** This 25-year-old soccer player experienced a severe crush injury of the hand with the disruption of circulation and a segmental bone defect. Debridement and vein grafting were performed to reconstruct the radial artery. **(b)** Intraoperative situs showing the three-dimensional defect. **(c)** Situs after the repair of all structures. **(d)** The patient's comminuted forearm fracture with a radial defect is shown (*continued*).

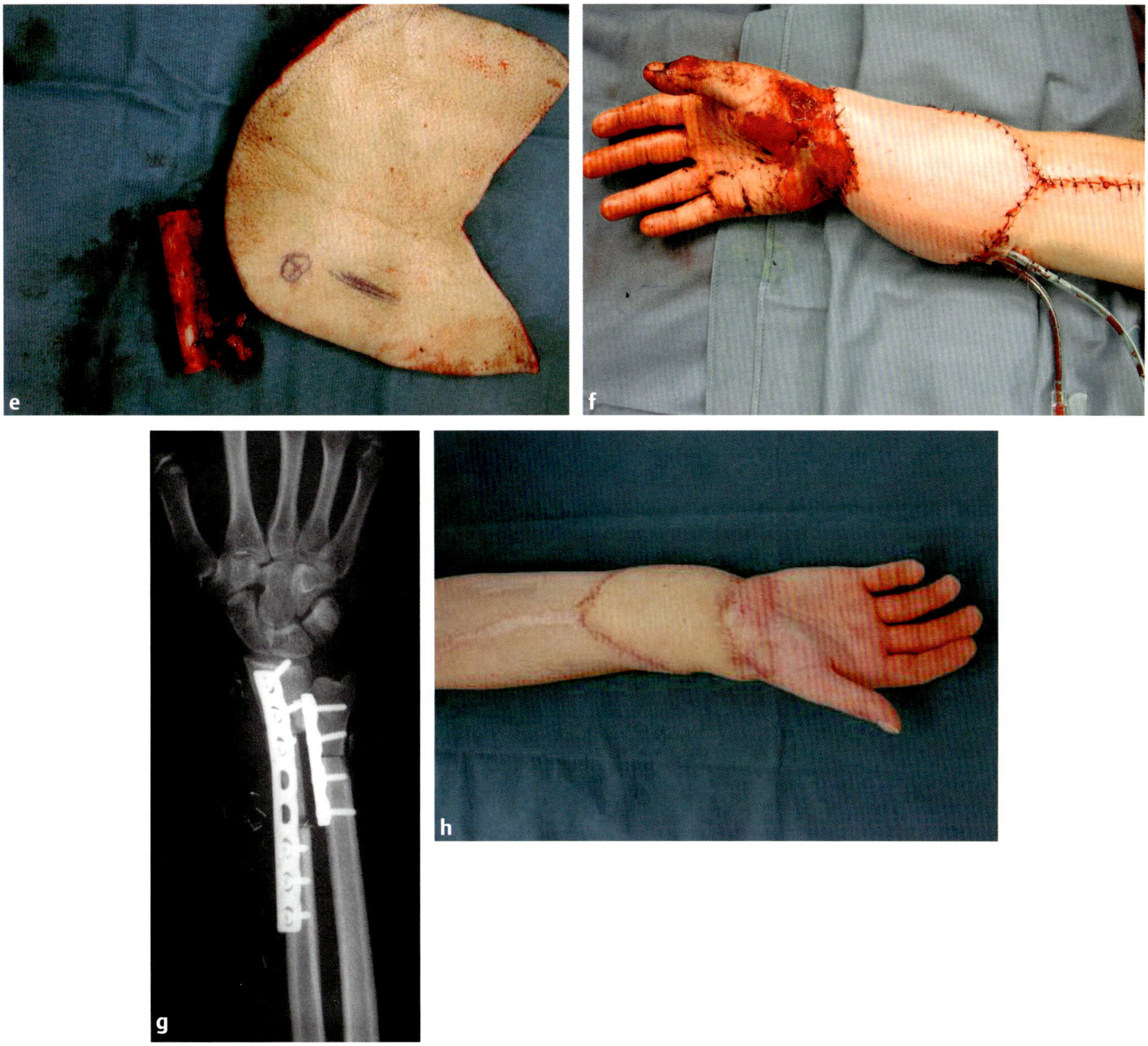

Fig. 46.2 (*continued*) **(e)** The patient's graft involved a scapular/parascapular flap with a vascularized scapula bone. **(f)** The postoperative situation after the reconstruction of all defects and the insetting of the flap. **(g)** A radiograph of the patient's arm immediately after surgery, with correct axial positioning of the forearm. **(h)** One year postoperatively.

Chapter 47

Anterolateral Thigh Flap

Table 47.1 Anterolateral thigh flap

Flap	
Tissue	Fasciocutaneous as perforator/myocutaneous
Course of the vessels	Base of the intermuscular space between the rectus femoris muscle and the vastus lateralis muscle
Dimensions	Maximum 20 × 10 cm; greatly dependent on the inclusion of the ABC perforators
Extensions and combinations	ALT/TFL, ALT/vastus lateralis, ALT/iliac crest, ALT/AMT
Anatomy	
Neurovascular pedicle	–
Artery	Descending branch of the lateral circumflex femoral artery
Veins	Two concomitant veins
Length and arc of rotation	8–16 cm depending on point
Diameter	2–2.5 cm below rectus femoris branch; 2.5–3.5 cm above rectus femoris branch
Nerve	Lateral femoral cutaneous/lateral branch
Surgical technique	
Preoperative examination and markings	Straight line drawn from the anterior superior iliac spine to the upper/outer margin of the patella; Doppler confirmation of perforator B just lateral to halfway point; Doppler confirmation of perforators A and C 5 cm above and below perforator B, respectively
Patient position	Supine neutral position feet straight up
Dissection	Begin with a curvilinear incision 1.5–2 cm medial to the anterior superior iliac spine/patellar line from a point proximal to perforator A to a point distal to perforator C; depth of dissection should be subfascial, moving from medial to lateral; retracting the rectus femoris medially will expose the descending branch of the lateral circumflex femoral pedicle; identify the appropriate perforators exiting the pedicle and determine their route to the surface; if confined to the septum, visualize their travel and ensure their continuity to the overlying skin paddle; in a majority of cases, the perforators will travel through the vastus lateralis and must be carefully dissected out of and away from the muscle; in this case, dissection is usually directed from superficial to deep; all intramuscular branches should be mechanically or thermally ligated
	When the perforators travel deeper within the muscle, it may be prudent to include a cuff of the muscle around the perforator; after concluding the dissection to the cutaneous island, the lateral curvilinear incision may be completed to the design needs of the recipient defect; the distal extent of the pedicle should be divided and the main vessels dissected proximally until sufficient length is attained; preservation of the co-located motor nerve is strongly recommended

Table 47.1, cont'd

Advantages	
Vascular pedicle	Generous length, large caliber, reliable location
Flap size and shape	Large, elliptical skin paddle
Combinations	May be raised with the TFL and/or the vastus lateralis muscle
Donor site	Minimal to no functional deficit; aesthetically favorable as compared with most other cutaneous flap donor sites
Disadvantages	
Donor site morbidity	Large flap donor sites may require skin graft closure
Dissection	Perforator continuity must be confirmed before cutaneous flap dissection can be completed; perforator and travel are highly variable
Flap	Thickness may present a problem in overweight patients
Pearls and pitfalls	
Dissection	Do not make the initial skin incision too laterally; be patient when determining the course and travel of the chosen perforator; do not isolate the cutaneous flap until the route of the perforators is ensured
Extensions and combinations	Including the TFL requires the inclusion of the transverse branch of the lateral circumflex femoral vessels
Contouring and correction	Thinning the flap is possible
Clinical applications	Wide variety of uses, including the head and neck, trunk, and upper and lower extremities

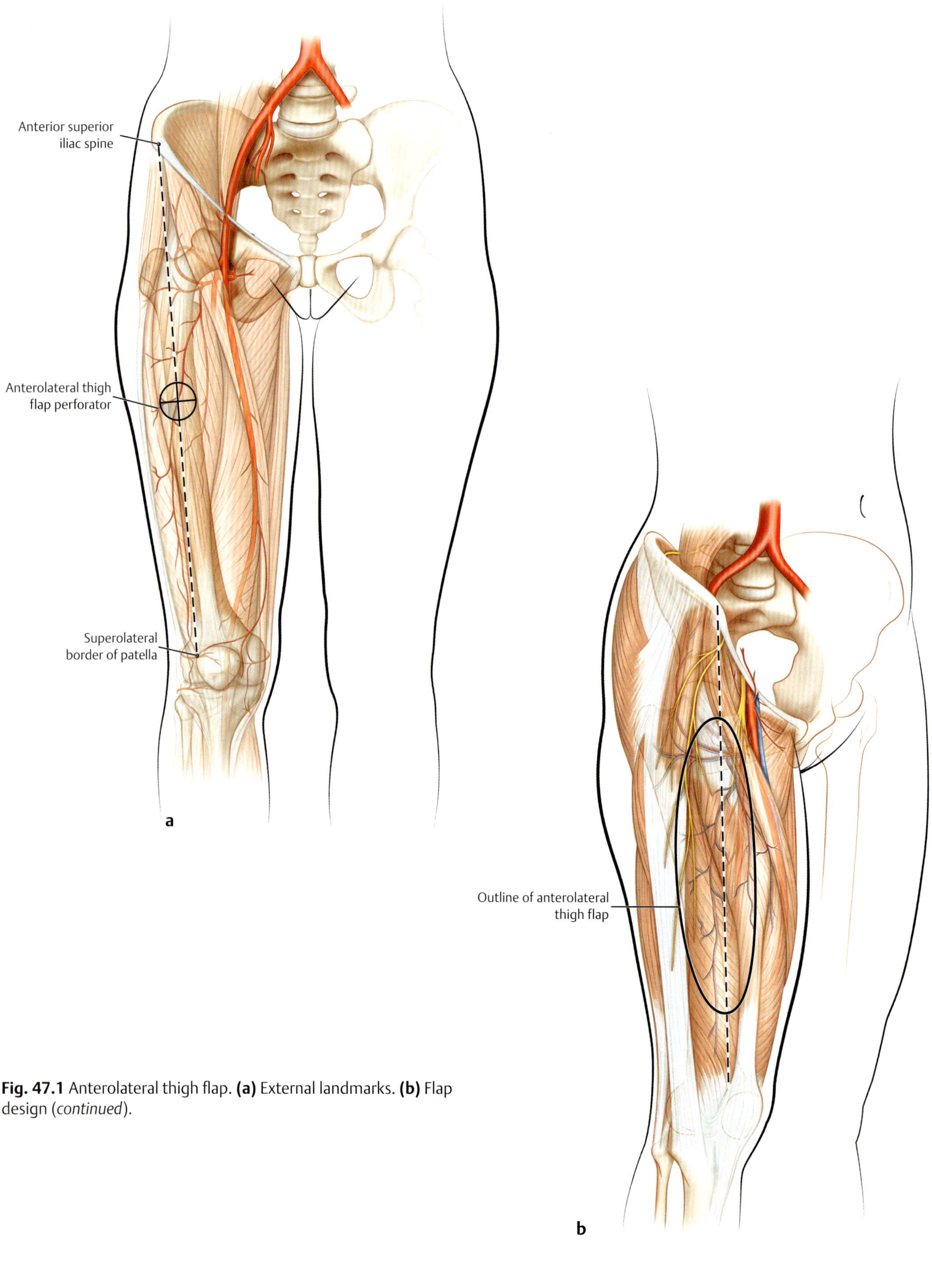

Fig. 47.1 Anterolateral thigh flap. **(a)** External landmarks. **(b)** Flap design (*continued*).

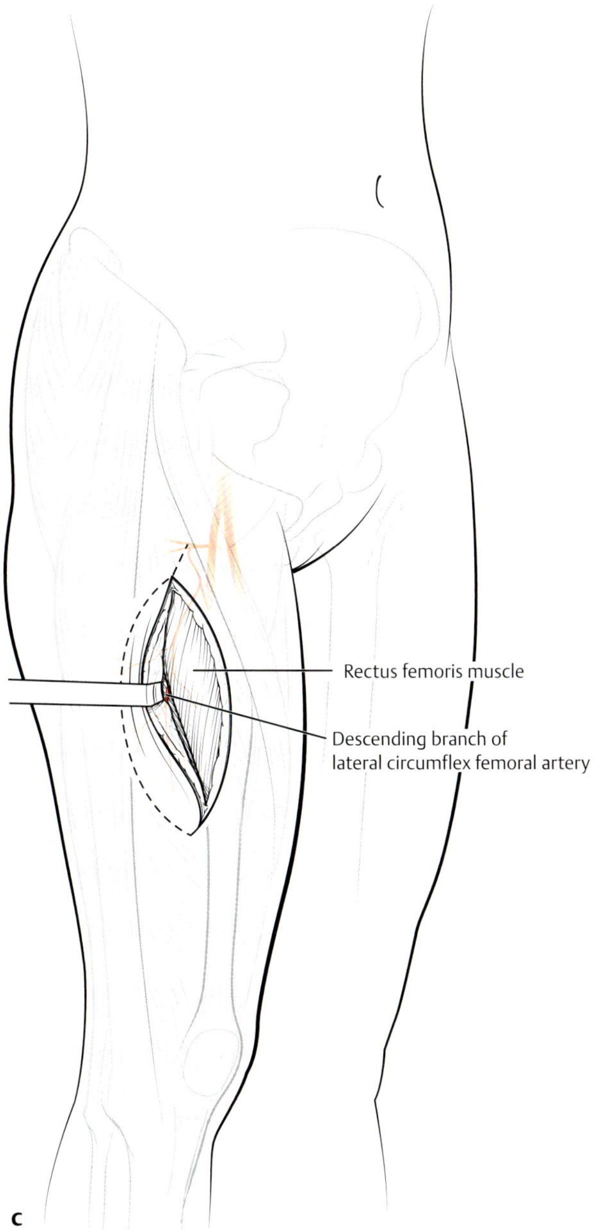

c

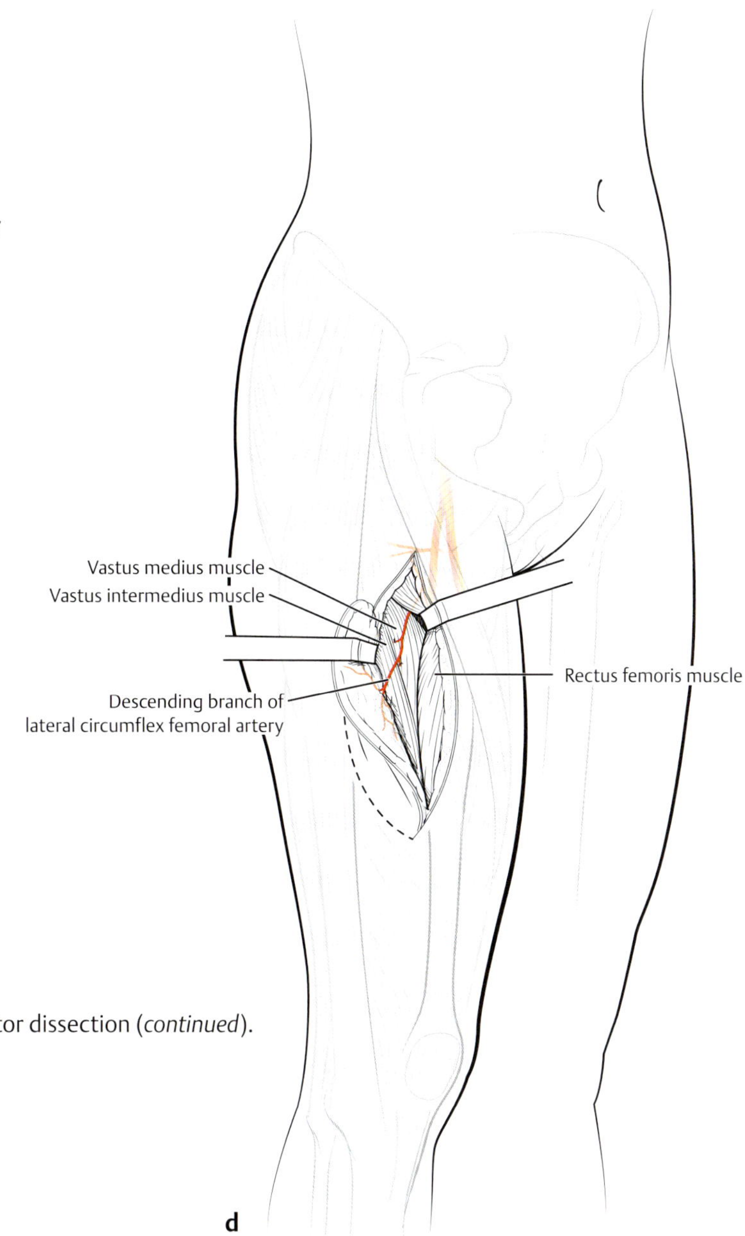

d

Fig. 47.1 (*continued*) **(c)** Pedicle identification. **(d)** Perforator dissection (*continued*).

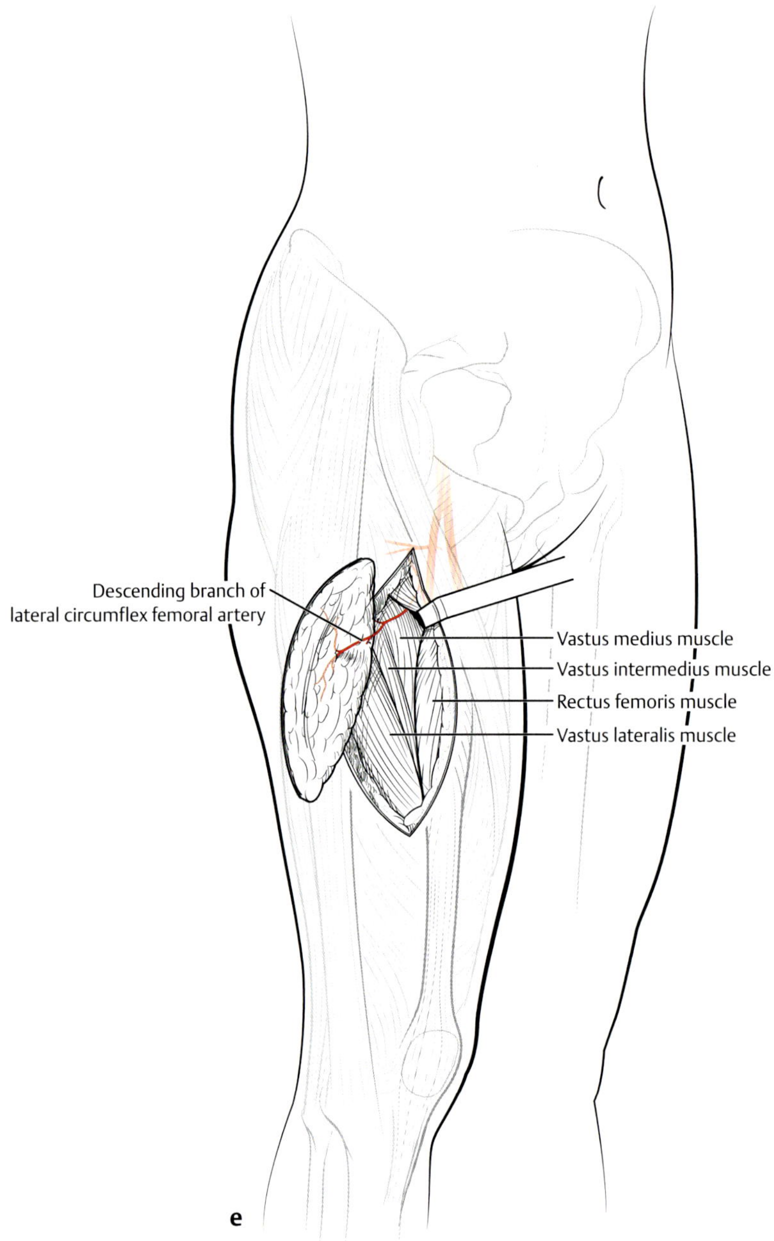

Fig. 47.1 (*continued*) **(e)** Flap elevated.

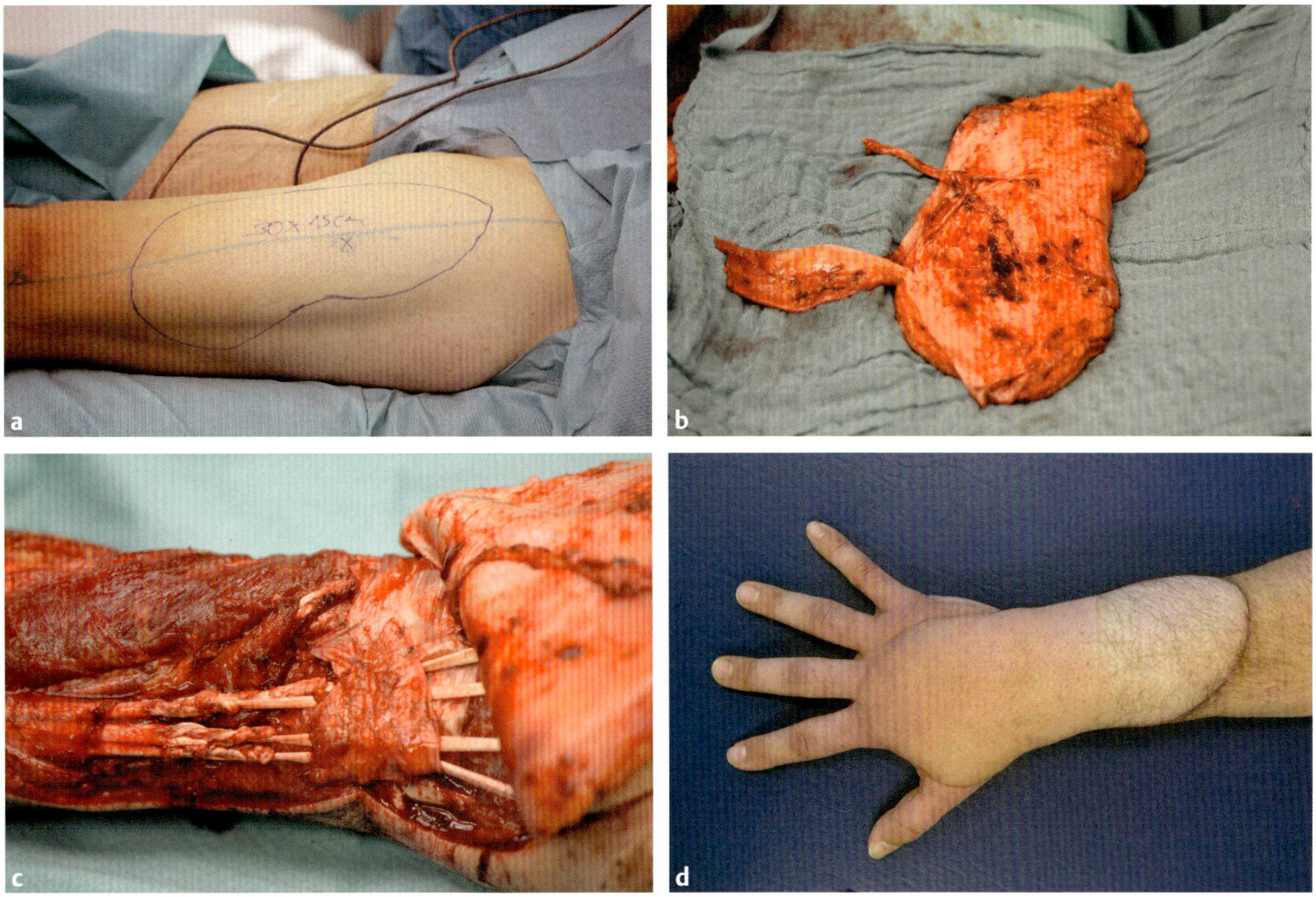

Fig. 47.2 Anterolateral thigh flap. **(a)** Reconstruction of tendons with PL and plantaris tendon from both sides. **(b)** Reconstruction of a soft tissue defect with a free fasciocutaneous ALT flap from the left thigh, with vascularized fascia lata. **(c)** Myxofibrosarcoma of the right hand after resection during inset, with fascial extensor retinacular reconstruction and soft tissue coverage. **(d)** The healed wound with the reconstructed flap is shown 6 months postoperatively.

Chapter 48

Latissimus Dorsi Flap

Table 48.1 Latissimus dorsi flap

Flap	
Tissue	Muscle or musculocutaneous flap, pedicle or free
Course of the vessels	From the axilla along the anterior border of the muscle: it enters the muscle from underneath and then spreads into the three major branches at the undersurface of the muscle
Dimensions	Can be tailored to almost any size; maximum dimensions, 20 × 35 cm
Extensions and combinations	Can be raised as muscle, musculocutaneous, and perforator flap; combinations are possible with any component from the subscapular system (i.e., bone, skin, fascia, or muscle)
Anatomy	
Neurovascular pedicle	Thoracodorsal artery
Artery	Usually one vein that originates from the subscapular vein
Veins	Up to 15 cm; branches of the subscapular system; anatomical variations in 3–5% of population
Length and arc of rotation	Artery, 2–4 mm; vein, 2–5 mm
Diameter	Motor nerve; some studies report deep sensation 18 months after coaptation to the sensory recipient
Nerve	
Surgical technique	
Preoperative examination and markings	No vessel identification necessary; in cases of previous axilla dissection or radiation, check muscle function; if muscle function is intact, vessels are usually not violated; mark the anterior muscle border and the tip of the scapula to outline the flap borders
Patient position	Midlateral; arm elevated 90 degrees
Dissection	Mark the flap dimensions; start with an incision along the muscle border; identify the muscle border and branch to the serratus muscle; identify the pedicle and follow the pedicle to its origin; free the anterior border of the muscle and raise the flap from ventral to dorsal toward the spine; take care to coagulate or ligate the perforating vessels; divide the muscle distally as required; divide the muscle at the spine insertions; raise the muscle in a cranial direction; ligate the serratus branches; check perfusion; divide the pedicle

Table 48.1, cont'd

Advantages	
Vascular pedicle	Long and reliable; large-caliber vessels
Flap size and shape	Any flap size is possible: the latissimus dorsi is the largest muscle in the body
Combinations	Numerous combinations are possible, including multicomponent flaps with other flaps from the subscapular system; vascularized bone can be harvested as rib grafts with the latissimus dorsi or on a connected pedicle from the scapula; fascia can be added from the serratus muscle
Further options	Scapular flaps are still available if the latissimus dorsi is harvested correctly; the serratus muscle is available, but vessels are small
Disadvantages	
Bulkiness	Muscle can be bulky; skin islands in musculocutaneous flaps are usually bulky and require secondary contour correction
Donor site morbidity	Donor scar is rather conspicuous; approximately 7% loss of shoulder function
Pearls and pitfalls	
Dissection	Watch out for constant large perforator vessels at the tip of the scapula (ligate); finalize the dissection of the pedicle by splitting the fascial leaf, which separates the latissimus dorsi from the teres muscles dorsally; ligate the branch to the scapula, and do not confuse it with the second branch to the muscle; take a skin island as a monitoring island, if desired.
Extensions and combinations	Dissect the pedicle up to the axillary artery to rule out anomalies of the vascular system so that all components are nourished by one pedicle; if there are anomalies, the operative strategy has to be adjusted to perform additional microanastomoses
Contouring and correction	Muscle flaps usually shrink, and contouring is required in approximately 50% of cases; musculocutaneous flaps almost all tend to sag and need contouring; in the case of functional muscle transfers, readjusting muscle tension is sometimes required
Clinical applications	Coverage of large surface area defects; functional free muscle transfer for loss of forearm flexor and extensor systems; pedicle muscle transfer for restoration of biceps function

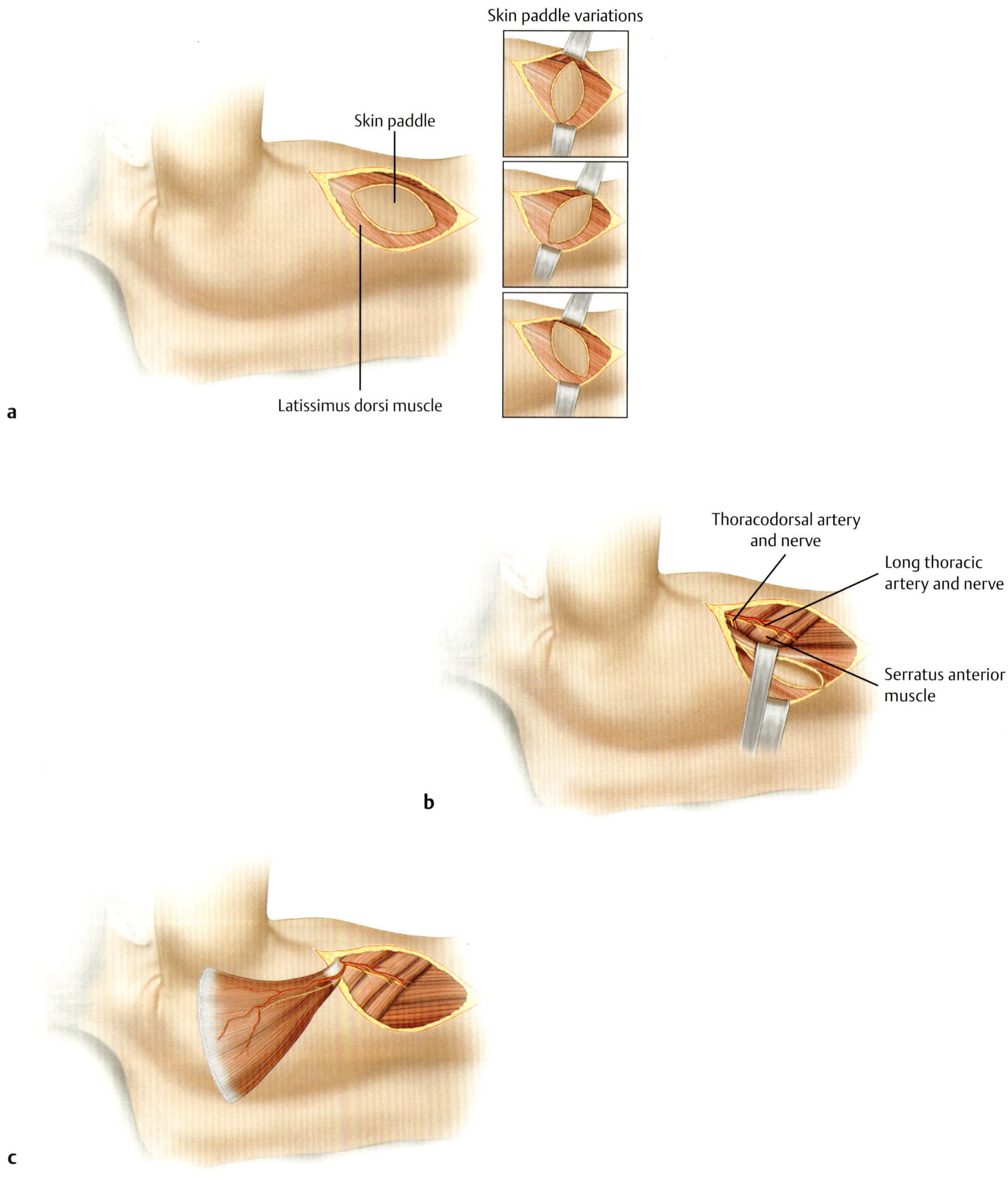

Fig. 48.1 Latissimus dorsi flap. **(a)** The medial border is always found more medially than projected. Make the skin island not too small to allow reliable clinical monitoring. **(b)** Identify the pedicle first. Proceed with dissection along the medial border. Divide distally and move toward the spine. Move up the anterior edge of latissimus dorsi or lateral. Re-orient the skin paddle. Accentuate borders between the latissimus dorsi serratus and teres major. **(c)** Leave the tendon insertion intact until the dissection is completed. Insert a suction drain into the axilla and lower donor site to prevent seromas. Coagulate all minor perforators, clip or ligate major perforators. Leave the circumflex scapular artery intact for possible future use. Mark the nerve with 5–0 suture; this facilitates manipulation of the pedicle during microsurgery. Clip branches of the pedicle to prevent bleeding after vascular microanastomosis.

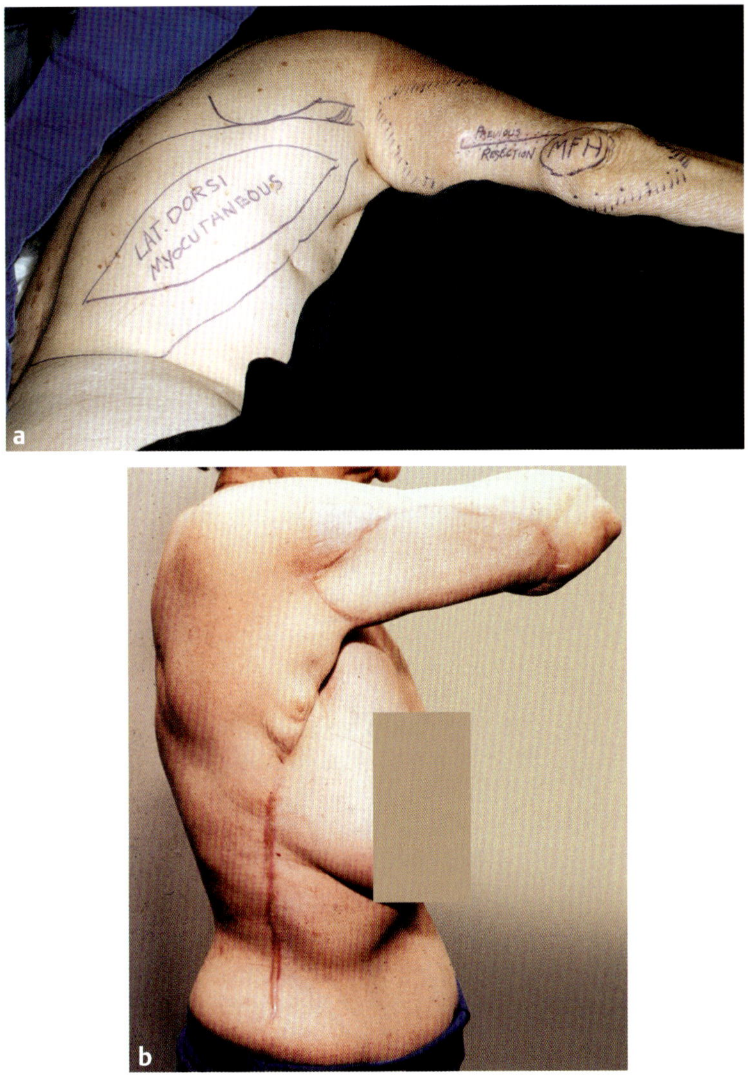

Fig. 48.2 Latissimus dorsi flap. **(a)** A latissimus dorsi subcutaneous flap was prepared before resection with a pedicle for the treatment of recurrent malignant fibrous histiocytoma. **(b)** The patient is shown 6 months after resection and reconstruction.

Chapter 49

Serratus Muscle/Fascial Flap

Table 49.1 Serratus muscle/fascial flap

Flap	
Tissue	Muscle or fascia (lower three muscle slips)
Course of the vessels	On the muscle surface
Dimensions	10 × 15 cm (muscle flap); 10 × 18 cm (fascial flap)
Extensions and combinations	Skin island; vascularized ribs
Anatomy	
Neurovascular pedicle	–
Artery	Serratus arcade as extension of the thoracodorsal pedicle; direct serratus branches of the thoracodorsal artery in > 97% of patients
Veins	Venae comitantes
Length and arc of rotation	≤ 16 cm (when a thoracodorsal pedicle is harvested)
Diameter	When thoracodorsal pedicle is harvested: artery, 3.5–4.5 mm; vein: 4–6 mm When only serratus arcade is taken: artery, 1–1.5 mm; vein, 1–1.5 mm
Nerve	Long thoracic nerve (does not always have to be included in the flap)
Surgical technique	
Preoperative examination and markings	Mark the anterior border of the latissimus dorsi muscle at the tip of the scapula and the 5th through 8th ribs
Patient position	Lateral, with the arm elevated at 90 degrees
Dissection	Muscle flap: make a slightly curved incision along the border of the latissimus muscle; identify the muscle border and the serratus arcade; check if the thoracodorsal pedicle is intact; determine the entrance points of motor fibers into the muscle; outline the flap size on the muscle surface; make a medial incision into the muscle; use ligation, coagulation, or clipping of the intercostal vessels to minimize bleeding; release the muscle from the thoracic wall; preserve three proximal slips to prevent wing scapula; dissect the thoracodorsal pedicle to the length required; check the flap for perfusion; transfer the flap Fascial flap: make a slightly curved incision along the border of the latissimus muscle; identify the muscle border and the serratus arcade; check if the thoracodorsal pedicle is intact; determine the entrance points of motor fibers into the muscle; outline the flap size on the muscle surface; raise the fascia from the muscle surface; coagulate the smaller vessels; preserve the motor nerve; dissect the thoracodorsal pedicle to the required length; check the flap for perfusion; transfer the flap

Table 49.1, cont'd

Advantages	
Vascular pedicle	Very long pedicle possible; extremely reliable
Flap size and shape	Thin and pliable as a fascial flap; minimal donor morbidity
Combinations	Vascularized ribs can be harvested with the flap; a small skin island can be included as a monitor island; any combination with other flaps from the subscapular system is possible
Disadvantages	
Flap	Dissection can be tedious due to many small intercostal connections; injury to the motor nerve may cause wing scapula; the fascia is delicate and can easily be perforated
Bulkiness	The muscle flap can be bulky
Donor site morbidity	Acceptable; no functional loss except when wing scapula occurs; donor scar is inconspicuous
Pearls and pitfalls	
Dissection	Identify where the motor fiber enters the muscle; avoid injury to the nerve; the nerve runs laterally from the vascular pedicle; preserve the upper muscle slips; the flaps tend to bleed profusely as fascial flaps; delayed secondary skin grafting is recommended
Extensions and combinations	Bone defects can be simultaneously reconstructed with vascularized rib grafts
Contouring and correction	Rarely required
Clinical applications	Perfect for mid-sized defects that require thin and pliable tissue; gliding tissue for tendon reconstruction; a fascial flap that is mechanically stable can be used for defects of the dorsum of the hand and forearm as well as exposed elbow joints

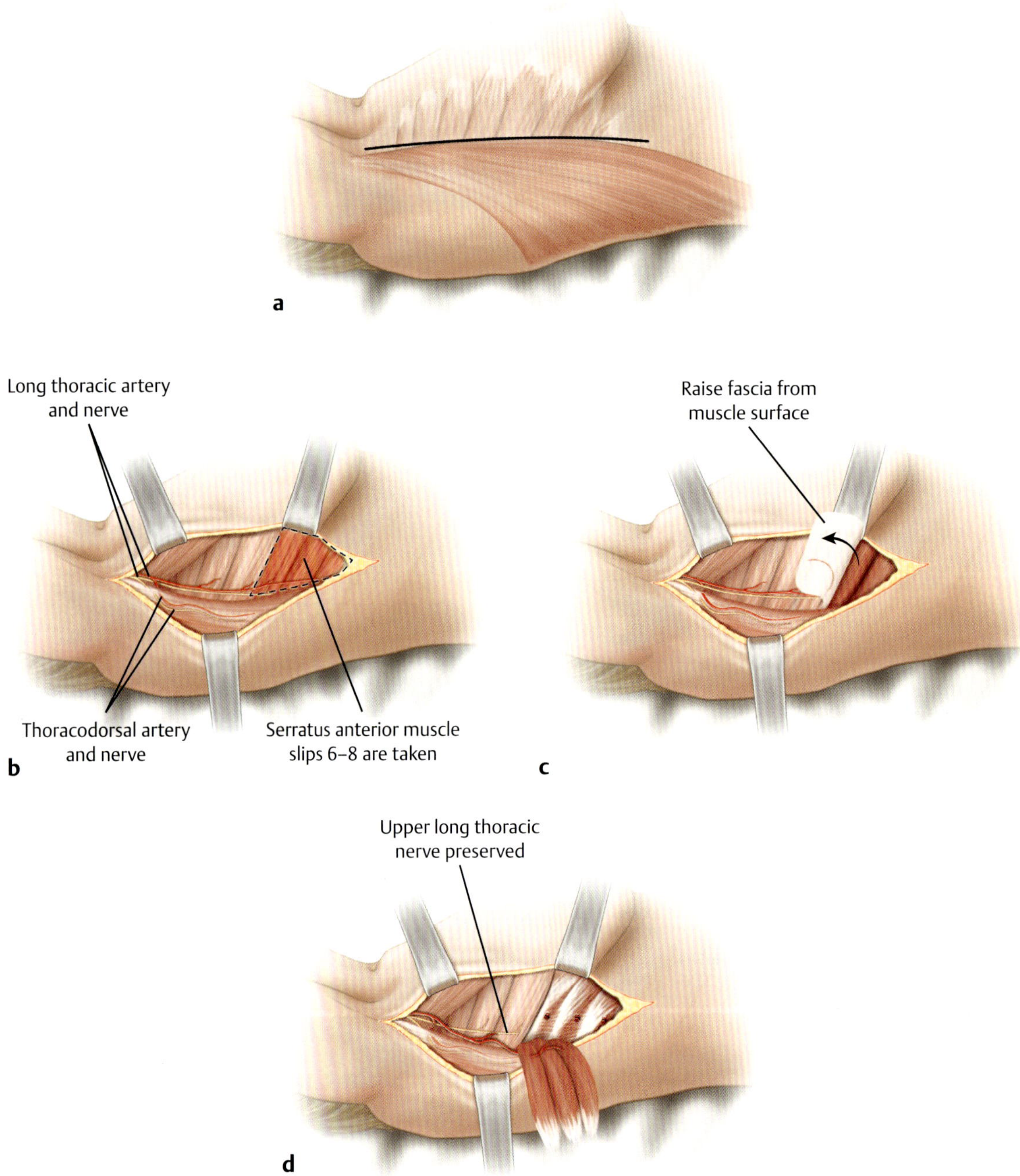

Fig. 49.1 Serratus muscle/fascial flap. **(a)** Use a straight incision along the medial latissimus border. **(b)** Start dissection distally. When the fascial flap is raised, take great care to maintain fascial integrity–defects will impair perfusion to distal parts. **(c)** Preserve the long thoracic nerve to avoid a winged scapula. Carefully coagulate perforators from intercostal vessels. The pedicle can include the entire length of the latissmus dorsi pedicle. Only take the lower slips (6–8) to preserve serratus function. **(d)** Flap elevated on pedicle.

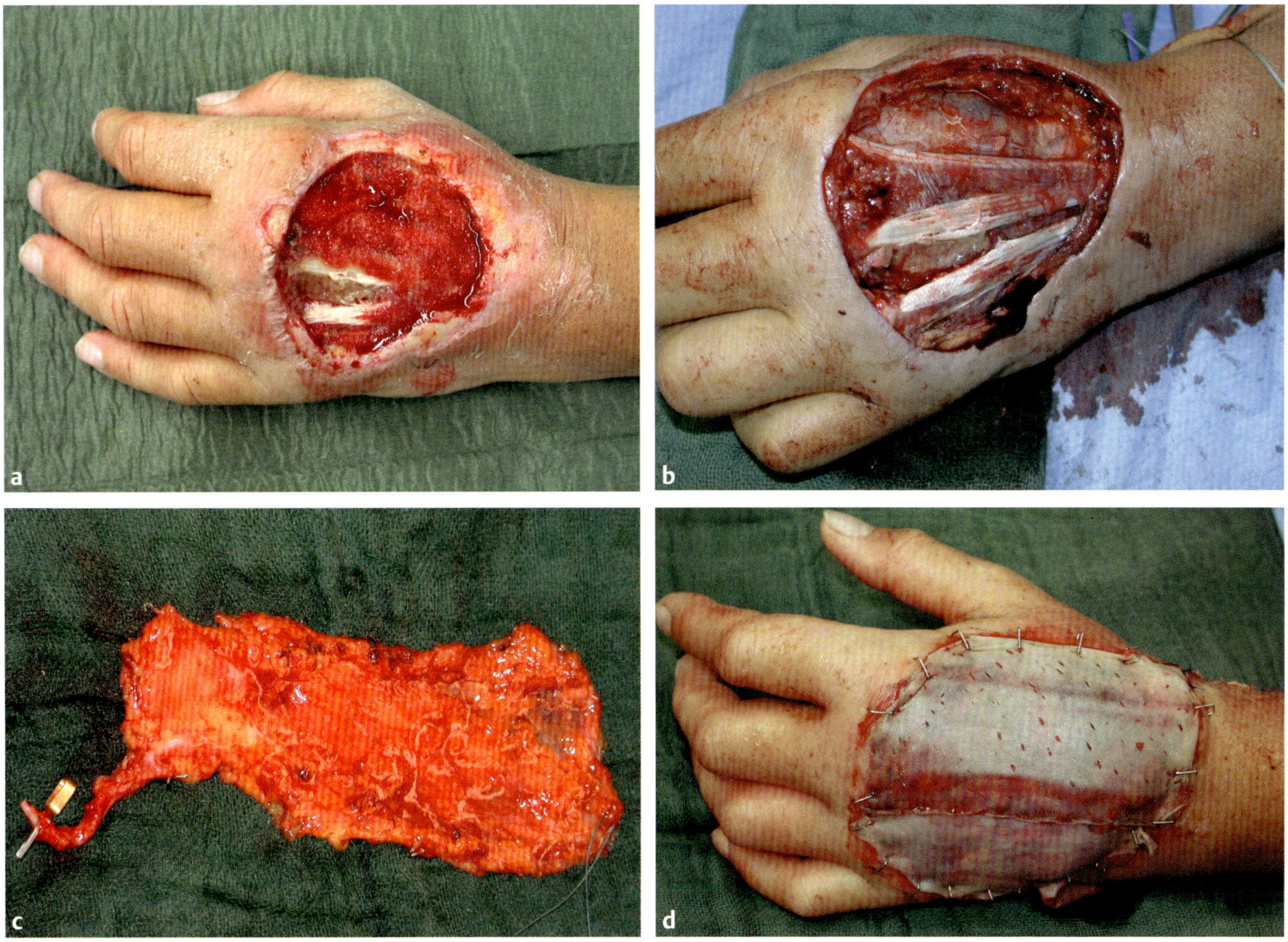

Fig. 49.2 Serratus muscle/fascial flap. **(a)** This patient had a granulating wound after primary treatment elsewhere. **(b)** Radical debridement. All vital structures were exposed, and the tendons still glided freely. **(c)** A free serratus fascial flap raised on the thoracodorsal pedicle. **(d)** The flap is shown after insertion and primary skin grafting (*continued*).

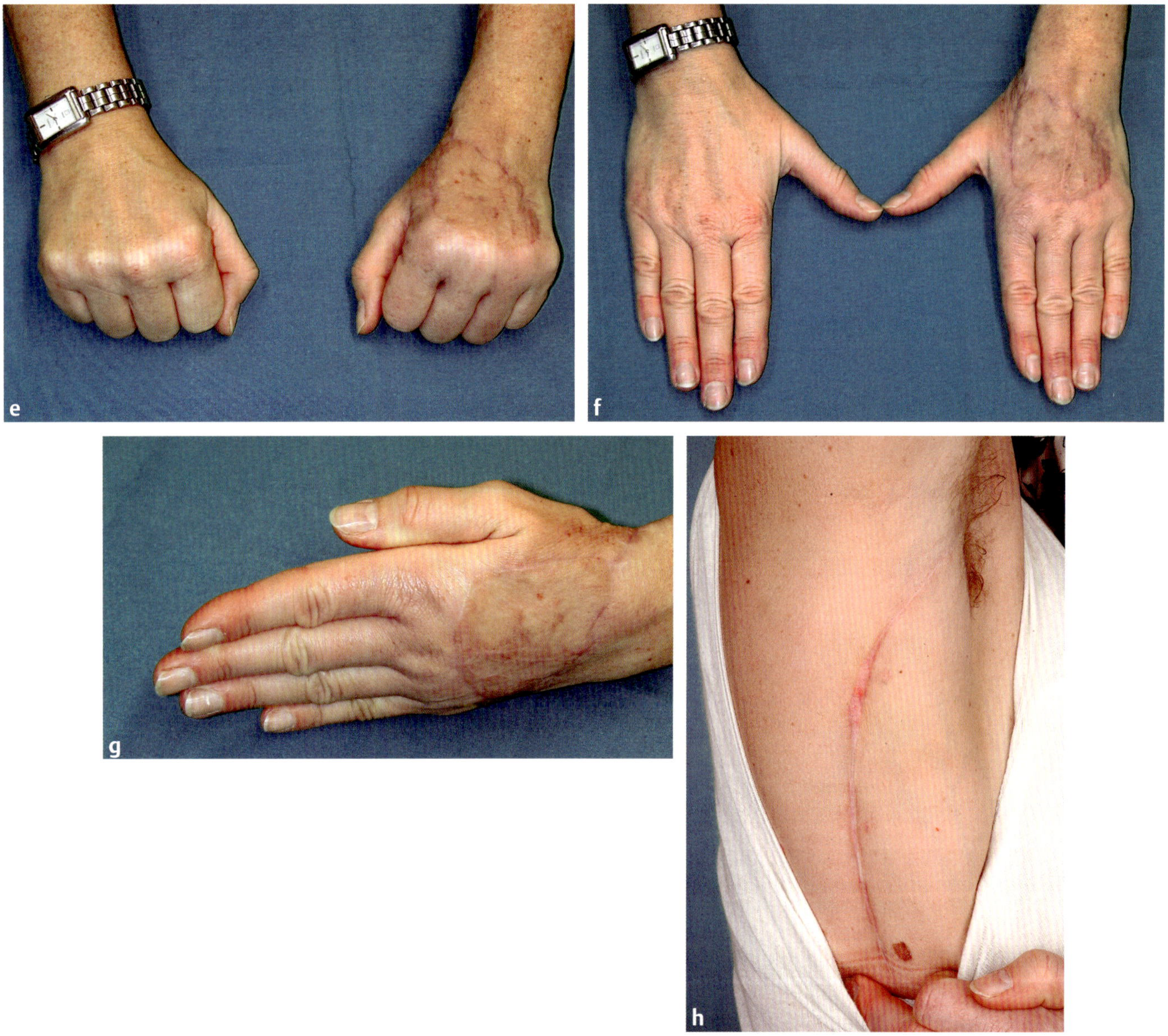

Fig. 49.2 (*continued*) **(e–g)** Function and aesthetics after 6 months. **(h)** Donor site scar.

Chapter 50

Temporal Fascial Flap

Table 50.1 Temporal fascial flap

Flap	
Tissue	Fascia (thickness, 1.5–3 mm)
Course of the vessels	Subcutaneously on the fascia, from preauricular into the temporal fossa
Dimensions	8 × 15 cm
Extensions and combinations	Can be combined with the deep fascial layer or calvarial bone
Anatomy	
Neurovascular pedicle	Common pedicle with deep fascia (proximal branch of superficial temporal vein/superficial temporal artery); there are no communicating vessels distal to the common pedicle
Artery	Superficial temporal artery (terminal branch of the carotid artery)
Veins	Superficial temporal vein
Length and arc of rotation	2–4 cm without incising the parotid gland
Diameter	Artery, 1.5–2.7 mm; vein, 2.0–3.2 mm
Nerve	Auriculotemporal nerve is included in the fascial layer, but the flap is not innervated
Surgical technique	
Preoperative examination and markings	Doppler identification of the course of the vessels; marking of the incision line parallel to the hair follicles; outline of flap dimensions
Patient position	Supine, with the head slightly tilted to the opposite side
Dissection	Use a T-shaped outline; start the incision by raising a pretragal skin flap; identify and spare the superficial temporal vein anterior and exterior to the superficial temporal artery; identify the superficial temporal artery; proceed with the dissection cephalad, deep to the hair follicles; avoid damage to the very superficial vein; use bipolar coagulation for terminal branches to subdermal plexus; do not damage the frontal branch of the facial nerve; after the cephalad completion of the dissection, incise the flap; lift the flap from the deep fascial plane toward the auricle; observe the flap for perfusion after the completed dissection
Advantages	
Vascular pedicle	Reliable pedicle with sufficient caliber and length
Flap size and shape	Considerable flap size that can cover, for example, the entire dorsum of the hand without bulk; dissection of the flap and donor site can be carried out simultaneously
Combinations	Can be combined with the deep temporal fascial layer: in this case, the middle temporal vessel at the level of the zygoma has to be preserved; possible combination with calvarial bone graft
Tissue	Flap is thin and pliable; cover without bulk
Donor site	Donor site completely inconspicuous; no functional loss

Continued

Table 50.1, cont'd

Disadvantages	
Flap size	—
Donor site morbidity	Frontal nerve may be damaged during dissection; alopecia may result if the superficial plane of the dissection is too close to the hair follicles
Dissection	—
Flap	Capillary bleeding may jeopardize graft take
Pedicle	Pedicle is short; vein is easy to damage due to it superficial location; sometimes vein is absent
Pearls and pitfalls	
Dissection	Watch out for the superficial temporal vein
Extensions and combinations	When combined with the deep layer, preserve the middle temporal vessel
Contouring and correction	Contour correction almost never indicated; delayed skin grafting recommended due to tendency for edema and capillary bleeding
Clinical applications	Dorsum of the hand; deep defects of the palm; degloving injuries of the digits; gliding tissue in scarred wound beds

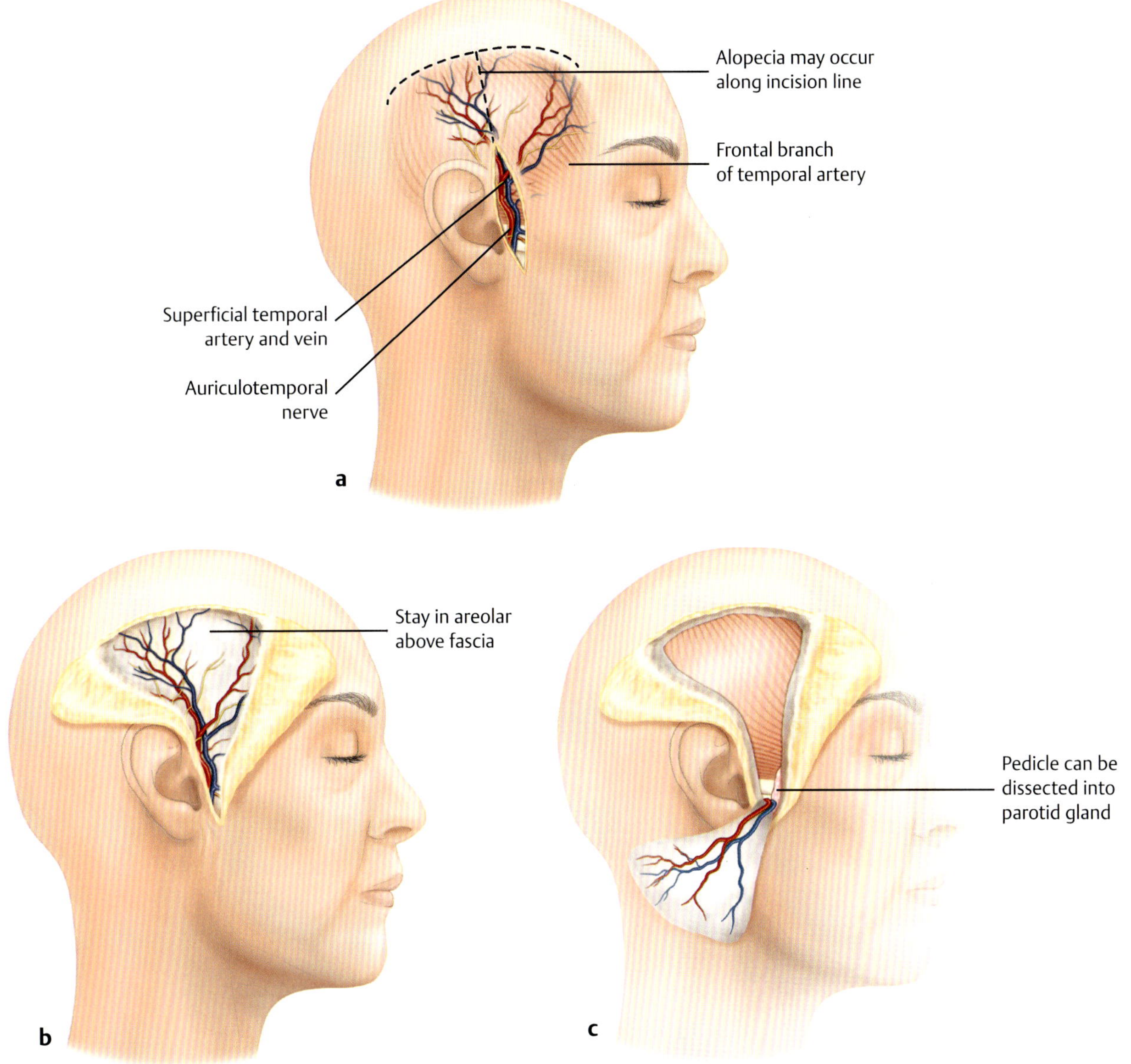

Fig. 50.1 Temporal fascial flap. **(a)** Define and mark the course of the pedicle by Doppler examination preoperatively. Inject the scalp donor site with xylocaine (0.5%) and epinephrine (1:200,000) before the dissection for better visualization and hemostasis. Alopecia may occur along the incision line. Vascular anomalies can be found. Try to identify draining veins by placing a slight touniquet around the head above the ear. Identify the vascular pedicle early in the dissection process. **(b)** Do not violate hair follicles to avoid alopecia. Stay in the areolar layer above the fascia. The frontalis branch can be identified by nerve stimulator. Avoid excessively deep skin incisions to prevent damage of the superficial temporal vessels. **(c)** Raise the flap from cephalad to caudad. The deep temporal fascia can be harvested along with the TPF to form a bilayer flap. The flap can be raised as a bilayer flap. Both flaps have a common pedicle, but no vascular connections after branching off the pedicle. A segment of calvarium can be raised with the flap, if the deep temporal layer is included. The pedicle can be dissected into the parotid gland.

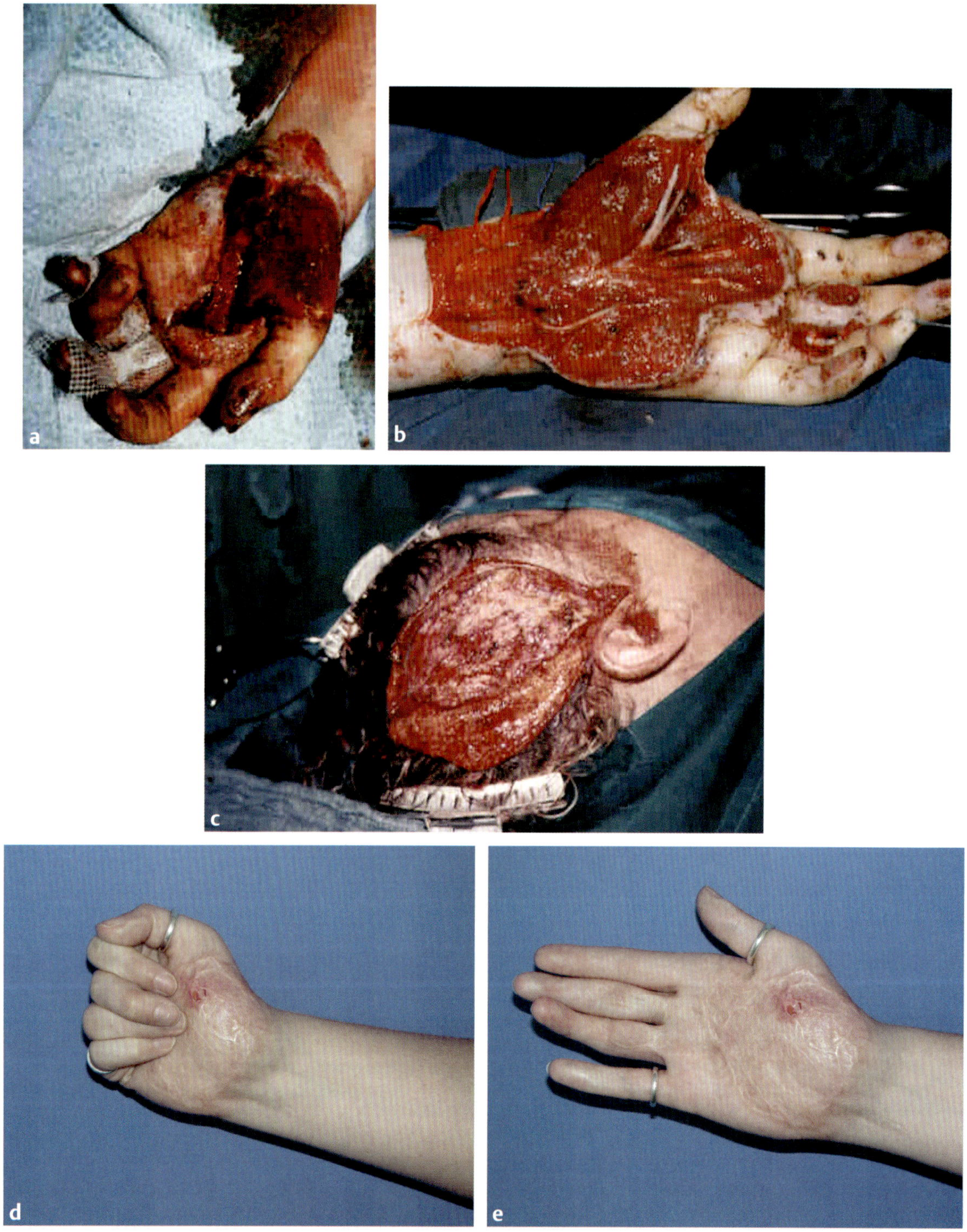

Fig. 50.2 Temporal fascial flap. **(a)** Volar avulsion injury. **(b)** After debridement. **(c)** Flap elevated. A patient with a similar injury is shown with her hand in **(d)** flexion and **(e)** extension. Excellent aesthetic appearance and function of the hand two years after the injury.

Chapter 51

Groin Flap

Table 51.1 Groin flap

Flap	
Tissue	Skin or dermal fat flap; can be used as a pedicle (most common) or free flap
Course of the vessels	Superficial to the Scarpa fascia, branching in the overlying skin toward the iliac crest
Dimensions	10 × 25 cm
Extensions and combinations	Usually no combinations with this type of flap; very experienced surgeons may raise the superficial inferior epigastric artery flap as a second skin paddle
Anatomy	
Neurovascular pedicle	—
Artery	Superficial circumflex iliac artery
Veins	Two venous systems: one parallels the superficial circumflex iliac artery and drains into the saphenous bulb, and the other runs deep and directly into the femoral vein
Length and arc of rotation	Artery, 1.5–2 cm; veins, 2.5–4 cm
Diameter	Artery, 0.8–1.8 mm; veins, 2–3 mm
Nerve	Flap is not innervated
Surgical technique	
Preoperative examination and markings	Create an outline of the flap so that one third is above and two thirds are below the inguinal ligament; the dividing line is drawn from the anterior superior iliac spine to the pubic tubercle
Patient position	Supine
Dissection	Lateral approach is preferable for a pedicle flap, which is raised from lateral superficial to deep muscle fascia; care must be taken to avoid injury to the pedicle Medial approach for free flaps: identify the superficial circumflex iliac artery approximately 5 cm below the inguinal line; use a medial incision; identify the superficial vein anterior to Scarpa's fascia; identify the femoral artery, the superficial inferior epigastric artery, and the superficial circumflex iliac artery; create a lateral skin incision, but leave the deep fascia intact; identify the lateral border of the sartorius muscle; ligate the muscle branches of the deep superficial circumflex iliac artery branch; divide the lateral cutaneous nerve; raise the flap and check for perfusion

Continued

Table 51.1, cont'd

Advantages	
Vascular pedicle	–
Flap size and shape	Large flap possible; non–hair-bearing flap
Combinations	Medial extensions for hair-bearing flap
Tissue	–
Dissection	–
Donor site	Perfect inconspicuous donor site, with primary wound closure when flap width does not exceed 10 cm
Further options	–
Disadvantages	
Bulkiness	Medial bulk
Donor site morbidity	Anesthesia in the lateral cutaneous nerve distribution area
Flap	Poor color match in exposed areas
Pedicle	Very short pedicle with variable arterial anatomy; arterial diameter is small, and vein grafts are frequently required
Pearls and pitfalls	
Dissection	Identification of pedicle should precede flap harvest when used as a free flap
Extensions and combinations	–
Contouring and correction	Correction and debulking are frequently indicated; color match
Clinical applications	Pedicle flap: dorsal hand and forearm defects in younger patients; free flap: dorsal hand and forearm defects in older patients when a short pedicle is possible; not recommended as a pedicle flap in older patients (risk of shoulder stiffness)

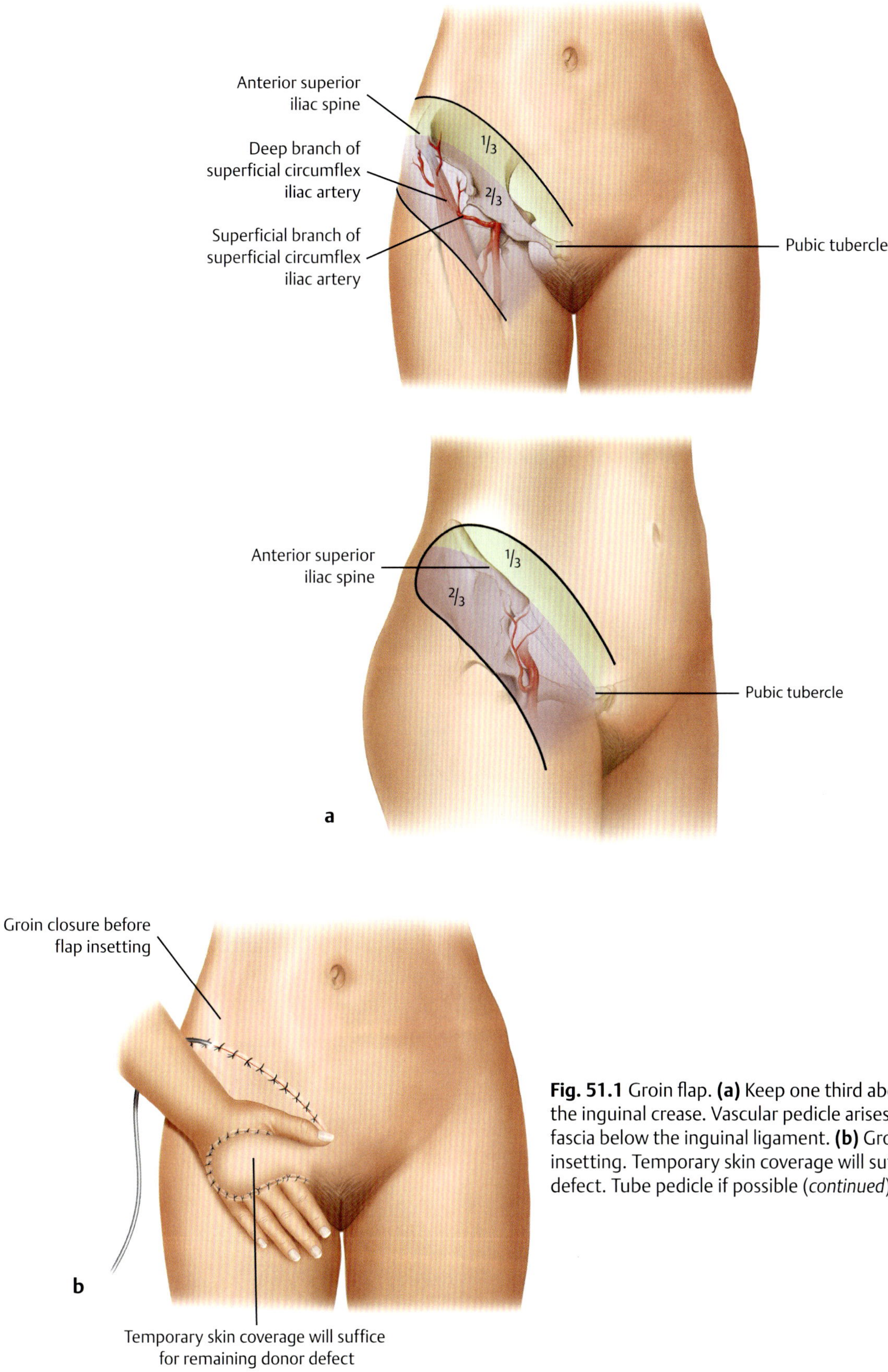

Fig. 51.1 Groin flap. **(a)** Keep one third above, two thirds below the inguinal crease. Vascular pedicle arises deep to the deep fascia below the inguinal ligament. **(b)** Groin closure before flap insetting. Temporary skin coverage will suffice for remaining donor defect. Tube pedicle if possible (*continued*).

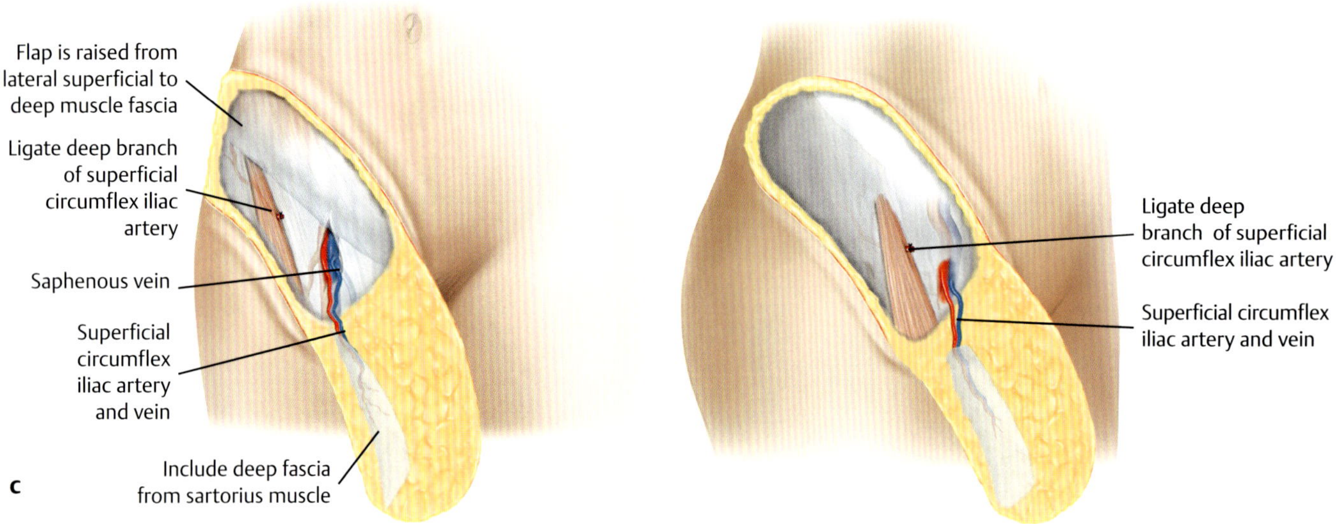

Fig. 51.1 (*continued*) **(c)** In free flaps a medial approach to identify the pedicle may be preferred. In pedicle flaps, a lateral approach is preferable. Identification and tracing of the saphenous vein will lead to the branching of the superior circumflex iliac vein. Do not include deep fascia until the sartorius muscle is encountered. From there the deep fascia is included.

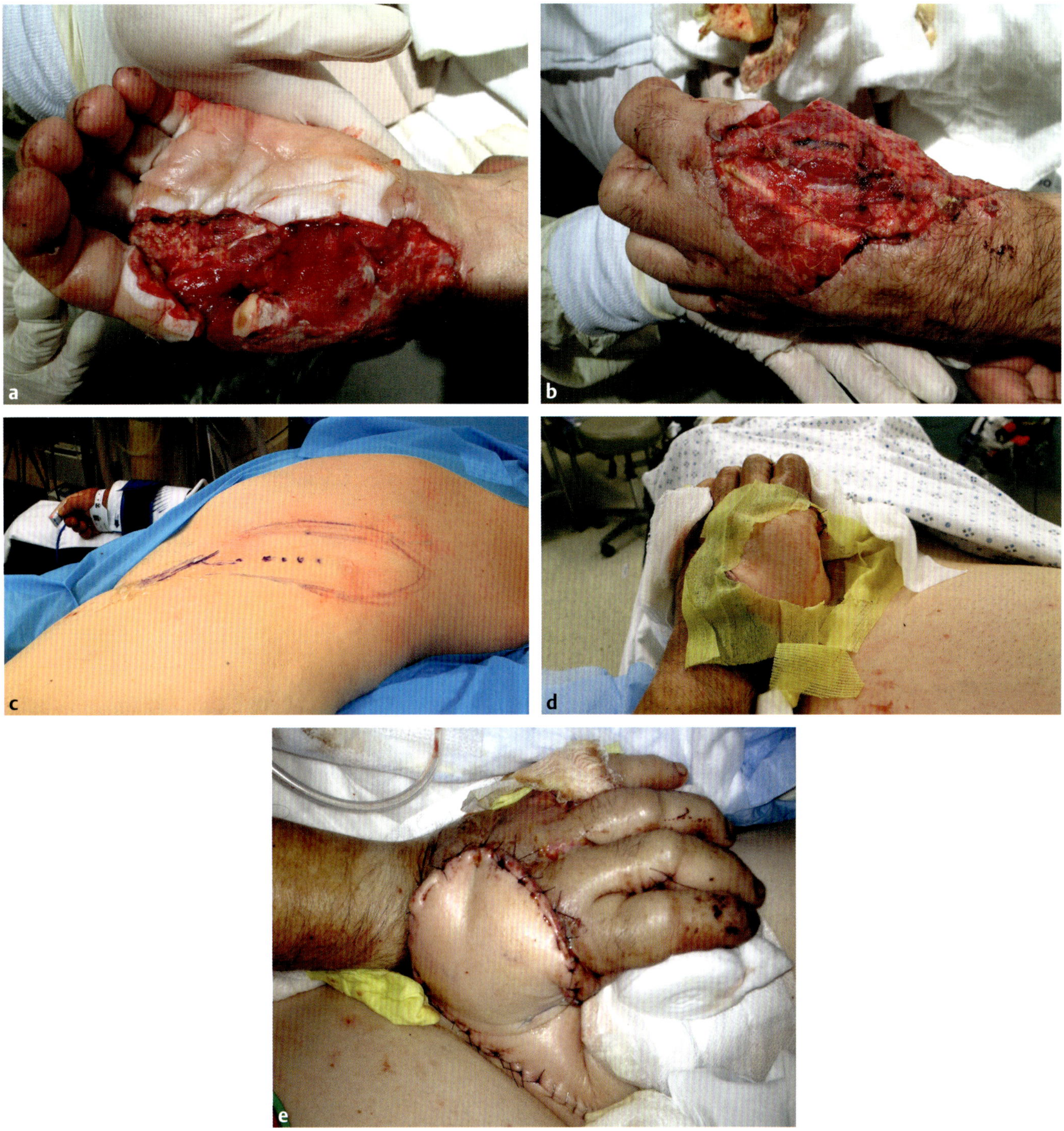

Fig. 51.2 Groin flap. **(a)** Crush avulsion of the thumb, volar view. **(b)** Crush avulsion of the thumb, dorsal view. **(c)** Groin flap with vascular axis. **(d)** Flap inset. **(e)** Flap inset, dorsal view (*continued*).

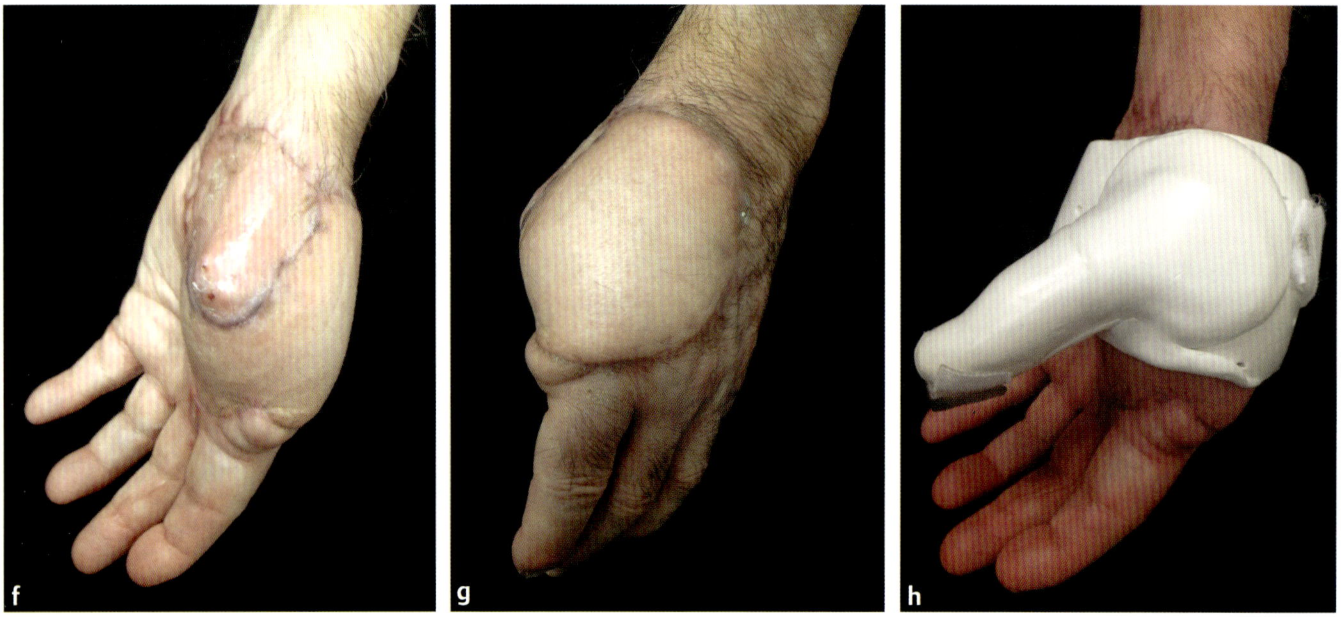

Fig. 51.2 (*continued*) **(f)** After release and insetting, volar view. **(g)** After release and insetting, dorsal view. **(h)** Prosthetic thumb opposition brace.

Chapter 52

Gracilis Muscle/Musculocutaneous Flap, Innervated Flap

Table 52.1 Gracilis muscle/musculocutaneous flap, innervated flap

Flap	
Tissue	Muscle or muscle with skin paddle
Course of the vessels	Underneath the muscle distally after entering the muscle laterally
Dimensions	4–6 × 20–25 cm (muscle); 6–8 × 10–12 cm (skin island)
Extensions and combinations	—
Anatomy	
Neurovascular pedicle	—
Artery	Terminal branch of the medial femoral circumflex artery
Veins	Concomitant veins of the medial femoral circumflex artery
Length and arc of rotation	6–7 cm
Diameter	Artery, 1.2–1.8 mm; vein, 1.5–2.5 mm
Nerve	Anterior motor branch from the obturator nerve
Surgical technique	
Preoperative examination and markings	Draw a line from the pubic tubercle to the medial condyle; the prominence of the adductor magnus marks the superior border of the gracilis
Patient position	Supine, with the hip and knee flexed and the leg abducted
Dissection	Incise 2 cm inferior and parallel to the line drawn preoperatively; do not violate the greater saphenous vein (anterior to the incision); incise the fascia; identify the gracilis muscle; divide the muscle distally; ligate the minor pedicle; proceed with the dissection cephalad; retract the adductor longus by moving proximally; expose the pedicle 6–12 cm distal to the pubic tubercle; protect the medial cutaneous nerve on the surface of the adductor magnus; clip or ligate small branches; divide the muscle superiorly; check for perfusion and then transfer the flap. NOTE: Center the skin island over the middle of the proximal portion; incise down to the fascia; include the fascia lata in the dissection; identify the muscle and proceed as above
Advantages	
Vascular pedicle	Short but reliable; vessel size is sufficient if the pedicle is dissected to maximal length
Flap size and shape	Long flat muscle with suitable cross-section area to serve as functional muscle transplant
Combinations	Skin island
Donor site	Minimal donor site morbidity with acceptable scar
Disadvantages	
Flap	Distal skin island is not reliable
Pearls and pitfalls	
Dissection	Do not confuse the gracilis and sartorius muscles; do not dissect the skin island too anteriorly; the gracilis is always more dorsal than projected; perform good muscle excursion for functional replacement
Extensions and combinations	—
Contouring and correction	Rarely required; sometimes needed with bulky skin islands
Clinical applications	Long narrow defects for coverage alone; functional muscle transfer for loss of muscle groups

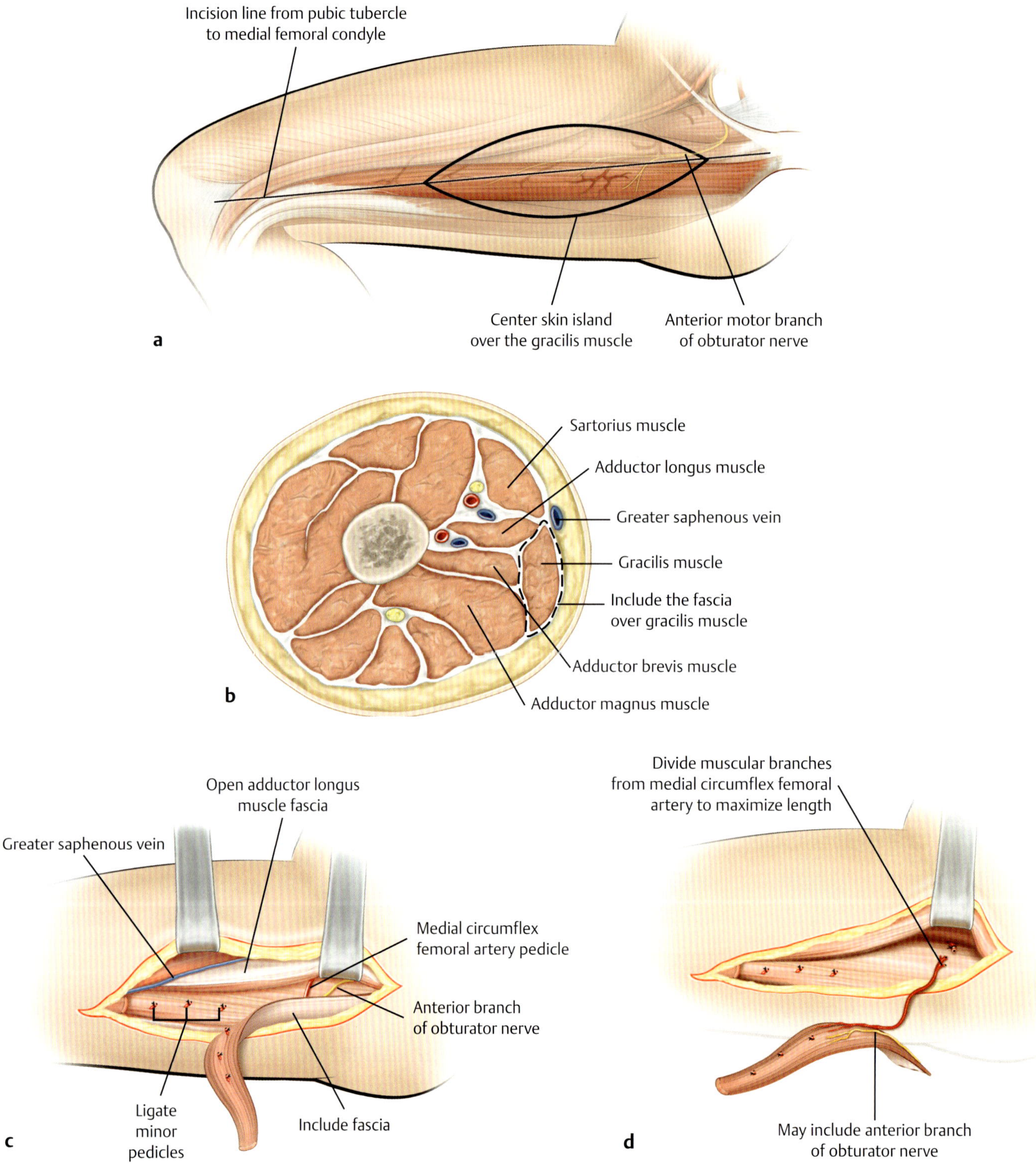

Fig. 52.1 Gracilis muscle/musculocutaneous flap, innervated flap. **(a)** Flap outline. **(b)** Cross-sectional anatomy. **(c)** Pedicle identification. **(d)** Flap isolated on pedicle (*continued*).

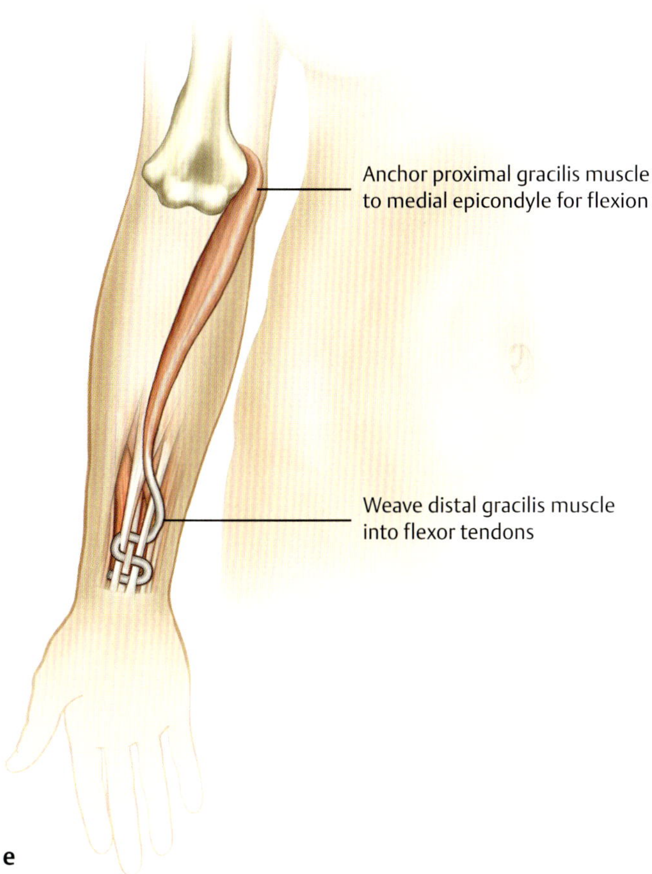

e

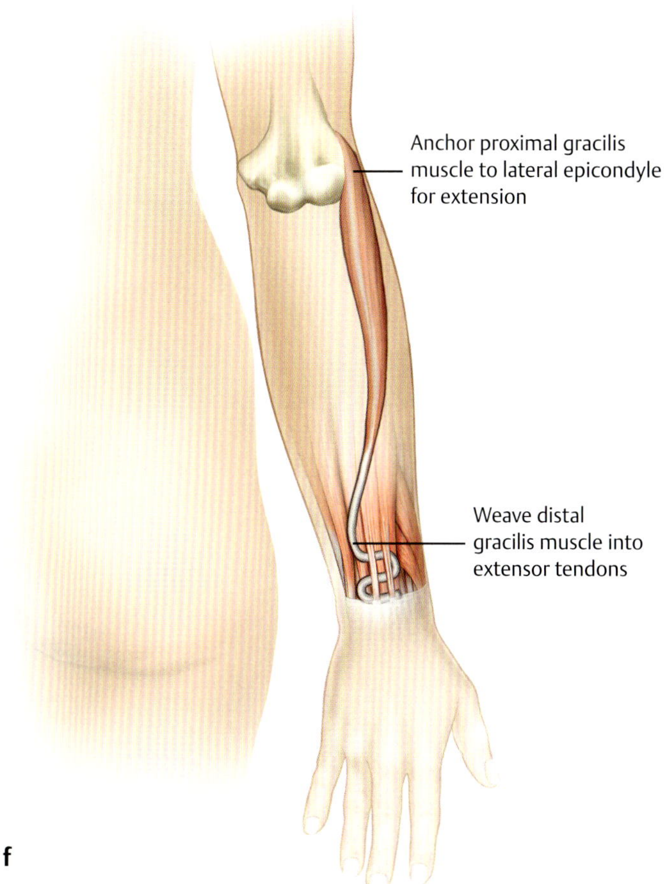

f

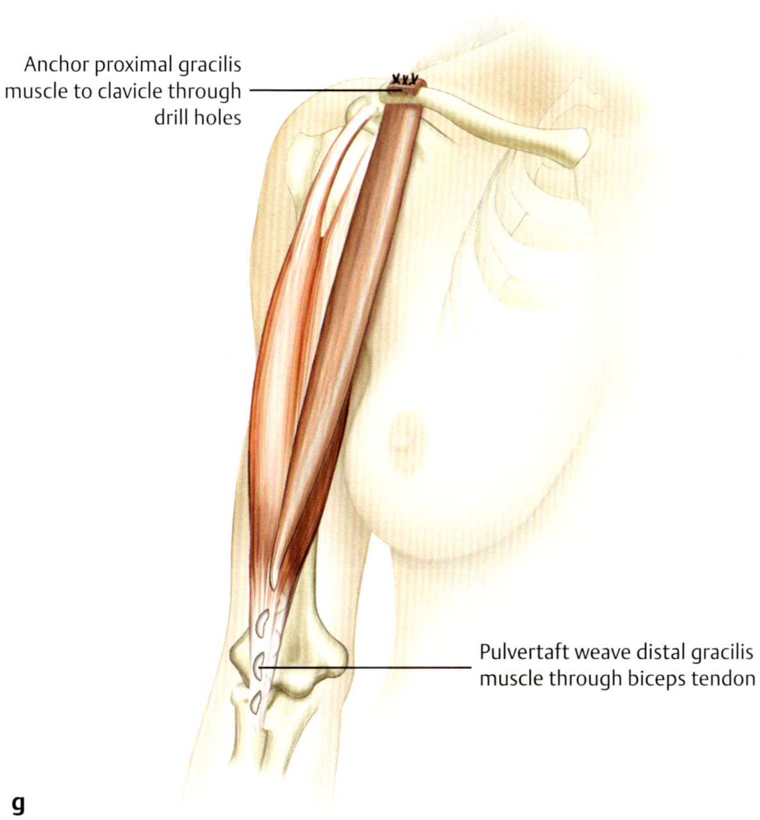

g

Fig. 52.1 (*continued*) **(e)** Use of gracilis as an innervated functional muscle transfer in flexion, and **(f)** extension. **(g)** Use of gracilis as a functional muscle for elbow flexion.

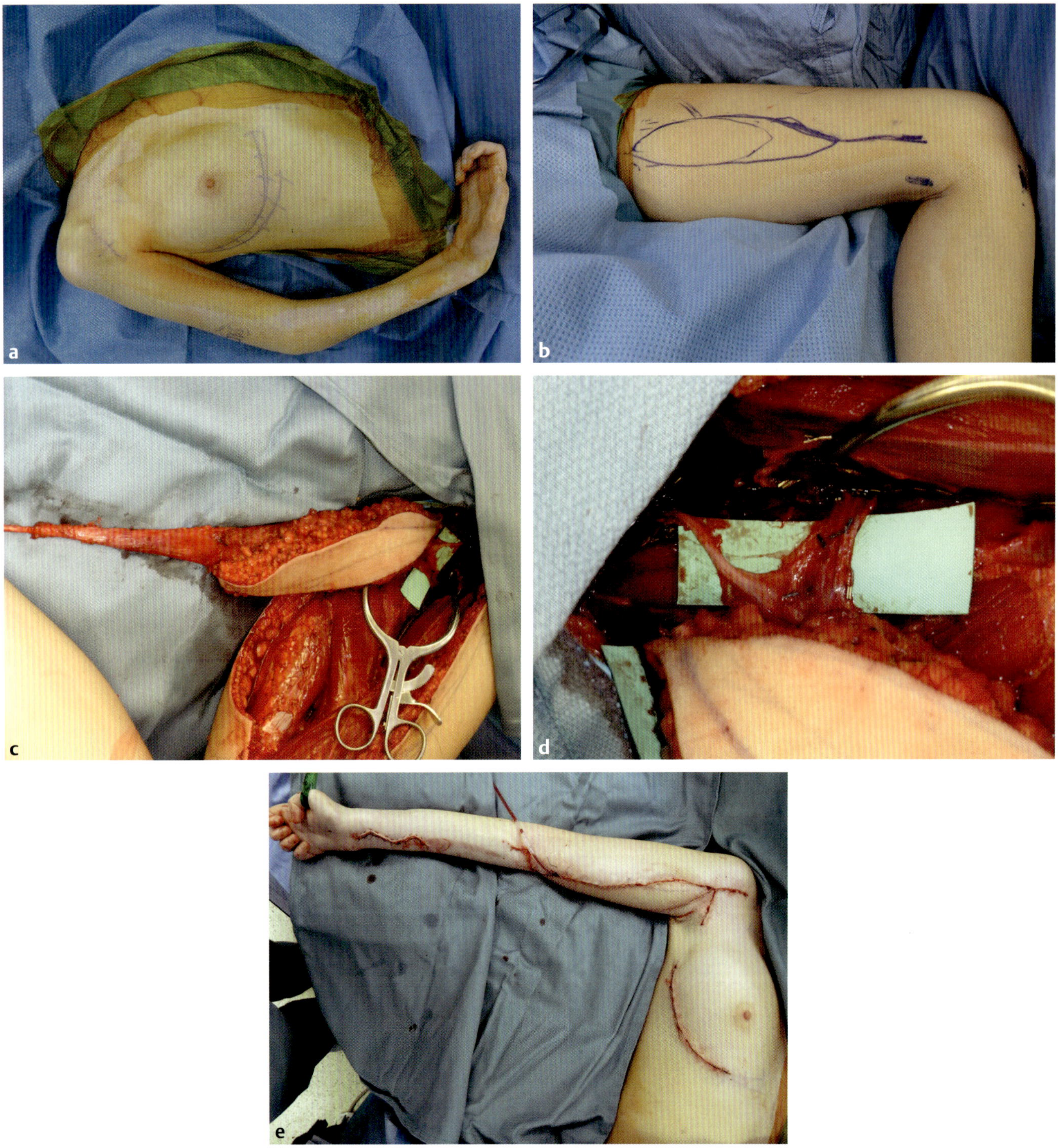

Fig. 52.2 Gracilis muscle/musculocutaneous flap, innervated flap. **(a)** Brachial plexus palsy, right arm. **(b)** Topical drawing of innervated myocutaneous gracilis. **(c)** Muscle in sheath with skin paddle. **(d)** Relationship of obturator nerve to vascular pedicle. **(e)** Final closure.

Chapter 53

Fibula Flap

Table 53.1 Fibula flap

Flap	
Tissue	Bone and skin paddle; bone, skin, and muscle flap
Course of the vessels	Posterior to the fibula, through or beneath the flexor hallucis muscle
Dimensions	Bone length, ≤ 26 cm; skin paddle 8 × 15 cm
Extensions and combinations	Parts of the soleus muscle can be included
Anatomy	
Neurovascular pedicle	—
Artery	Peroneal artery
Veins	Peroneal veins
Length and arc of rotation	2–4 cm
Diameter	Artery, 1.5–2.5 mm; vein, 2–4 mm
Nerve	—
Surgical technique	
Preoperative examination and markings	Draw a line from the fibula head to the lateral malleolus posterior to the peroneal tendons; mark the midpoint approximately 15–17 cm from the fibula head; identify skin perforators
Patient position	Supine, with a tourniquet on the thigh
Dissection	Lateral approach is preferred for both flaps; create the anterior incision of the designed skin paddle through the crural fascia to the peroneus muscles; make a subfascial dissection toward the posterior intermuscular septum; incise through the posterior margin of the skin paddle; make a subfascial dissection of the soleus muscle to the posterior intermuscular septum; the septum is traced to the fibula; the dissection proceeds anteriorly to detach the anterior septum from the fibula; the posterior dissection moves toward the flexor hallucis muscle; identify the vessels (a cuff of the flexor hallucis muscle may have to be incorporated); create a distal osteotomy (insert retractors close to the fibula to protect the vessels); the distal end of the fibula is distracted cephalad with a clamp; divide the interosseous membrane; expose the peroneal vessels; create a proximal osteotomy; trace the vessels back to the origin; open the tourniquet and check for perfusion

Continued

Table 53.1, cont'd

Advantages	
Vascular pedicle	Reliable, large-caliber vessels; loss of donor vessels is usually tolerable
Flap size and shape	Skin paddle is mobile; many defect variations can be reconstructed with a combined osteocutaneous flap; the fibula provides ideal bone for the replacement of the radius, ulna, and humerus
Combinations	Soleus muscle can be included to fill larger dead spaces
Donor site	Despite a slight torsion instability, donor morbidity is minimal if taken as a bone flap only
Disadvantages	
Donor site morbidity	Donor scar is conspicuous; risk of nerve injury to peroneal nerve or motor nerve of the flexor hallucis muscle; possible exposure of peroneal tendons
Dissection	Dissection is tedious and technically difficult; pedicle is short
Flap	Skin island may be too small in complex injuries with major soft tissue loss
Pearls and pitfalls	
Dissection	Do not confuse peroneal vessels with posterior tibial vessels; take a muscle cuff (1–2 mm) to ensure bone perfusion; preserve the proximal and distal 6 cm of the fibula to maintain stability; in children, the distal 10 cm should be preserved
Extensions and combinations	When part of the soleus muscle is included, be sure to include a muscle perforator, otherwise risk of muscle necrosis is high
Contouring and correction	Rarely required
Clinical applications	Complex segmental defects of the wrist, forearm, humerus, and shoulder (arthrodesis)

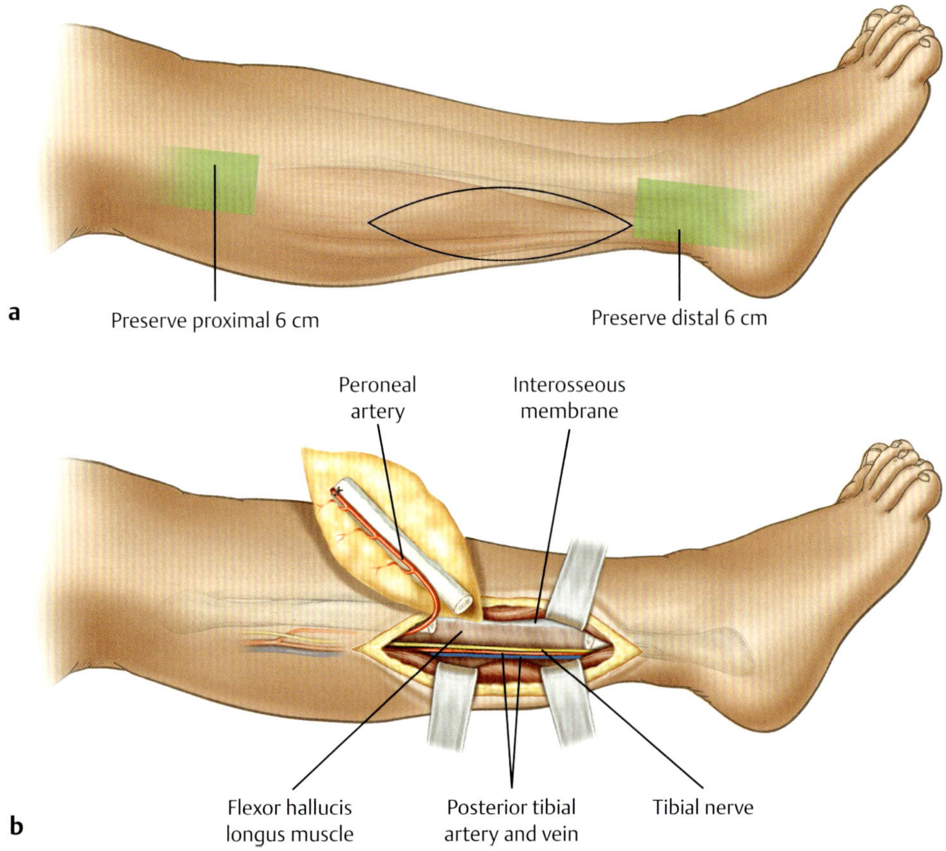

Fig. 53.1 Fibula flap. **(a)** Locate the skin island over the perforator vessel. The proximal and distal 6 cm of the fibula have to be preserved to reduce donor site moribidity. Identify perforator vessels by preoperative Doppler examination. **(b)** Do not confuse the peroneal vessels with the posterior tibial vessels. The distal pedicle is ligated. Dissection proceeds cephalad after distal osteotomy.

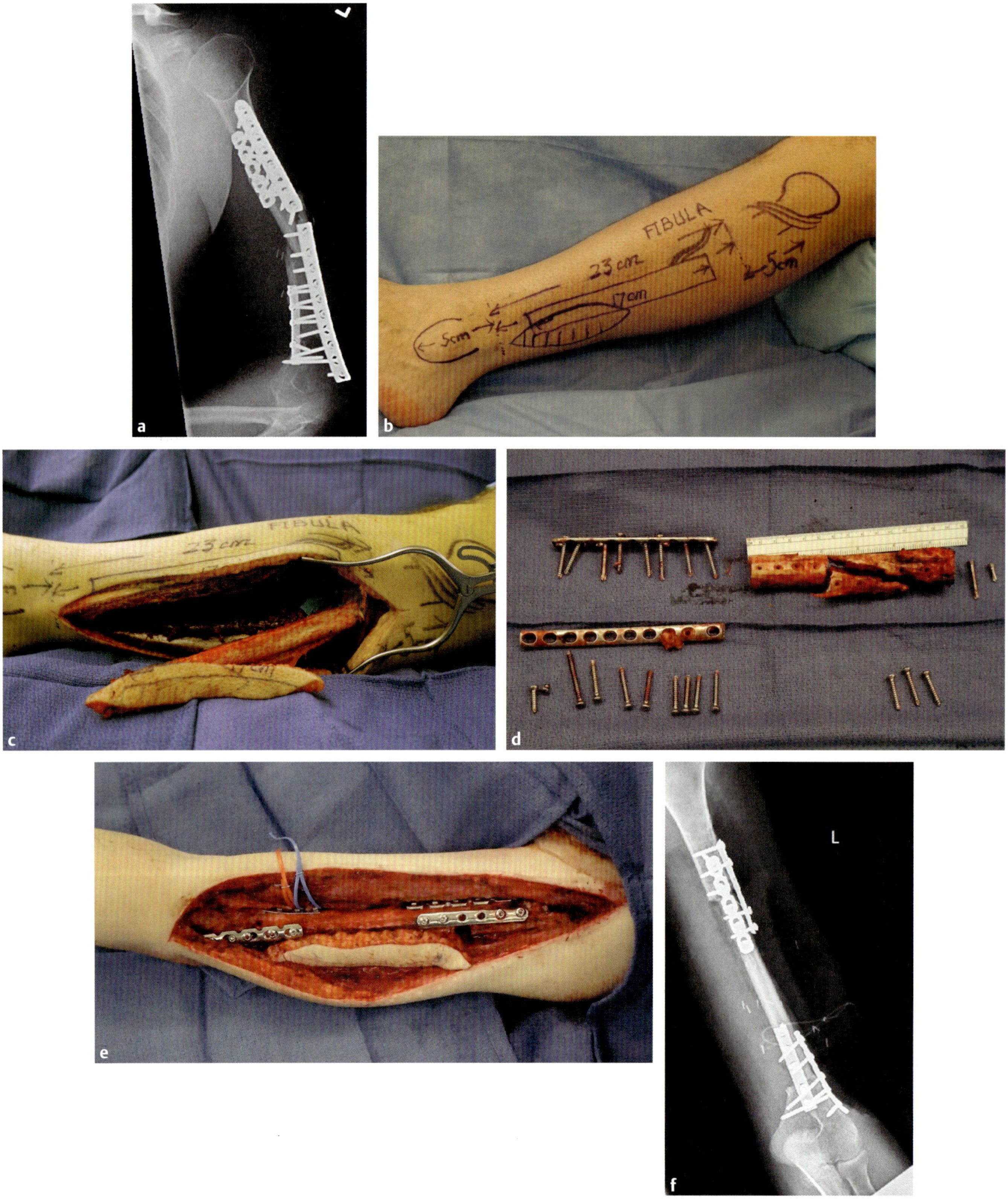

Fig. 53.2 Fibular flap. **(a)** Radiograph revealing failed, comminuted allograft intercalary reconstruction after multiple revisions. **(b)** Design of fibular osteocutaneous flap. **(c)** Fibular flap raised and isolated on peroneal vessels. **(d)** Debrided hardware and allograft. **(e)** Inset, ORIF and revascularization of fibular flap. **(f)** Radiograph shows excellent incorporation after bone healing.

Chapter 54

Additional Free Vascularized Bone Grafts

Table 54.1 Medial geniculate artery flap

Flap	
Tissue	Reliable vascular pedicle that is based on the medial geniculate artery; descending branch originates from the femoral artery in Hunter's canal; variation includes the superior geniculate artery, which courses posterior to the medial femoral condyle; skin flap can be based on the saphenous artery perforators or the perforating vessels that originate directly from the medial geniculate artery
Course of the vessels	—
Dimensions	—
Extensions and combinations	—
Anatomy	
Neurovascular pedicle	—
Artery	—
Veins	—
Length and arc of rotation	—
Diameter	—
Nerve	—
Surgical technique	—
Preoperative examination and markings	—
Patient position	—
Dissection	—
Advantages	
Vascular pedicle	—
Flap size and shape	Versatile source of small vascularized bone grafts; may be harvested as a periosteal flap only, a corticocancellous bone flap, an osteocutaneous flap, or an osteomyocutaneous flap; long pedicle possible; muscle can be included; hyaline cartilage can be harvested from the trochlear non-articular portion of the knee as a substitute for articular surface defects (i.e., as a replacement for the proximal pole of the scaphoid)
Combinations	—
Tissue	—
Dissection	—
Donor site	—
Further options	—

Continued

Table 54.1, cont'd

Disadvantages	
Flap size	—
Donor site morbidity	—
Dissection	—
Flap	—
Pedicle	—
Pearls and pitfalls	
Dissection	Dissection should proceed distal to proximal, with a tourniquet in place; periosteal vessels and optimal condylar vascularity will be found in the distal inferior quadrant of the knee; begin with a longitudinal incision over the mid portion of the medial femoral condyle; divide the skin and dissect to the vastus medialis oblique fascia; incise the fascia and reflect the vastus medialis anteriorly; identify the periosteal perforators on the condylar surface (more superficial layers of fascia that contain vessels can be confused for the medial geniculate artery, but these are not the periosteal perforators); follow the vessels from distal to proximal along the adductor longus tendon; the medial geniculate artery and vein originate from the femoral artery and vein; saphenous branch for skin flap posterior in thigh is a possibility to use as an osteocutaneous flap.
Extensions and combinations	—
Contouring and correction	—
Clinical applications	Use cautery to incise the rich periosteum around bone, being sure to leave the periosteum attached to the cortical surface of the condyle; use an oscillating saw or an osteotome to cut the bone flap; leverage bone from the condyle, and keep it attached to the periosteal sleeve from the surface of the femoral diaphysis; trace the vessels proximally for the pedicle length desired; close the donor site over a drain; bone putty or allograft paste may be placed in the femoral condyle to augment the local site after the harvest of living bone

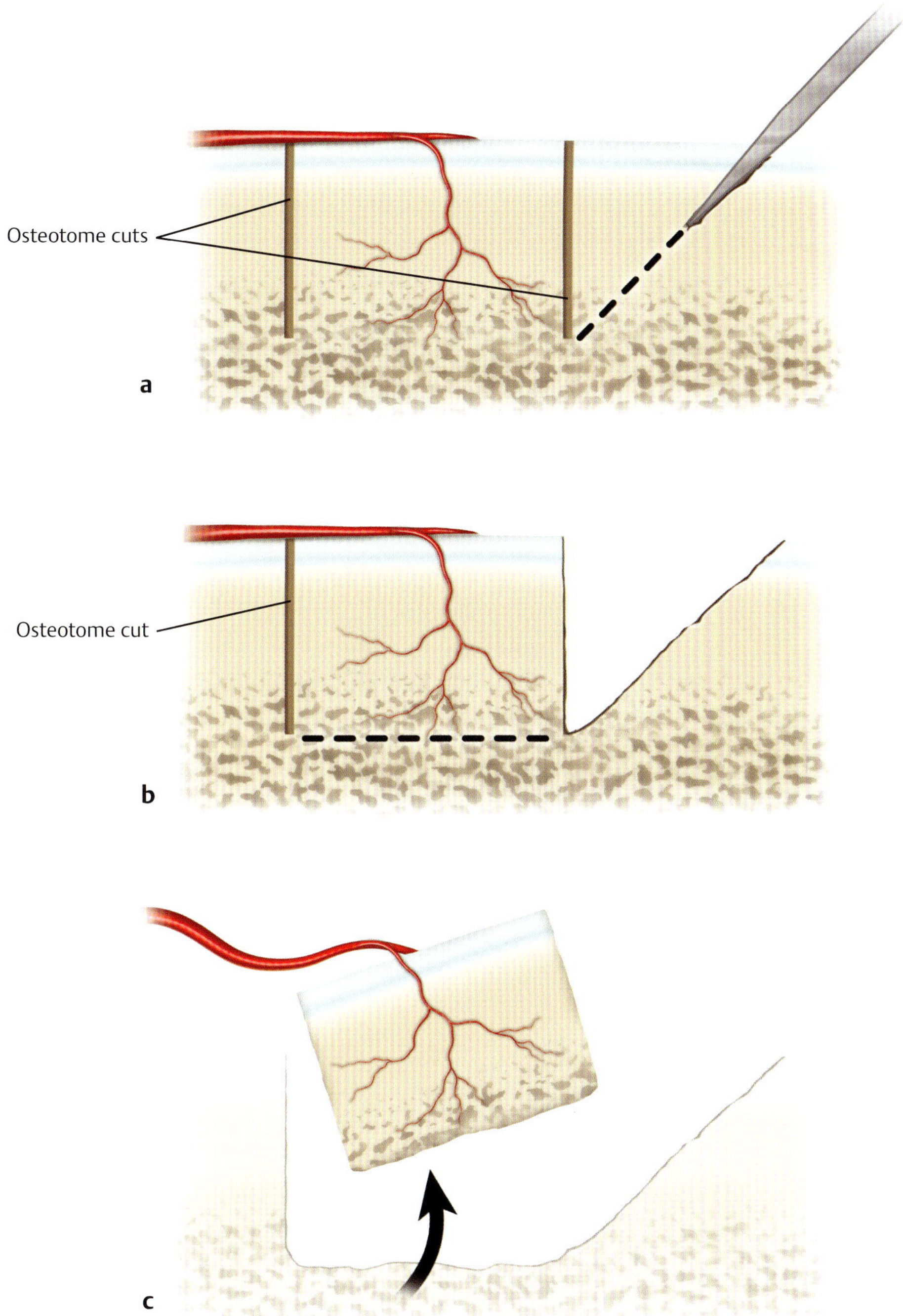

Fig. 54.1 Additional free vascularized bone grafts. **(a)** Removal of a wedge of bone with osteotome so that **(b)** osteotomy can include cancellous bone. **(c)** Wedge of bone removed.

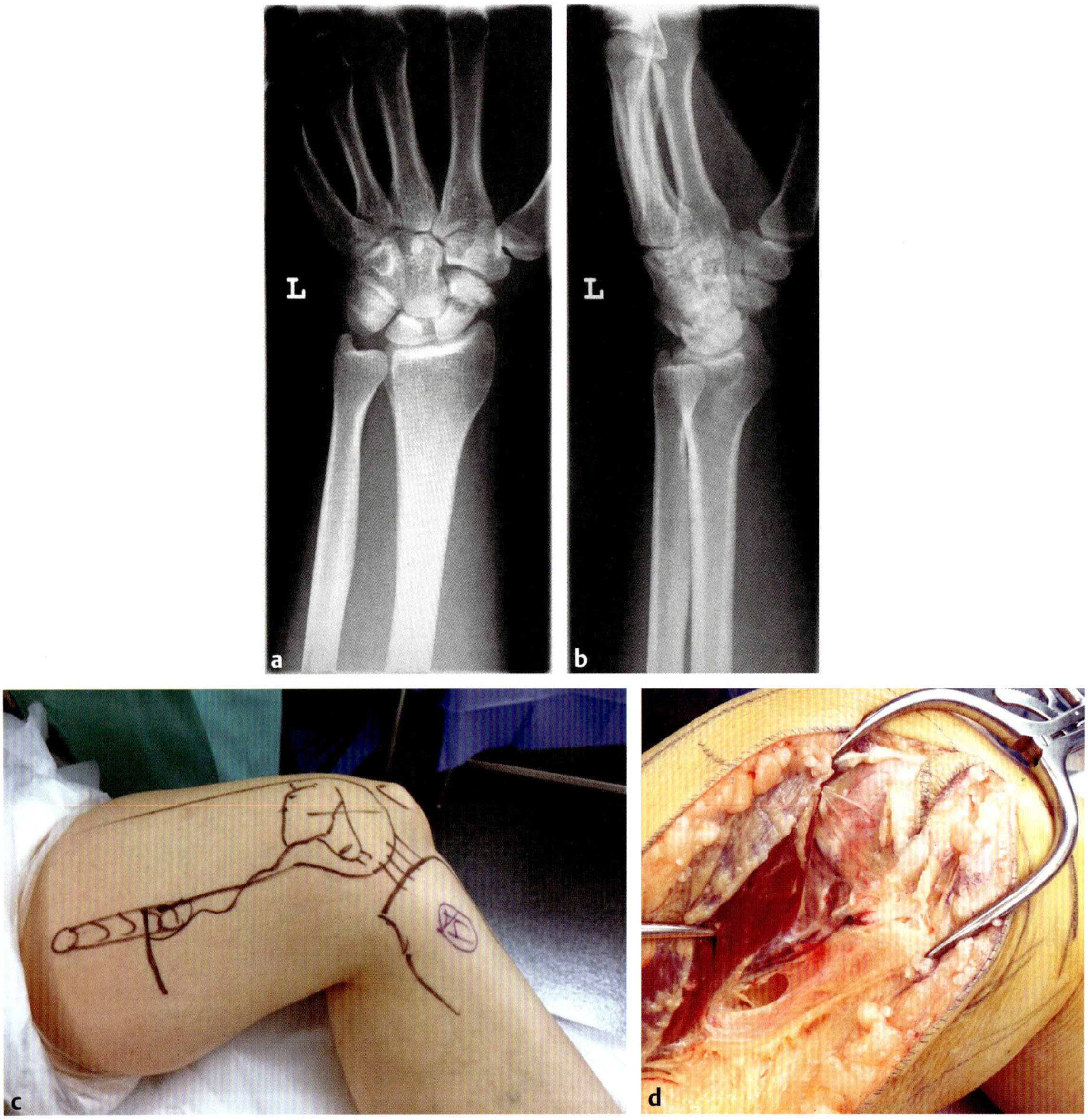

Fig. 54.2 PA **(a)** and lateral **(b)** views of long-lasting scaphoid non-union. One surgical attempt with a nonvascularized bone graft failed already. **(c)** Marking for the harvest of a medial femur condyle vascularized graft. **(d)** Medial genicular artery and concomitant veins (*continued*).

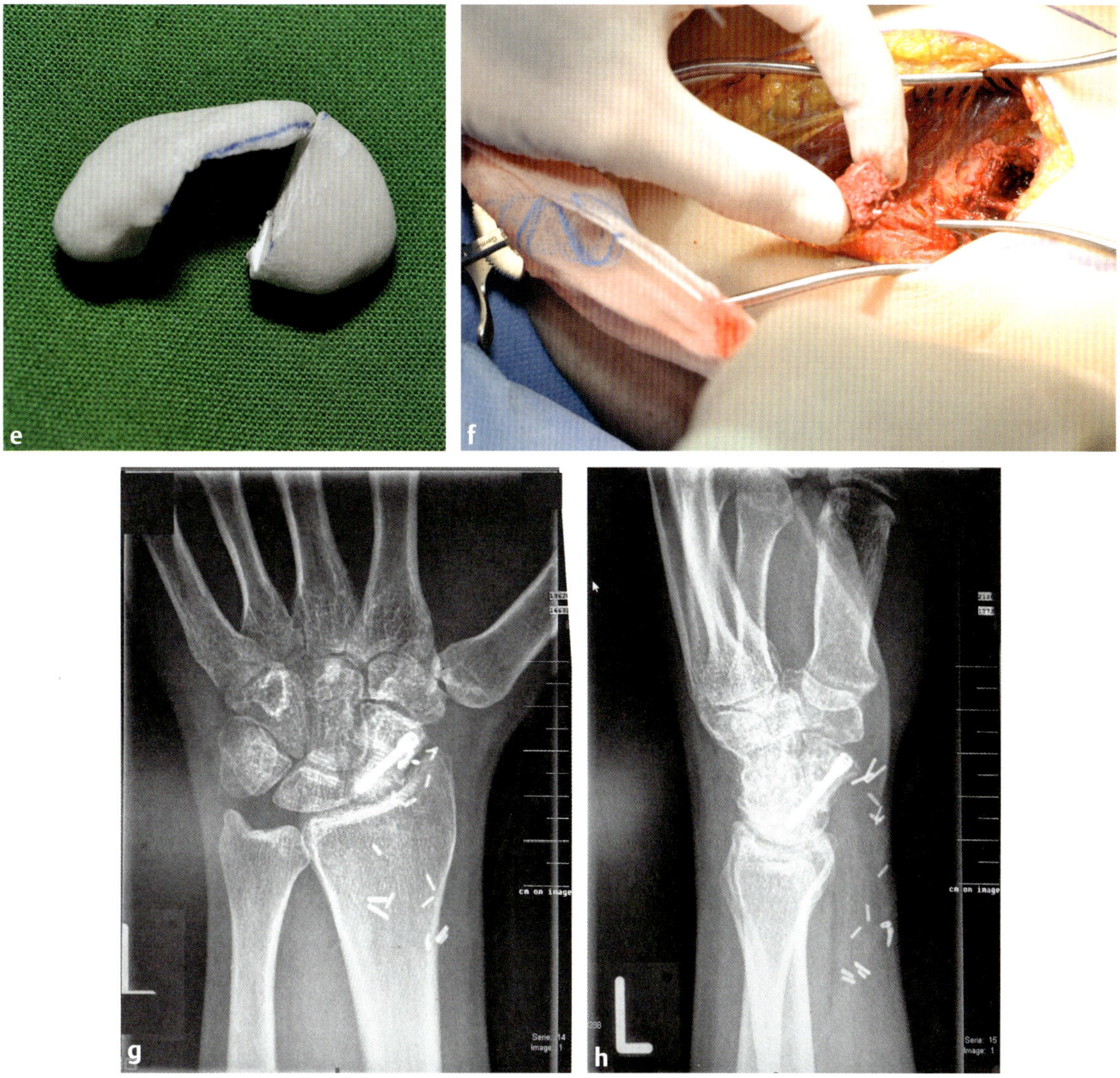

Fig. 54.2 (*continued*) **(e)** 3D printed model of the scaphoid after a CT scan. The first time in hand surgery such a model was used as a mold for the in situ shaping of a vascularized graft from the medial femur condyle. **(f)** Graft harvested from the medial femur condyle. PA **(g)** and lateral **(h)** views two years after scaphoid reconstruction with the vascularized medial femur condyle graft and a headless compression screw.

Chapter 55

Tendon Transfer

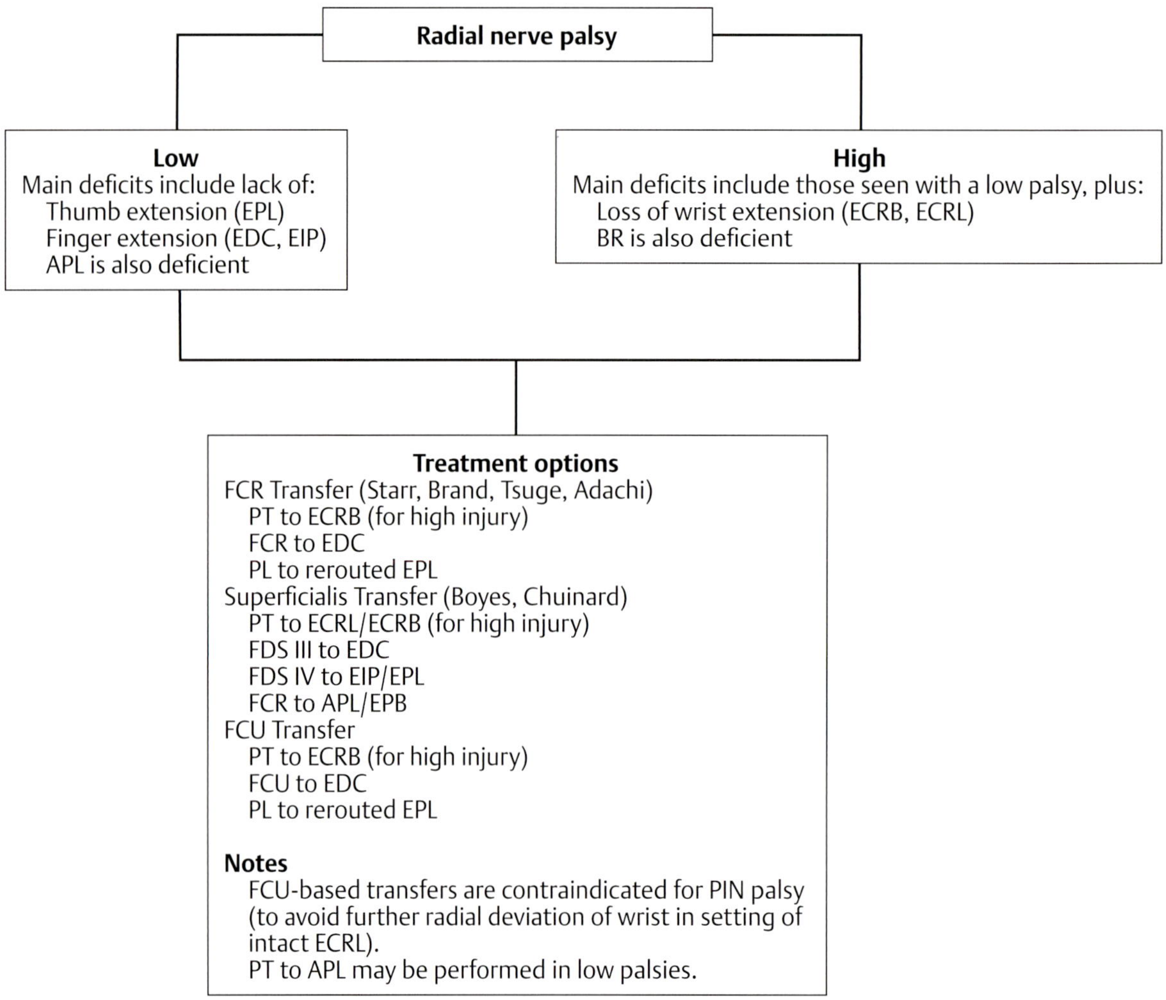

Algorithm 55.1

Median nerve palsy

Low (distal to AIN origin)
Main deficits include lack of:
- Thumb opposition (opponens pollicis)
- Thumb palmar abduction (APB)
- Thumb flexion (FPL and superficial head of FPB)

High (proximal to AIN origin)
Main deficits include those for low palsy, plus:
- All FDS and PL
  - Limits opponensplasty options
- FDP to index and long
- PT

Treatment options
- Opponensplasty
- FDS (Royle-Thompson or Bunnell)
- EIP (Burkhalter)
- ADM (Huber)
- PL (Camitz)
- Other (ECU, ECRL, EDM, FPL, EPL)

Treatment options
- Opponensplasty
- EPL
- EIP
- EDM
- Index finger flexion
- ECRL to index FDP
- Index and long FDP to ring/small FDP (side-to-side)
- Thumb flexion
- BR to FPL

Caveats
- Sensation is critical for overall hand function, and transfers in an insensate hand may lead to overall poor function.

Algorithm 55.2

Ulnar nerve palsy

Low (distal to motor origins of FCU, FDP to ring/small)
Clinical issues include:
- Weak thumb pinch
- Loss of normal finger flexion pattern
  - Pathologic sequence: DIP → PIP → MP flexion
- Loss of hand dexterity and strength
- Claw deformity

High (proximal to motor origins of FCU, FDP to ring/small)
Clinical issues include those for low palsy, plus:
- Loss of active ring/small DIP joint flexion (FDP to ring/small)
- Weak wrist flexion (FCU)
- Clawing tends to be less severe

Treatment approaches, high
Similar approaches as for low palsy to address claw deformity, restoration of thumb adduction, restoration of transverse metacarpal arch, and correction of small finger abduction deformity
Weak FDP must be avoided as a donor
Restoration of ring and small finger flexion
Brand advocated for similar treatment as for low palsies, because loss of FCU and FDP to small/ring deemed insignificant
Anderson advocated for restoration of extrinsic flexion power before addressing weak intrinsics
May consider suturing of small and ring FDP to middle FDP

Treatment approaches, low

Claw deformity	**Static techniques to prevent MP hyperextension** Zancolli technique Riordan static tenodesis Parkes static tenodesis Fowler wrist tenodesis Fasciodermadesis or bone block (rarely performed) **Dynamic techniques (tendon transfer)** FDS transfers Stiles and Forrester-Brown Bunnell Littler Burkhalter Shah	**EIP and EDM transfers** Riordan Anderson **Wrist flexor/extensor and BR transfers** ECRB/ECRL dorsal route transfer (Burkhalter, Strait) ECRL flexor route transfer (Brand) FCR transfer (Riordan) PL four-tail transfer
Restoration of thumb adduction	ECRB (Smith, Omer) FDS ring (Edgerton and Brand) EIP (Brown) Combined EIP/EDC to small Other donors: BR, ECU, ECRL	
Index finger abduction (transfers to first dorsal interosseous)	EIP transfer PL transfer EPB transfer (Bruner)	
Restoration of transverse metacarpal arch	Bunnell T operation (FDS to thumb P1 and small MC neck with graft) EDM transfer (Ranney) Modified ECRL flexor route transfer (Palande)	
Correction of small finger abduction deformity	Split EDM transfer Juncturae tendinum and medial EDC slip of ring finger transfer	

Algorithm 55.3

Part VI

Rehabilitation Protocols

Chapter 56

Flexor Tendon Repair

Underlying Principles

- At least four core strands are recommended to allow for early active motion rehabilitation protocols.
- Eight strands may be stronger than four strands from time zero through 6 weeks after treatment.
- Although 3–0 suture is stronger than 4–0 suture, the choice of suture caliber may be influenced by the size of the tendon.
- Nonlocked epitendinous repair improves strength and reduces gliding resistance.
- Locking loops result in greater time zero tensile strength as compared with grasping loops.

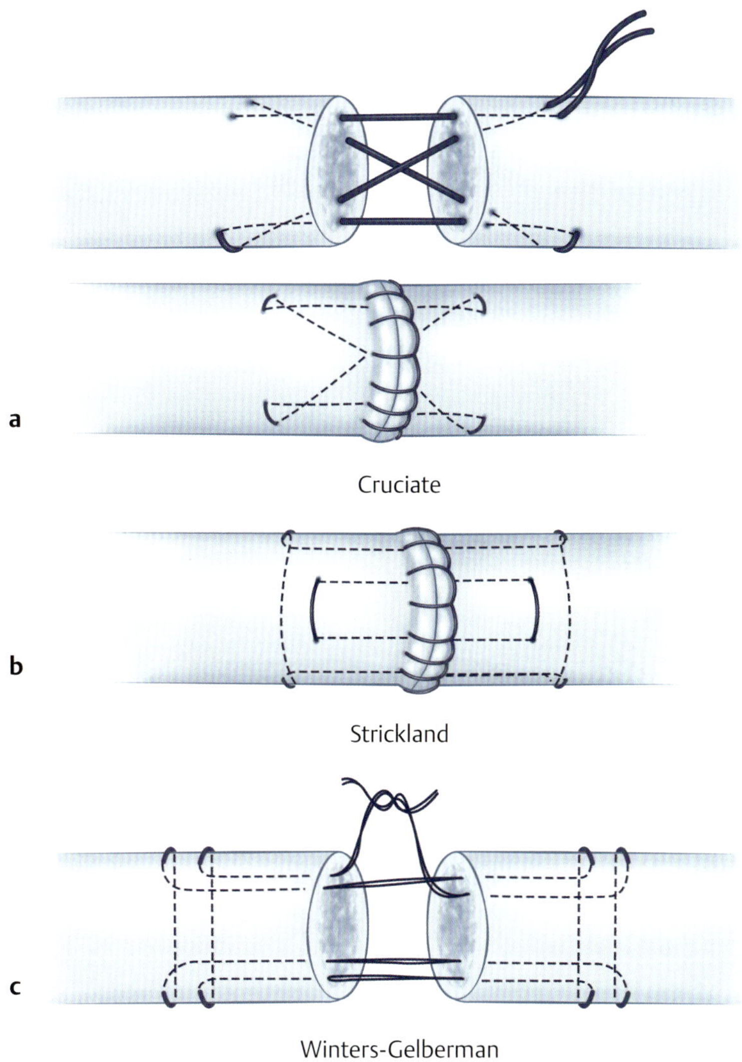

Fig. 56.1 Common suture techniques. **(a)** Cruciate. **(b)** Strickland. **(c)** Winters-Gelberman.

Chapter 57

Repair of Long Finger Flexor Tendon

Evaluation

- Patient should be seen by postoperative day 3

History

- Date of injury
- Date of surgery
- Mechanism of injury
- Tendons repaired
- Zone
- Status of tendon(s)
- Status of pulleys
- Status of digital nerve

Physical presentation

- Edema
- Incision status

Measurable tests

- Pain level
- PROM measurements
- Two-point discrimination

Table 57.1 Flexor tendon mobilization: early passive

	Precautions	Splint	Exercises	Other considerations
Weeks 1–2 *Therapy 2–3 times/ week*	Splint full time No wrist and digit extension beyond the splint No use of hand No resistance	Dorsal blocking splint Wrist 20 degrees of flexion MPs 50–70 degrees of flexion IPs full extension. If digital nerve is repaired, ask MD about amount of tension on the nerve IP extension strap when not exercising (based on therapist and MD preference)	Perform in the following sequence: Modified Duran exercises 2 times/day, 5 repetitions each Passive composite flexion 5 times/day, 10 repetitions Active extension to limits of the DBS, with MPs held in maximal flexion Wrist tenodesis out of the splint while in therapy (Duran)	**Scar management** Initiate scar massage when stitches are removed and incision is healed Initiate use of silicone when incision is healed **Edema control** Elevation Coban Retrograde massage

Table 57.1, cont'd

	Precautions	Splint	Exercises	Other considerations
Week 3	Wrist tenodesis at home	Discontinue splint Wrist tenodesis at home Initiate full digit extension with wrist in neutral Initiate tendon gliding Initiate light use with no resistance	Continue present program Continue splint, increase extension to neutral	Continue present program
Week 4	Initiate blocking Initiate FDS glides Add light resistance	No changes in present program	Discontinue splint Wrist tenodesis at home Initiate digit extension with wrist in neutral Initiate tendon gliding Initiate light use with no resistance	Continue present program
Week 5	Gradually increase resistance	Initiate blocking Initiate FDS glides Initiate light resistance	No changes in present program	Discontinue splint Initiate full active extension of digits with wrist in neutral Initiate tendon glides Initiate wrist tenodesis at home Initiate light use with no resistance
Week 6	Heavy resistance	Gradually increase resistance	Initiate blocking Initiate FDS glides Initiate light resistance	Continue present program
Week 7	Continue	Heavy resistance	Gradually increase resistance	Light resistance
Week 8	Continue	Continue	Heavy resistance	Hold heavy resistance until week 10

Source: Courtesy Good Shepherd Penn Partners, Philadelphia, Pennsylvania.

Table 57.2 Flexor tendon mobilization: early active

	Precautions	Splint	Exercises	Other considerations
Weeks 1–2 *Therapy 2–3 times/ week*	Splint full time No simultaneous wrist and digit extension No use of hand No resistance	Dorsal blocking splint Wrist in neutral MPs 50–70 degrees of flexion IPs full extension. If digital nerve is repaired, ask MD about amount of tension on the nerve IP extension strap when not exercising (based on therapist and MD preference)	Edema control measures before active exercise: Retrograde massage Compression Elevation Perform in the following sequence: Modified Duran exercises 2 times/day, 5 repetitions each Passive composite flexion 5 times/day, 10 repetitions "Place and hold flexion" 5 times/day, 3–5 repetitions, hold 3–5 seconds Gradually increase to active flexion as tolerated by patient without straining to obtain motion Active extension to limits of the DBS, with MPs held in maximal flexion Wrist tenodesis out of the splint while in therapy (Duran)	**Scar management** Initiate scar massage when stitches are removed and incision is healed Initiate use of silicone when incision is healed **Edema control** Elevation Coban Retrograde massage

Table 57.2, cont'd

	Precautions	Splint	Exercises	Other considerations
Week 3		Discontinue splint Wrist tenodesis at home Initiate full digit extension with wrist in neutral Initiate tendon gliding Initiate light use with no resistance	Continue present program	Continue present program
Week 4	Initiate blocking Initiate FDS glides Add light resistance	No changes in present program	Discontinue splint Wrist tenodesis at home Initiate digit extension with wrist in neutral Initiate tendon gliding Initiate light use with no resistance	Continue present program
Week 5	Gradually increase resistance	Initiate blocking Initiate FDS glides Initiate light resistance	No changes in present program	Discontinue splint Initiate full active extension of digits with wrist in neutral Initiate tendon glides Initiate wrist tenodesis at home Initiate light use with no resistance
Week 6	Heavy resistance	Gradually increase resistance	Initiate light resistance	Continue present program
Week 7	Continue	Heavy resistance	Gradually increase resistance	Light resistance
Week 8	Continue	Continue	Heavy resistance	Hold heavy resistance until week 10

Source: Courtesy Good Shepherd Penn Partners, Philadelphia, Pennsylvania.

Bibliography

Bainbridge LC, Robertson C, Gillies D, Elliot D. A comparison of post-operative mobilization of flexor tendon repairs with "passive flexion-active extension" and "controlled active motion" techniques. J Hand Surg Br 1994;19:517–521

Evans RB, Thompson DE. The application of force to the healing tendon. J Hand Ther 1993;6:266–284

Hatanaka H, Kojima T, Mizoguchi T, Ueshin Y. Aggressive active mobilization following zone II flexor tendon repair using a two-strand heavy-gauge locking loop technique. J Orthop Sci 2002;7:457–461

Kitsis CK, Wade PJ, Krikler SJ, Parsons NK, Nicholls KD. Controlled active motion following primary tendon repair: a prospective study over 9 years. J Hand Surg Br 1998;23:344–349

May EJ, Silfverskiöld KL, Sollerman CJ. Controlled mobilization after flexor tendon repair in zone II: a prospective comparison of three methods. J Hand Surg Am 1992;17:942–952

Riaz M, Hill C, Khan K, Small JO. Long term outcome of early active mobilization following flexor tendon repair in zone II. J Hand Surg Br 1999;24:157–160

Silfverskiöld KL, May EJ. Flexor tendon repair in zone II with a new suture technique and an early mobilization program combining passive and active flexion. J Hand Surg Am 1994;19:53–60

Stewart Pettengil K, van Strien G. Postoperative management of flexor tendon injuries. In: Hunter J, Mackin EJ, Callahan AD, Skirven TM, Schneider LH, Osterman AL, eds. Rehabilitation of the Hand and Upper Extremity. 5th ed. St Louis, MO: Mosby; 2002:431–456

Wang AW, Gupta A. Early motion after flexor tendon surgery. Hand Clin 1996;12:43–54

Chapter 58

Extensor Tendon Repair: Zone III

A boutonnière's deformity is caused by disruption of the central slip of the extensor tendon mechanism at the PIP joint. Disruption of the central slip results in a change in pull of the interosseous and lumbrical muscles from the central slip to the lateral bands, which over time causes the lateral bands to migrate volarly and eventually contract if not treated. This volar migration of the lateral bands pulls the PIP joint into a flexed posture. Additionally, secondary shortening of the oblique retinacular ligaments results in hyperextension of the distal phalanx.

History

- Date of injury
- Mechanism of injury

Physical presentation

- Edema
- Incision status

Measurable tests

- Pain level
- PIP extension lag
- DIP flexion: AROM or contractor
- Edema (circumferential)

Table 58.1 Extensor tendon zone III

	Precautions	Frequency of treatment	Splint	Exercises
Weeks 1–5	No PIP flexion Splint full time	1 time/week as needed Check: Splint position Skin integrity Exercises	Finger-based splint PIP in full extension DIP and MP free If lateral bands are lacerated, include DIP in splint, full extension	DIP flexion and extension (AROM/PROM): 10 times/hour Full MP ROM
Week 6	If extensor lag becomes noticeable once ROM is allowed: Stop all PIP ROM Wear splint full time for 2 additional weeks Resume exercises (after the 2 additional weeks) as if patient is beginning at week 6, and progress	1–3 times/week as needed Monitor motion Adjust program	Continue splint except when exercising	Introduce gentle PIP flexion while maintaining ability to fully extend the PIP after flexion (goal: 30 degrees of PIP flexion) Continue DIP and MP ROM

Continued

Table 58.1, cont'd

	Precautions	Frequency of treatment	Splint	Exercises
Week 7	If extensor lag becomes noticeable once ROM is allowed: Stop all PIP ROM Wear splint full time for 2 additional weeks Resume exercises (after the 2 additional weeks) as if patient is beginning at week 6, and progress	1–3 times/week as needed Monitor motion Adjust program	Gradually wear splint less as flexion of PIP increases and extension is maintained Continue splint	Continue to increase PIP flexion while maintaining full extension (goal: 50 degrees) Gradually add light functional use and strengthening
Weeks 8–11	If extensor lag becomes noticeable once ROM is allowed: Stop all PIP ROM Wear splint full time for 2 additional weeks Resume exercises (after the 2 additional weeks) as if patient is beginning at week 6, and progress	1–3 times/week as needed Monitor motion Monitor strength Adjust program	Discontinue splint during the day as long as full extension of PIP is maintained Continue to splint at night for 4 weeks after the splint is discontinued during the day	Continue to increase PIP flexion while maintaining full extension (goal: obtain full fist) Gradually increase use of hand with heavy resistance as needed
Week 12	If extensor lag becomes noticeable once ROM is allowed: Stop all PIP ROM Wear splint full time for 2 additional weeks Resume exercises (after the 2 additional weeks) as if patient is beginning at week 6, and progress	Discharge to home program unless continued strengthening is required to get back to work and is ordered by the physician Consider: Refer to work hardening if more strengthening is required to return to work Job site evaluation		

Source: Courtesy Good Shepherd Penn Partners, Philadelphia, Pennsylvania.

Bibliography

Coons MS, Green SM. Boutonniere deformity. Hand Clin 2005;11:387–402

Doyle JR. Extensor tendons: acute injuries. In: Green DP, ed. Operative Hand Surgery. 2nd ed. New York, NY: Churchill Livingstone; 1988:1925–1955

Evans R. Clinical management of extensor tendon injuries. In: Hunter J, Mackin EJ, Callahan AD, Skirven TM, Schneider LH, Osterman AL, eds. Rehabilitation of the Hand and Upper Extremity. 5th ed. St Louis, MO: Mosby; 2002:542–575

Purcell T, Eadie PA, Murugan S, O'Donnell M, Lawless M. Static splinting of extensor tendon repairs. J Hand Surg Br 2000;25:180–182

Chapter 59

Extensor Tendon Repair: Zones IV–VIII

Evaluation
- Patient should be seen by postoperative day 3

History
- Date of injury
- Mechanism of injury
- Date of surgery
- Tendons repaired
- Zone
- Status of tendon(s)

Physical presentation
- Incision status
- Edema
- Current immobilization device

Measurable tests
- Edema
- Pain level
- Visual Analog Scale
- ROM (protective positioning)
- Outcome measures
- Two-point discrimination

Table 59.1 Early active

	Precautions	Frequency of treatment	Splint	Exercises
Days 1–5	No digit flexion No wrist ROM Splint full time No resistance No PROM	1 time/week as needed Check splint position Check skin integrity Review and adjust program	Static forearm-based splint Wrist extension 30 degrees MPs 30 degrees of flexion IPs full extension	5 times/hour Full MP and IP extension while in the splint
Days 6–7	No simultaneous MP and IP flexion No wrist ROM Splint between exercises No resistance No PROM	1–2 times/week as needed Check splint position Check skin integrity Review and adjust program	Continue splint except when exercising	Continue previous exercises Remove splint: support wrist in extension, begin AROM Flexion/extension MPs to 45 degrees with IPs in extension Flexion/extension IPs with MPs in extension

Table 59.1, cont'd

	Precautions	Frequency of treatment	Splint	Exercises
Week 2	No simultaneous MP and IP flexion No wrist ROM Splint between exercises No resistance No PROM	1–2 times/week as needed Check splint position Check skin integrity Review and adjust program	Continue splint except when exercising	Continue previous exercises, increase MP flexion to 60 degrees Add active wrist extension/wrist flexion
Week 3	No resistance No PROM	1–2 times/week as needed	Continue splint except when exercising	Continue previous exercises, increasing to full MP flexion Add active fist exercises
Weeks 4–6	No resistance	2–3 times/week as needed	Discontinue splint during the day Continue splint during the night until week 6	Continue previous exercises Add PROM Light functional use Add light resistance at week 6
Weeks 7–8		2–3 times/week as needed Begin to prepare patient for discharge to home program Refer to work hardening if needed for return to work		Increase to heavy resistance at week 8

Source: Courtesy Good Shepherd Penn Partners, Philadelphia, Pennsylvania.

Table 59.2 Early passive

	Precautions	Orthosis	Exercises	Other considerations
Weeks 1–2 *Therapy 1–2 times/ week*	Spint full time No active digit extension No use of hand	Dynamic forearm-based splint for daytime use Wrist in 45 degrees of extension Dynamic outrigger to maintain MPs at 0 degrees with volar block allowing approximately 30 degrees of MP flexion Static volar-based splint for nighttime use Wrist 45 degrees of extension MPs and IPs in full extension	20 times/hour Active flexion of MPs to 30 degrees with passive extension to 0 degrees	**Scar management** Initiate scar massage when stitches are removed and incision is healed Initiate use of silicone when incision is healed **Edema management** Elevation Coban Retrograde massage
Week 3 *Therapy 2–3 times/ week*	Continue dynamic splint No resistance	Remove volar block on dynamic splint and continue use during the day Continue static volar splint at night	Progress to digit flexion ROM with dynamic extension splint	Continue present scar management program
Weeks 4–5 *Therapy 2–3 times/ week*	No resistance to extensors No simultaneous WF and digit flexion Stop ROM and return to splint if extension lag develops	Gradually discontinue as long as extension is maintained	Progress to full digit flexion while maintaining digit extension Progress to full wrist ROM Gradually introduce light functional use	Continue present scar management program as needed
Weeks 6–7 *Therapy 2–3 times/ week*	No heavy resistance to extensors	May begin flexion splinting as needed to gain full ROM	Add simultaneous digit and wrist flexion Add light resistive strengthening to extensors	Continue present scar management program as needed
Weeks 8–12 *Therapy 2–3 times/ week*	No precautions	Continue flexion splinting if needed	Continue to increase digit and wrist flexion Add heavy resistance	Continue present scar management program as needed

Source: Courtesy Good Shepherd Penn Partners, Philadelphia, Pennsylvania.

Table 59.3 Immediate controlled active motion (ICAM)

	Precautions	Orthosis	Exercises	Other considerations
Phase I: Days 0–21	Wear both orthoses 24/7 No heavy activity No strengthening AROM within confines of orthoses	Wrist/hand orthosis (WHO, aka volar wrist splint) in 20–25 degrees of extension Relative motion orthosis (RMO) holding involved digit in 15–25 degrees of relative extension	Digit AROM within confines of both orthoses Goal: full-digit AROM within confines of both orthoses	Edema management Pain management Wound and scar management
Phase II: Days 22–35	Must have full digit AROM within confines of both orthoses before starting Phase II Must wear both components for medium to heavy activity See orthosis weaning schedule	Must wear RMO at all times Discontinue WHO for light activity only once patient regains wrist ROM Must wear both components for medium to heavy activity and for sleep	Digit AROM within confines or RMO Wrist AROM tendonysis pattern with wrist component removed If no lag develops, begin reverse tenolysis	Edema management Pain management Wound and scar management
Phase III: Days 36–49	No heavy activity	Discharge WHO Continue RMO or buddy strapping except for exercises Discharge RMO once full wrist and digit ROM achieved	AROM out of all orthoses Consider: TGE, digit extension, EDC glides, digit ABD/ADD, FMC Light to moderate functional task	PRN: Edema management Pain management Wound and scar management
Phase IV: 4 months	No restrictions	Discharge splint	Exercises PRN	

Source: Courtesy Good Shepherd Penn Partners, Philadelphia, Pennsylvania.

Table 59.4 Immobilization

	Precautions	Orthosis	Exercises	Other considerations
Weeks 1–4 *Therapy 1 time/week*	No ROM Splint full time	Forearm-based splint: Wrist in 30–45 degrees of extension MPs in 0–20 degrees of extension IPs in full extension If only the EI or EDM is lacerated, splint only the injured finger If repair is distal to the juncturae tendinum, splint adjacent MPs in 30 degrees of flexion	No exercises	**Scar management** Initiate scar massage when stitches are removed and incision is healed Initiate use of silicone when incision is healed **Edema management** Elevation Coban Retrograde massage
Weeks 4–6 *Therapy 2–3 times/week*	No resistance No simultaneous wrist flexion and digit flexion Stop ROM and return to splint if extensor lag develops	Gradually discharge splint at postoperative week 4 Full extension is maintained	Progress to full digit flexion while maintaining digit extension Progress to full wrist ROM Gradually introduce light functional use	Continue present scar management program
Weeks 4–5 *Therapy 2–3 times/week*	No heavy resistance to extensors	Extension splint should be fully discharged May begin flexion splinting as needed to gain full ROM	Add simultaneous digit and wrist flexion Add light resistive strengthening to extensors	Continue present scar management program as needed
Weeks 6–7 *Therapy 2–3 times/week*	No heavy resistance to extensors	Extension splint should be fully discharged May begin flexion splinting as needed to gain full ROM	Add simultaneous digit and wrist flexion Add light resistive strengthening to extensors	Continue present scar management program as needed
Weeks 8–12 *Therapy 2–3 times/week*	No precautions	Continue flexion splinting if needed	Continue to increase digit and wrist flexion Add heavy resistance	Continue present scar management program as needed

Source: Courtesy Good Shepherd Penn Partners, Philadelphia, Pennsylvania.

Bibliography

Chester DL, Beale S, Beveridge L, Nancarrow DJ, Titley OG. A prospective, controlled, randomized trial comparing early active extension with passive extension using a dynamic splint in the rehabilitation of repaired extensor tendons. J Hand Surg Br 2002;27:283–288

Evans R. Clinical application of controlled stress to the healing extensor tendon: A review of 112 cases. Phys Ther 1989;69(12):1041–1049

Evans R. Clinical management of extensor tendon injuries. In: Hunter J, Mackin EJ, Callahan AD, Skirven TM, Schneider LH, Osterman AL, eds. Rehabilitation of the Hand and Upper Extremity. 5th ed. St Louis, MO: Mosby; 2002: 542–575

Ip WY, Chow SP. Results of dynamic splintage following extensor tendon repair. J Hand Surg Br 1997;22:283–287

Howell JW, Merritt WH, Robinson SJ. Immediate controlled active motion following zone 4–7 extensor tendon repair. J Hand Ther 2005;18:182–190

Chapter 60

Injuries to the Digital Joints

Conservative and Postoperative Treatment

Metacarpophalangeal collateral ligament injury (digits II–V)

Collateral ligaments of the MP joint support the joint, especially during grip and pinch. Taut in flexion and lax in extension, these ligaments are most frequently injured as a result of hyperextension or extreme lateral force. The radial ligament is more vulnerable than the ulnar collateral ligaments. Partial tears are usually treated conservatively, whereas complete tears are corrected surgically. Conservative management and postoperative management are nearly similar and have been consolidated here.

History
- Date of injury
- Mechanism of injury
- Pain
- Functional status

Physical presentation
- Ecchymosis at MP joint
- Joint deformity
- Lateral joint tenderness

Measurable tests
- ROM
- Outcome measures
- Edema measures
- Visual Analog Scale
- Sensation
- Pain level

Goals
- Stable MP joint
- Pain reduction
- Prevent adhesions of extensor mechanism with IP ROM
- Stable, mobile MP joint
- Avoid rotation or angulation
- Return of function

Table 60.1 Metacarpophalangeal collateral ligament injury (digits II–V): conservative and postoperative treatment

	Precautions	Orthosis	Exercises	Other considerations
Weeks 0–3	No lateral stress No key pinch if index finger injured	Wear orthosis full time Hand-based splint: MP at 50 degrees, IP free	3–5 times/day, 5–10 repetitions IP AROM	Edema management Pain management Scar management Monitor for digital nerve symptoms
Week 3	Avoid lateral stress Avoid hyperextension No strengthening	Buddy strap during the day Splint as above at night	3–5 times/day, 5–10 repetitions Tendon glides Digital AROM extension	Edema management Pain management Scar management Monitor for digital nerve symptoms
Week 6	No heavy resistance or strong pinch	Static progressive or dynamic splint for ROM deficits	PROM/stretching if necessary Light strength	Edema management Pain management Scar management Monitor for digital nerve symptoms
Week 8	No restrictions	Tape/buddy strap for contact support	Grip/pinch strength as tolerated	Edema management Pain management Scar management Monitor for digital nerve symptoms

Source: Courtesy Good Shepherd Penn Partners, Philadelphia, Pennsylvania.

Proximal interphalangeal collateral ligament injury

The PIP collateral ligament consists of the proper collateral ligament and the accessory collateral ligament. The primary stabilizer, the PCL, is taut in flexion and lax in extension, whereas the ACL is taut in extension and lax in flexion. Grade I sprains are stable through AROM and PROM. Stress testing may be painful, but stable. Grade II indicates a complete tear of at least one collateral ligament. It is stable through AROM and demonstrates less than 20 degrees of angulation. Grade III injuries include at least one collateral ligament and some aspect of the volar or dorsal structures. It is unstable in both AROM and PROM and usually requires surgical correction.

History

- Date of injury
- Mechanism of injury
- Pain
- Functional status

Physical presentation

- Ecchymosis at MP joint
- Joint deformity
- Lateral joint tenderness

Measurable tests

- ROM
- Outcome measures
- Edema measures
- Visual Analog Scale
- Sensation
- Pain level

Goals

- Stable joint
- Pain reduction
- Prevent adhesions of extensor mechanism with IP ROM
- Avoid rotation or angulation
- Resume function

Table 60.2 Proximal interphalangeal collateral ligament injury: conservative and postoperative treatment

	Precautions	Orthosis	Exercises	Other considerations
Initial stage Grade I: 0–10 days Grade II: 2–4 weeks	Immobilization No lateral stress No resistance	Immobilize in static PIP 0–20 degrees	Gentle AROM digit flexion as tolerate	Edema management Scar management
Intermediate stage Grade III: 6 weeks Duration of 3–4 weeks after immobilization	No lateral stress No resistance No pinch with involved digit	Daytime: Buddy strap except if radial collateral ligament and small finger ulnar collateral ligament require splint Nighttime: Continue immobilization splint	AROM digit flexion	Edema management Scar management
Late stage	Activity as tolerated	Extension splint to regain any motion loss	Flexion and extension blocking PROM and splinting PRN for extension lag or flexion contractures Strength as tolerated and necessary for patient's ADLs	Edema management Scar management

Source: Courtesy Good Shepherd Penn Partners, Philadelphia, Pennsylvania.

Fracture Protocol

History
- Date of injury
- Mechanism of injury
- Pain
- Functional status

Physical presentation
- Ecchymosis
- Joint deformity
- Joint tenderness

Measurable tests
- ROM
- Outcome measures
- Edema measures
- Visual Analog Scale
- Sensation
- Pain level

Table 60.3 Metacarpophalangeal and proximal interphalangeal injury: fracture protocol

	Precautions	Orthosis	Exercises	Other considerations
Weeks 0–3	No resistance to fracture site No strengthening Orthosis	Worn full time MP fracture: MP in 70 degrees of flexion, IPs free, MD to determine forearm- versus hand-based PIP fracture: Include PIP and DIP, finger-based	3–5 times/day, 5–10 repetitions AROM Extensor tendon gliding Digital flexion tendon gliding	Edema management Scar management Pain management Activity modification Monitor for digital nerve symptoms
Weeks 4–6	No strengthening	Decrease wearing schedule based on fracture healing per MD Consider buddy straps for PIP fractures	3–5 times/day, 5–10 repetitions Tendon glides Digit AROM extension	Edema management Scar management Pain management Activity modification Monitor for digital nerve symptoms
Week 7	No heavy resistance	Discharge once cleared by MD	PROM if necessary Light strength	Edema management Scar management Pain management Activity modification Monitor for digital nerve symptoms
Week 8	None		Increase to heavier strengthening	Edema management Scar management Pain management Activity modification Monitor for digital nerve symptoms

Source: Courtesy Good Shepherd Penn Partners, Philadelphia, Pennsylvania.

Volar Plate Injury

Dorsal dislocation proximal interphalangeal

History
- Date of injury
- Mechanism of injury
- Pain
- Functional status

Physical presentation
- Ecchymosis at MP joint
- Joint deformity
- Lateral joint tenderness
- Edema
- Pain

Measurable tests
- ROM
- Outcome measures
- Edema measures
- Visual Analog Scale
- Sensation
- Pain level

Table 60.4 Volar plate injury: dorsal dislocation proximal interphalangeal joint

	Precautions	Orthosis	Exercises	Other considerations
Weeks 0–4	No resistance	Worn full time PIP extension block orthosis Degree of PIP blocked extension determined by MD	3–5 times/day, 5–10 repetitions Full PIP flexion AROM/PROM PIP extension to limits of the orthosis	Edema management Scar management Pain management Activity modification Monitor for digital nerve symptoms
Weeks 5–6	No strengthening	Buddy strap worn during the day Orthosis (as above) worn at night	3–5 times/day, 5–10 repetitions Tendon glides Digit AROM extension (determined by MD)	Edema management Scar management Pain management Activity modification Monitor for digital nerve symptoms
Week 7	No heavy resistance Light resistance allowed	Discharge	Continue tendon glides as needed Light strength	Edema management Scar management Pain management Activity modification Monitor for digital nerve symptoms
Week 8	None	Discharge	Grip/pinch strength as tolerated	Edema management Scar management Pain management Activity modification Monitor for digital nerve symptoms

Source: Courtesy Good Shepherd Penn Partners, Philadelphia, Pennsylvania.

Volar dislocation proximal interphalangeal joint

History
- Date of injury
- Mechanism of injury
- Pain
- Functional status

Physical presentation
- Ecchymosis at MP joint
- Joint deformity
- Lateral joint tenderness
- Edema
- Pain

Measurable tests
- ROM
- Outcome measures
- Edema measures
- Visual Analog Scale
- Sensation
- Pain level

Table 60.5 Volar plate injury: volar dislocation proximal interphalangeal joint

	Precautions	Orthosis	Exercises	Other considerations
Weeks 0–4	No resistance	Worn full time PIP extension gutter orthosis DIP free	3–5 times/day, 5–10 repetitions DIP flexion and extension	Edema management Scar management Pain management Activity modification Monitor for digital nerve symptoms
Weeks 5–6	No strengthening	Dynamic PIP extension orthosis during the day as long as extension is maintained Finger gutter at night	Patient may flex PIP while in dynamic extension orthosis as long as PIP extension is maintained	Edema management Scar management Pain management Activity modification Monitor for digital nerve symptoms
Week 7	No heavy resistance Light resistance allowed	Wean from dynamic orthosis during the day as long as PIP extension is maintained Continue figure gutter at night	Gradual increased digit flexion while maintaining extension Light strength	Edema management Scar management Pain management Activity modification Monitor for digital nerve symptoms
Week 8	None	Wean from all orthoses	Grip/pinch strength as tolerated	Edema management Scar management Pain management Activity modification Monitor for digital nerve symptoms

Source: Courtesy Good Shepherd Penn Partners, Philadelphia, Pennsylvania.

Bibliography

Belsky MR, Leibman M. Extra-articular hand fractures, Part II: therapist's management. In: Skerven TM, Osterman AL, Fedorczyk JM, Amadio PC, eds. Rehabilitation of the Hand and Upper Extremity. 6th ed. Philadelphia, PA: Mosby; 2011:377–385

Blazar PE. Dislocations/instability. In: Beredjiklian PK, Bozentka DJ, eds. Review of Hand Surgery. Philadelphia, PA: Saunders; 2004:139-150

Campbell PJ, Wilson RL. Management of joint injuries and intraarticular fractures. In: Hunter J, Mackin EJ, Callahan AD, Skirven TM, Schneider LH, Osterman AL, eds. Rehabilitation of the Hand and Upper Extremity. 5th ed. St Louis, MO: Mosby; 2002:382–395

Gaffney Gallagher K, Blackmore SM. Extra-articular hand fractures and joint injuries, Part II: therapist's management. In: Skerven TM, Osterman AL, Fedorczyk JM, Amadio PC, eds. Rehabilitation of the Hand and Upper Extremity. 6th ed. Philadelphia, PA: Mosby; 2011:417–436

Mannarino S. Skeletal injuries. In: Stanley BG, Tribuzi SM, eds. Concepts in Hand Rehabilitation. Philadelphia, PA: FA Davis; 1992:275–321

Chapter 61

Locking Plate Principles

Locking Versus Nonlocking Plates: Advantages to a Locking Plate/Screw System

There are several advantages to a locking plate/screw system:

- Locking plate and screw systems have advantages over the conventional screw systems. Conventional plate/screw systems require precise adaptation of the plate to the underlying bone. Without this intimate contact, tightening of the screws will draw the bone segments toward the plate, resulting in alterations in the position of the osseous segments and the occlusal relationship. Locking plate/screw systems offer certain advantages over other plates in this regard. The most significant advantage may be that it becomes unnecessary for the plate to intimately contact the underlying bone in all areas. As the screws are tightened, they "lock" to the plate, thus stabilizing the segments without the need to compress the bone to the plate. This makes it impossible for the screw insertion to alter the reduction.
- Another potential advantage in locking plate/screw systems is that they do not disrupt the underlying cortical bone perfusion as much as conventional plates, which compress the undersurface of the plate to the cortical bone.
- A third advantage to the use of locking plate/screw systems is that the screws are unlikely to loosen from the plate. This means that even if a screw is inserted into a fracture gap, loosening of the screw will not occur. Similarly, if a bone graft is screwed to the plate, a locking screw will not loosen during the phase of graft incorporation and healing. The possible advantage to this property of a locking plate/screw system is a decreased incidence of inflammatory complications from loosening of the hardware. It is known that loose hardware propagates an inflammatory response and promotes infection. For the hardware of a locking plate/screw system to loosen, loosening of a screw from the plate or loosening of all of the screws from their bony insertions would have to occur.
- Locking plate/screw systems have been shown to provide more stable fixation than conventional nonlocking plate/screw systems.

Plate Design

Locking plates 2.0 are available in four thicknesses, with or without center space (**Fig. 61.1**):

1. Small profile
2. Medium profile
3. Large profile
4. Extra-large profile

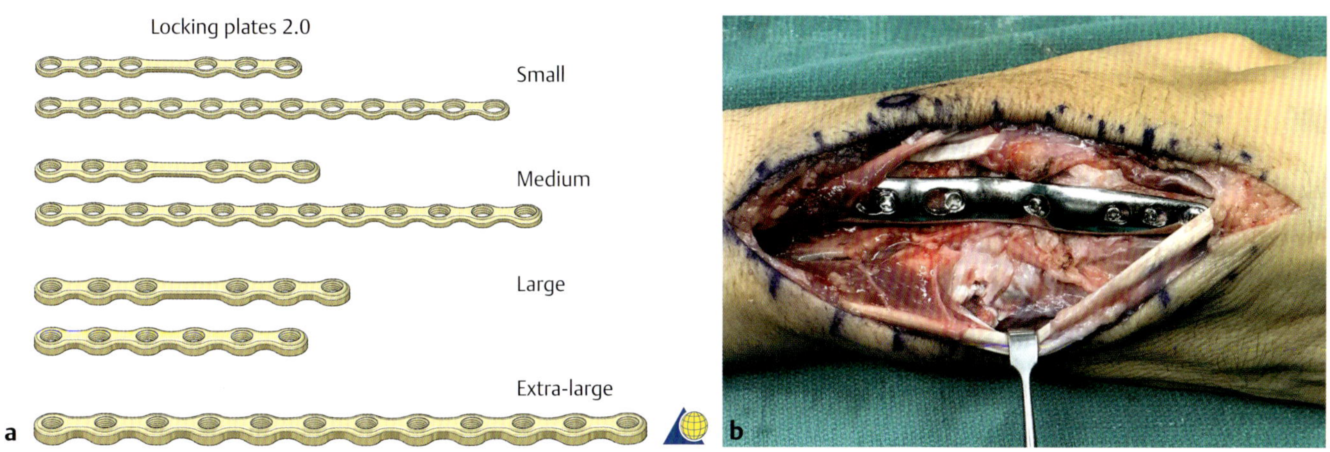

Fig. 61.1 (a) Locking plates 2.0. **(b)** Locking plate used for wrist arthrodesis.

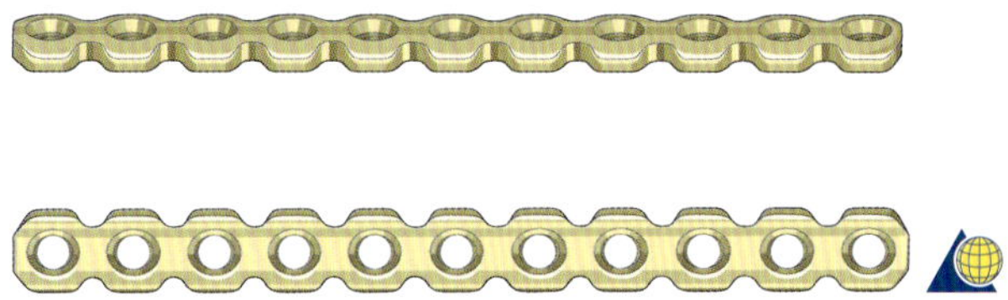

Fig. 61.2 Locking reconstruction plate 2.4.

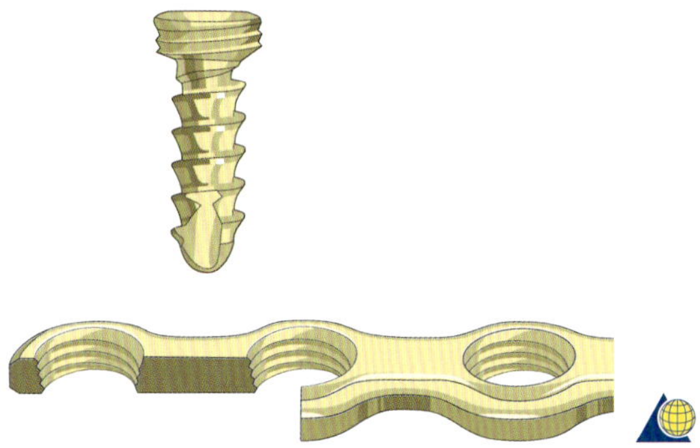

Fig. 61.3 Locking head screws.

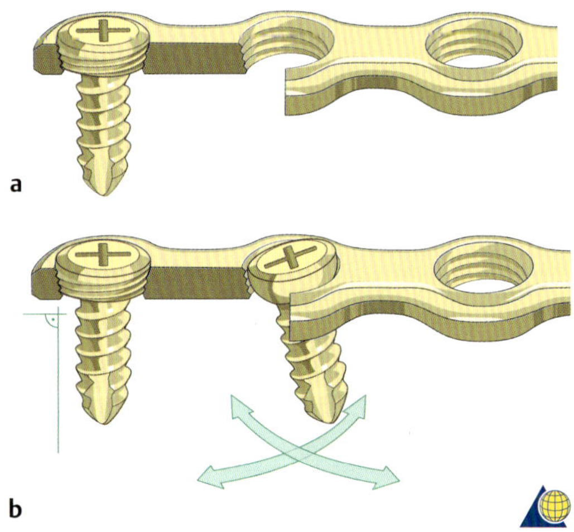

Fig. 61.4 Insertion of a locking head screw **(a)** and a conventional screw **(b)**.

They are also available in multiple shapes to meet a variety of clinical applications. The threaded head of the 2.0 mm locking head screws is conical. It is therefore possible to insert locking head screws at small angles. A threaded drill guide is not necessary.

There is only one thickness of the locking reconstruction plate (LRP) 2.4 (**Fig. 61.2**). However, there are multiple plate configurations to meet a variety of clinical applications.

The threaded head of the 2.4 mm locking head screws is cylindrical. Therefore, a threaded drill guide is mandatory to assure the correct perpendicular insertion of 2.4 mm locking head screws (**Fig. 61.3**). Angulation is not possible.

The locking plate has a corresponding threaded plate hole. During insertion the locking head screw engages and locks into the threaded plate hole (**Fig. 61.4, a**). If necessary the threaded plate hole also accepts nonlocking screws, which permit greater angulation (**Fig. 61.4, b**).

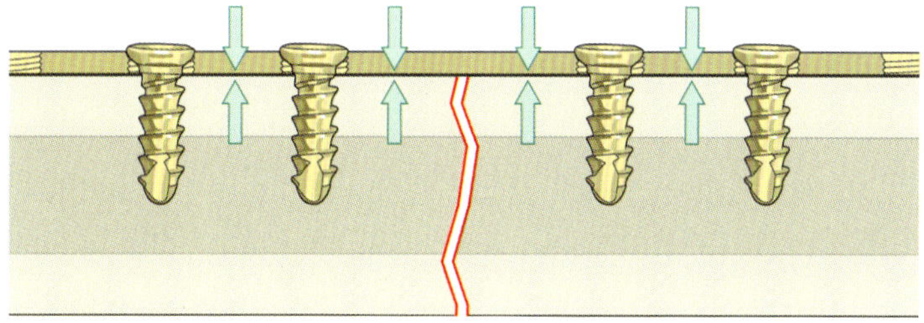

Fig. 61.5 Fixation of plate to bone using conventional screws.

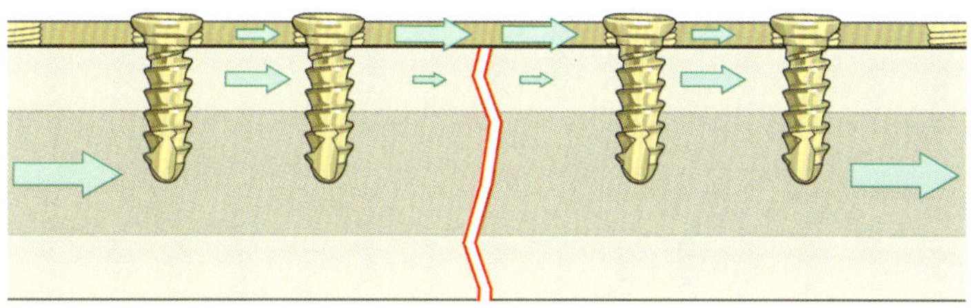

Fig. 61.6 Loading forces with conventional screws.

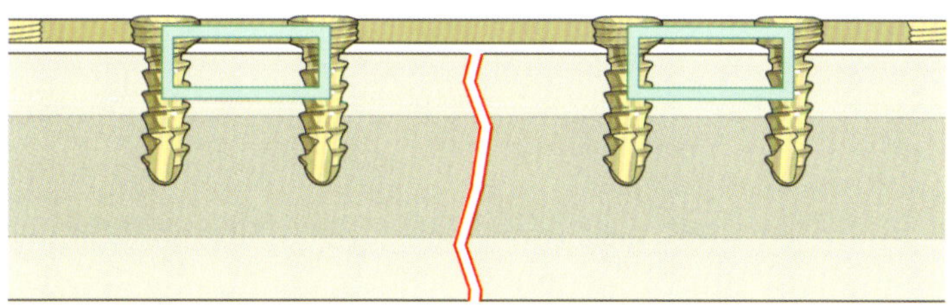

Fig. 61.7 Fixation and loading forces with locking head screws.

Biomechanics

With the conventional technique, the tightening of the screws presses the plate against the bone. This pressure generates friction, which contributes significantly to primary stability (**Fig. 61.5**). Loading forces are transmitted from the bone to the plate, across the fracture, and back into the bone. Friction between plate and bone is necessary for stability using conventional screws.

However, with the locking head screws engaged in the plate, the plate is not pressed onto the bone. This reduces the blood supply to the bone underlying the plate. Loading forces are transmitted directly from the bone to the screws, then onto the plate, across the fracture, and again through the screws into the bone (**Fig. 61.6**). Friction between plate and bone is not necessary for stability.

The plate and screws provide adequate rigidity and do not depend on the underlying bone (load-bearing osteosynthesis) when using a locking reconstruction plate 2.4. On each side of the fracture, the screws are locked into the plate as well as into the bone (**Fig. 61.7**). The result is a rigid frame construct with high mechanical stability (internal external fixator).

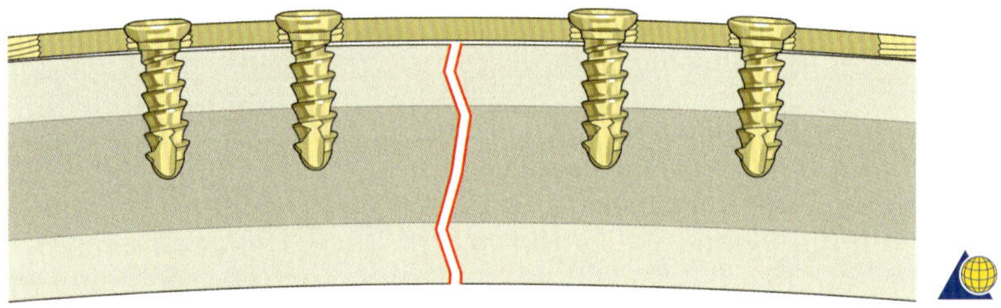

Fig. 61.8 Conventional plate system.

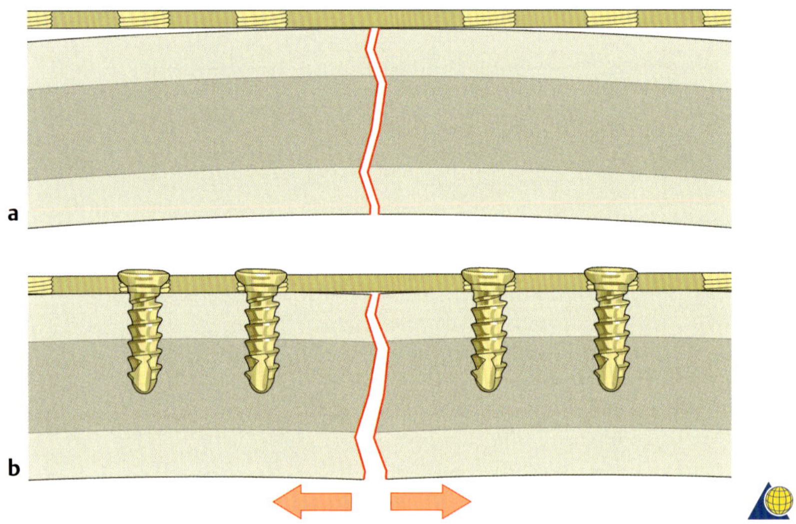

Fig. 61.9 Primary loss of reduction with a conventional plate system.

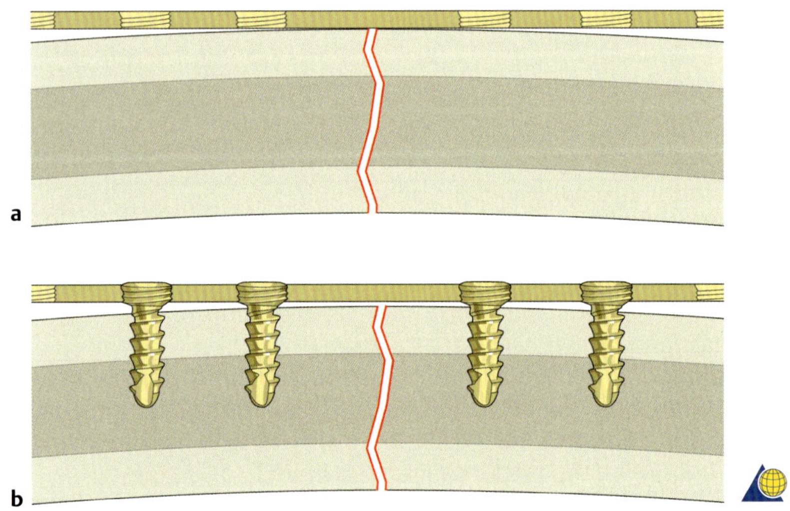

Fig. 61.10. No loss of reduction with a locking plate system.

Primary Loss of Reduction

When using conventional plates and screws it is essential to contour the plate precisely to the bone surface (**Fig. 61.8**).

When using a conventional plate and screws the plate must be precisely adapted to the bone, otherwise the tightening of the screws will lead to a primary loss of reduction (**Fig. 61.9**).

Note how in **Fig. 61.10, a**, the plate is not well adapted to the outer cortex. **Fig. 61.10, b**, shows that when the screws are inserted, the bone will be pulled to the plate,

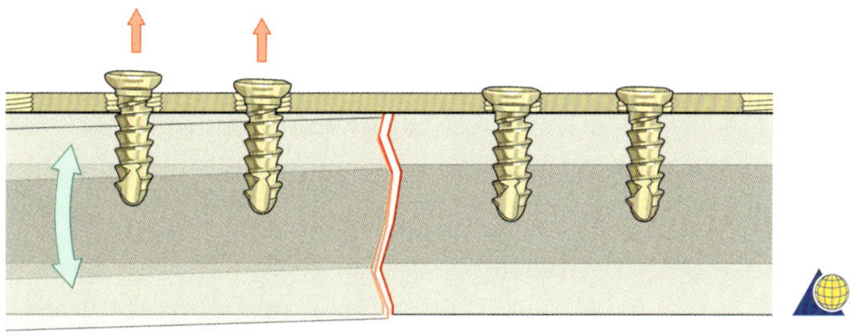

Fig. 61.11 Secondary loss of reduction (*left*) when conventional screws loosen.

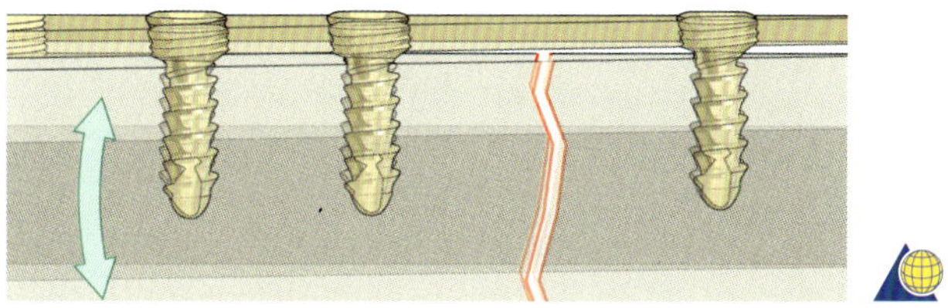

Fig. 61.12. Screw loosening rarely occurs with locking screws.

causing malreduction of the fracture. When using a locking plate/screw system, the plate does not have to be precisely adapted to the bone. When tightening a locking head screw, the screw will not cause a primary loss of reduction as it tightens into the threaded plate hole and will not draw the bone fragments to the plate.

Secondary Loss of Reduction

In conventional plate systems, screw loosening may lead to loss of reduction (**Fig. 61.11**).

In a locking system, screw loosening rarely occurs, because the screw head is locked to the plate (**Fig. 61.12**).

Part VII

Classification and Zones of Injury

Chapter 62

AO/ASIF Fracture Classification

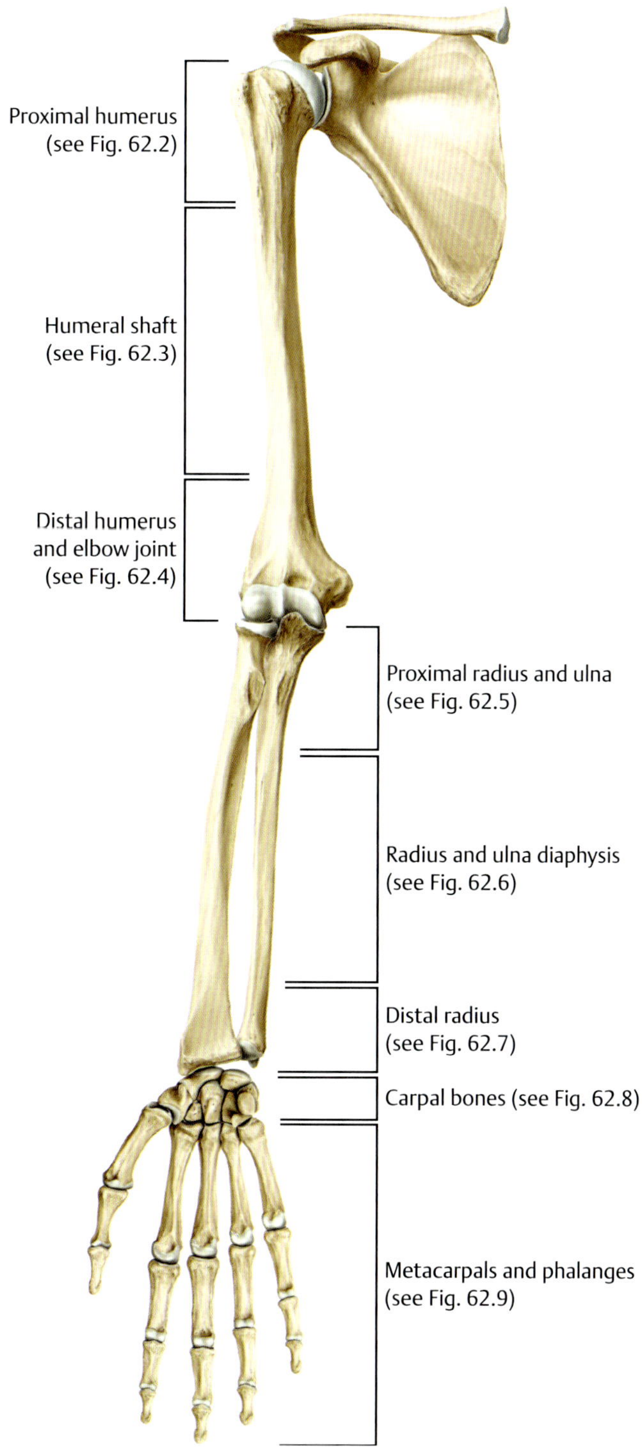

Fig. 62.1 AO/ASIF fracture classification.

Proximal Humerus

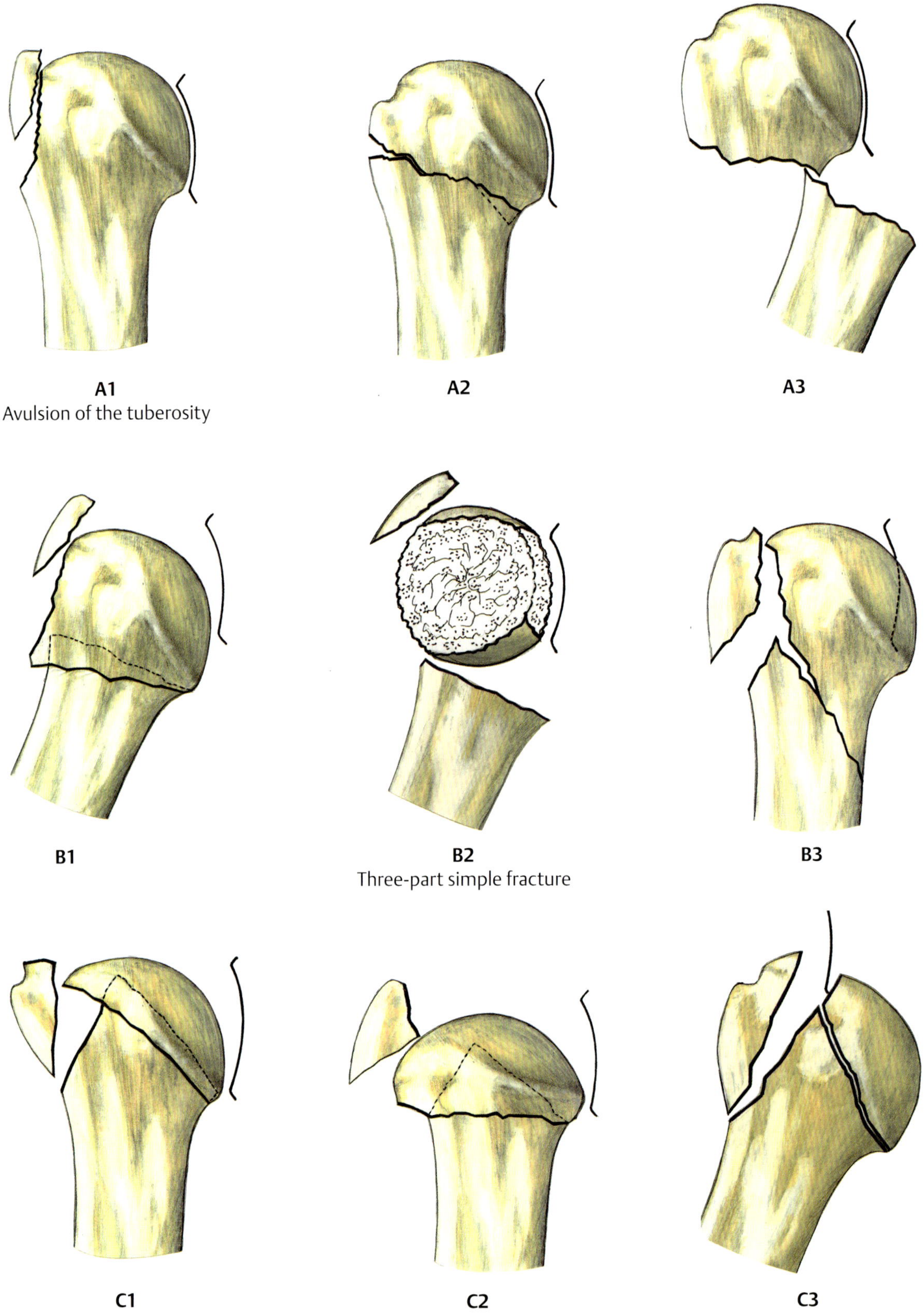

Fig. 62.2 AO/ASIF fracture classification: proximal humerus.

Humeral Shaft

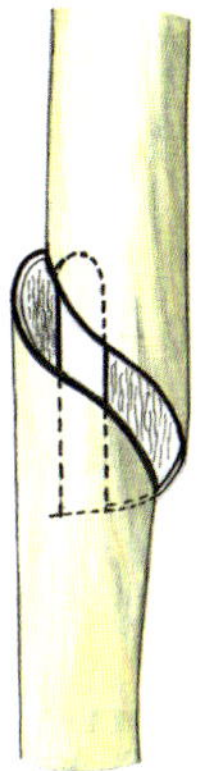

A1
Spiral diaphyseal fracture

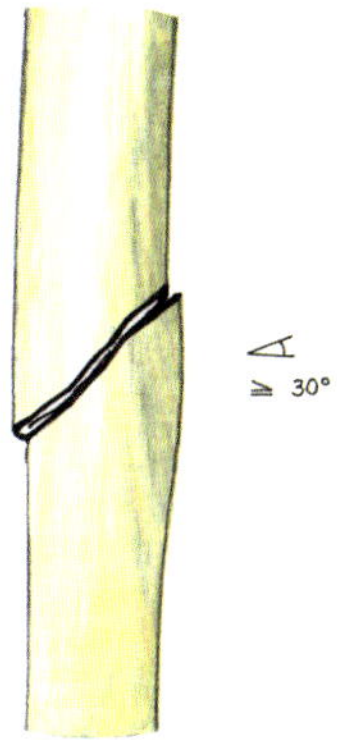

A2
Oblique diaphyseal fracture

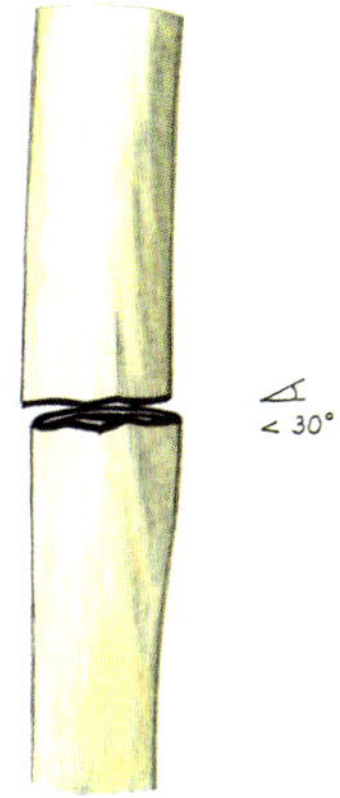

A3
Transverse diaphyseal fracture

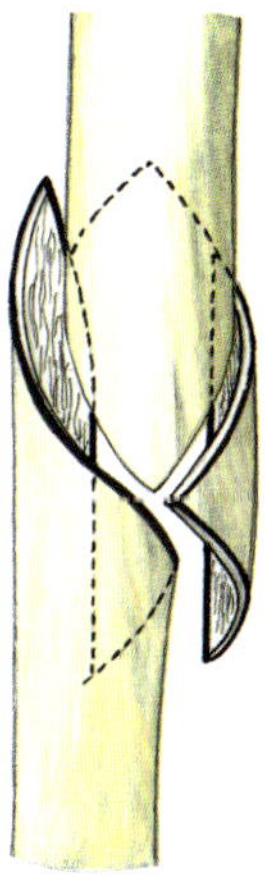

B1
Spiral diaphyseal butterfly fracture

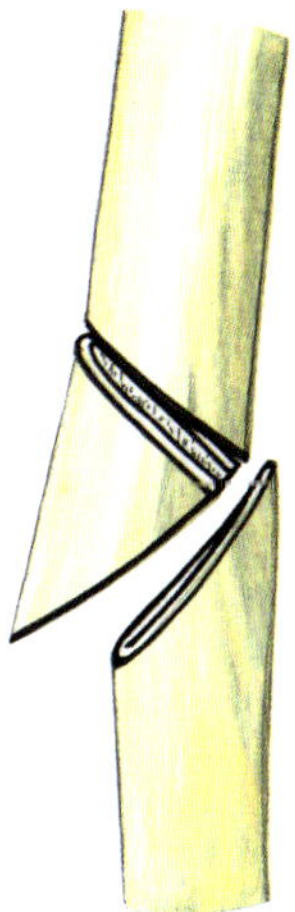

B2
Oblique diaphyseal butterfly fracture

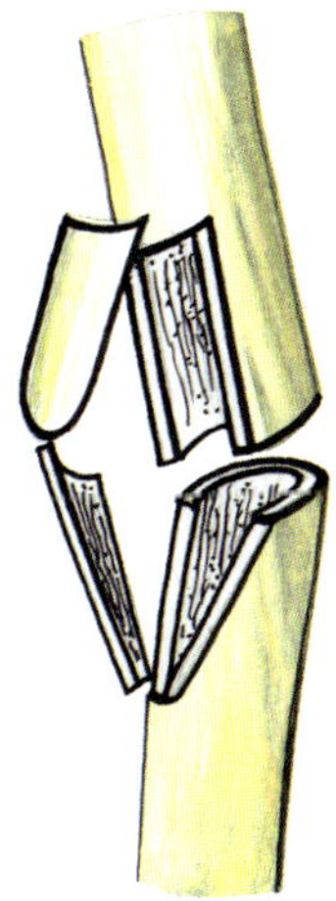

B3
Transverse diaphyseal butterfly fracture

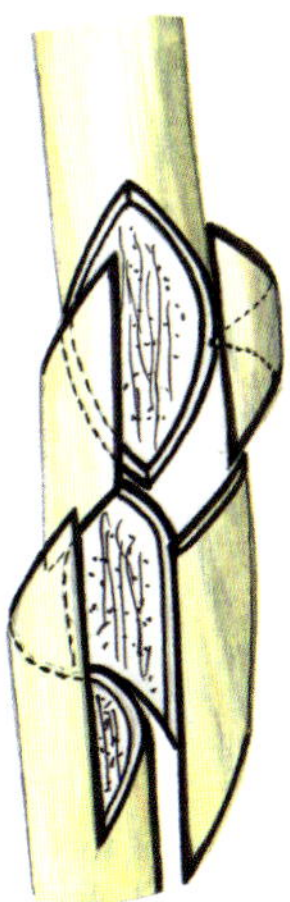

C1

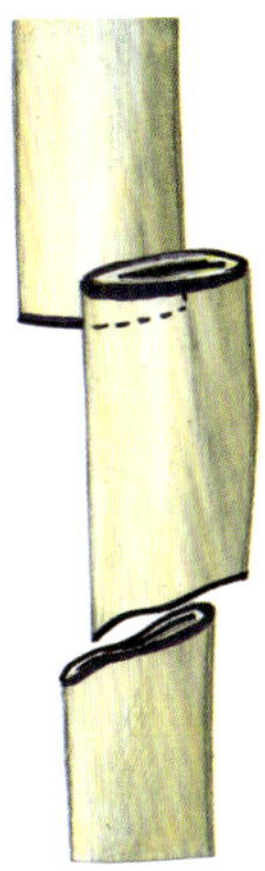

C2

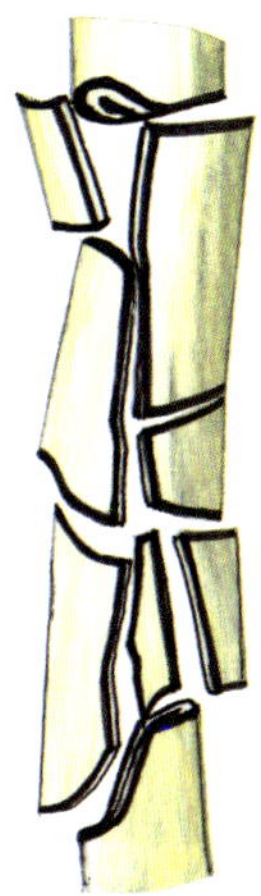

C3

Segmental or comminuted diaphyseal fracture

Fig. 62.3 AO/ASIF fracture classification: humeral shaft.

Distal Humerus and Elbow Joint

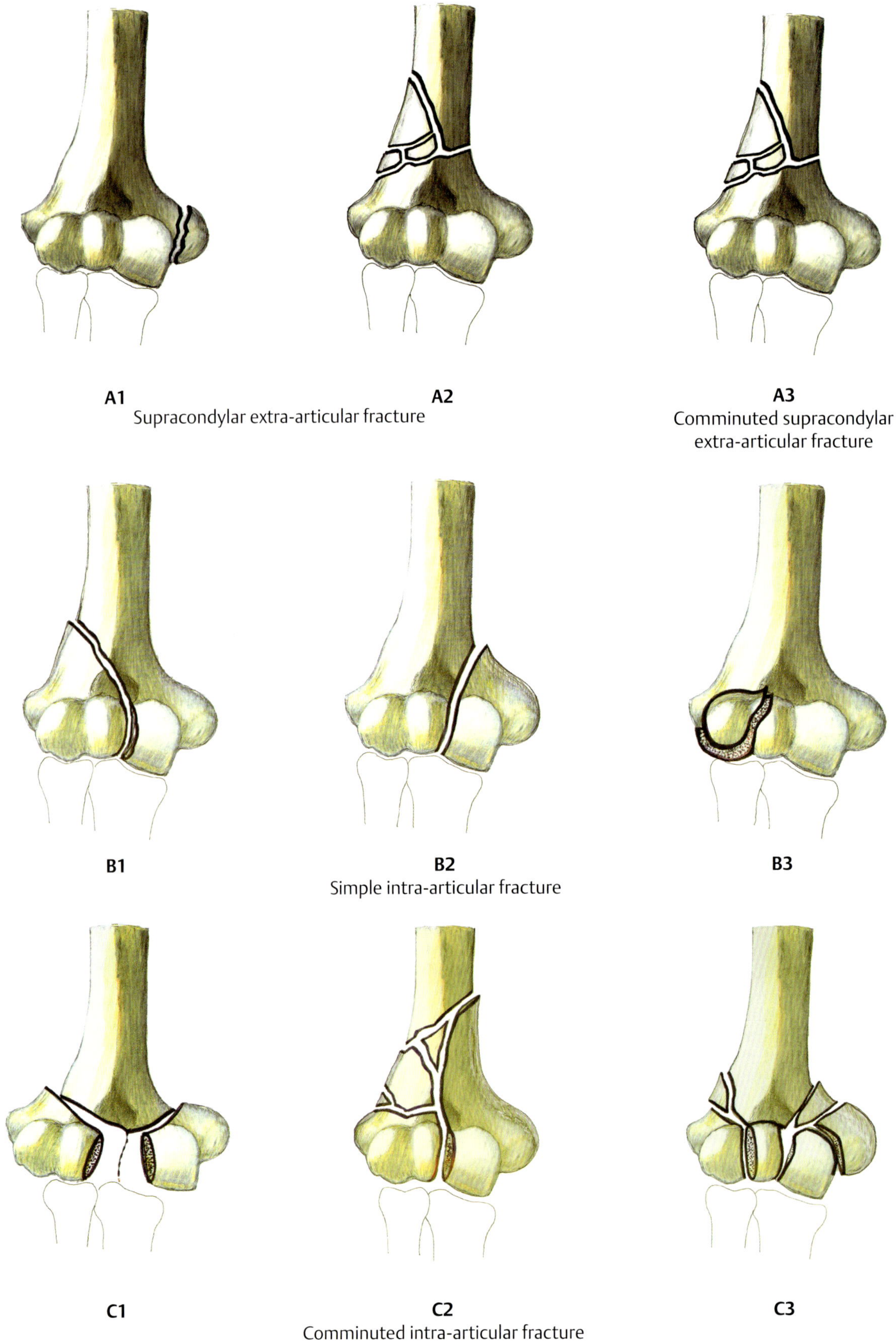

Fig. 62.4 AO/ASIF fracture classification: distal humerus and elbow joint.

Proximal Radius and Ulna

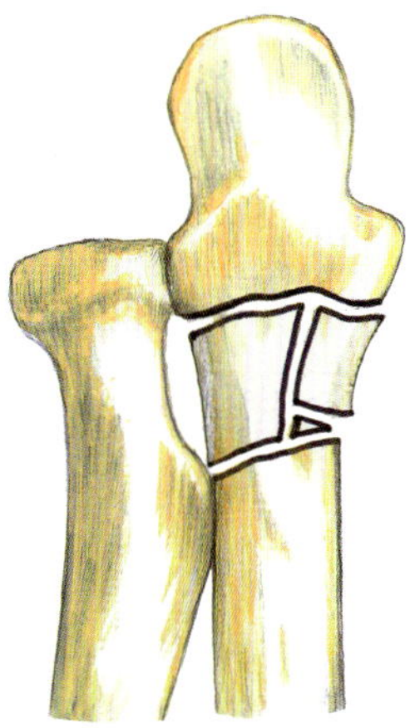

A1
Extra-articular ulnar fracture

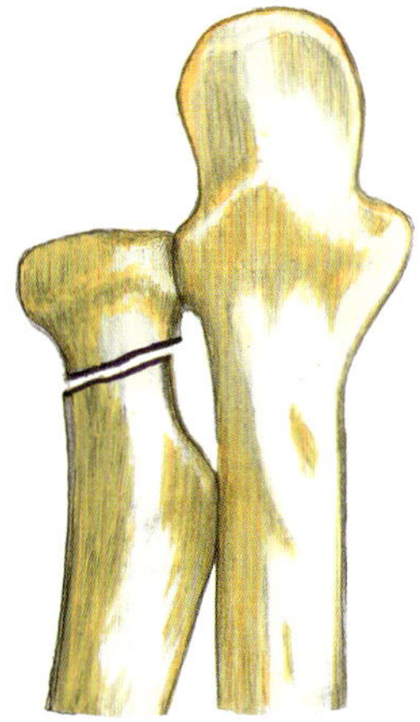

A2
Extra-articular radial head fracture

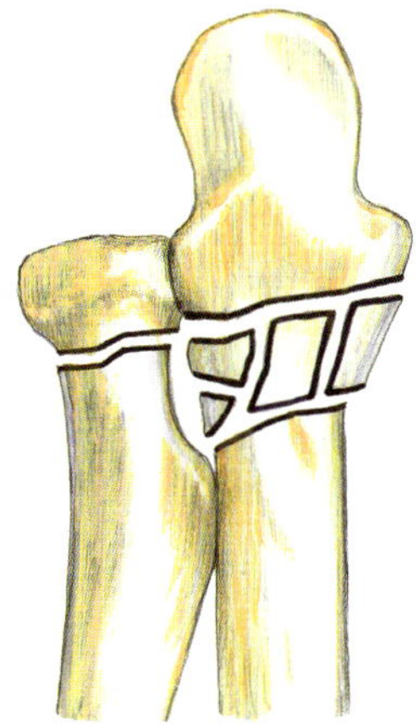

A3
Both bones extra-articular fracture

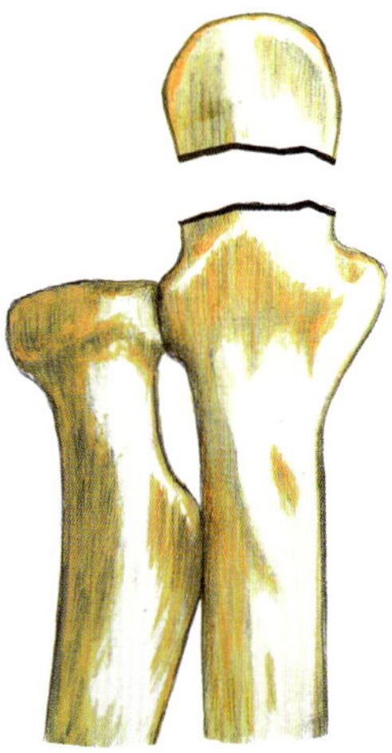

B1
Simple olecranon fracture

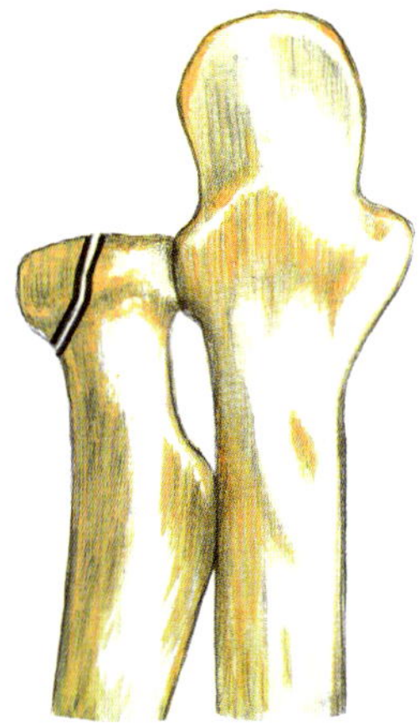

B2
Radial head fracture

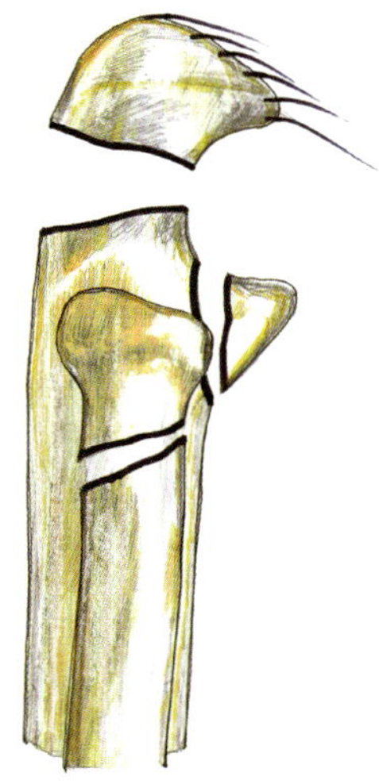

B3
Dislocated olecranon fracture with radial head fracture

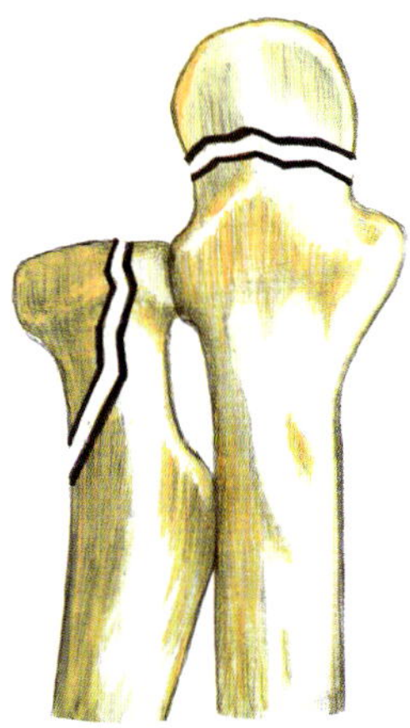

C1

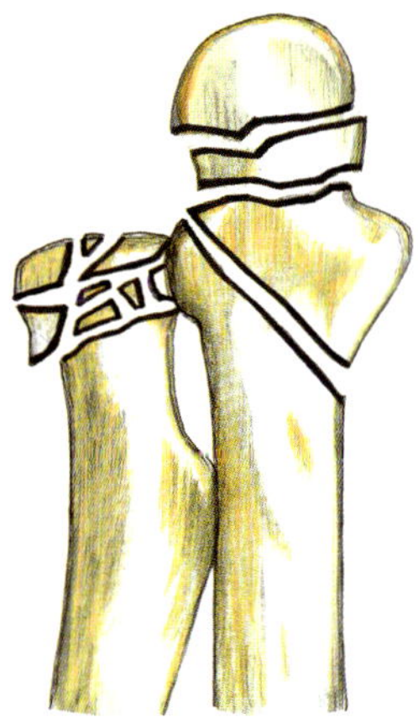

C2

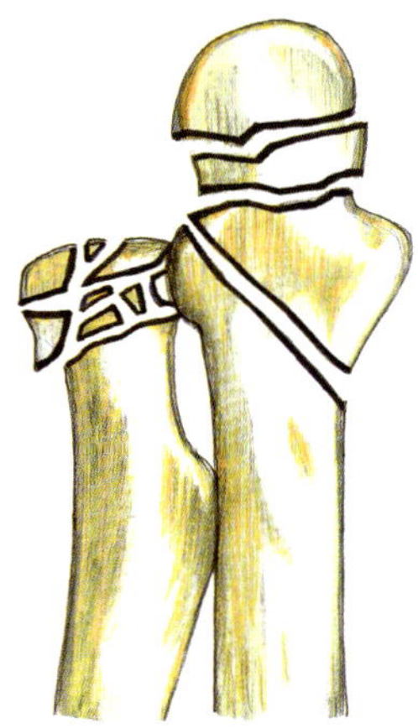

C3

Comminuted both bones intra-articular fracture

Fig. 62.5 AO/ASIF fracture classification: proximal radius and ulna.

Radius and Ulna Diaphysis

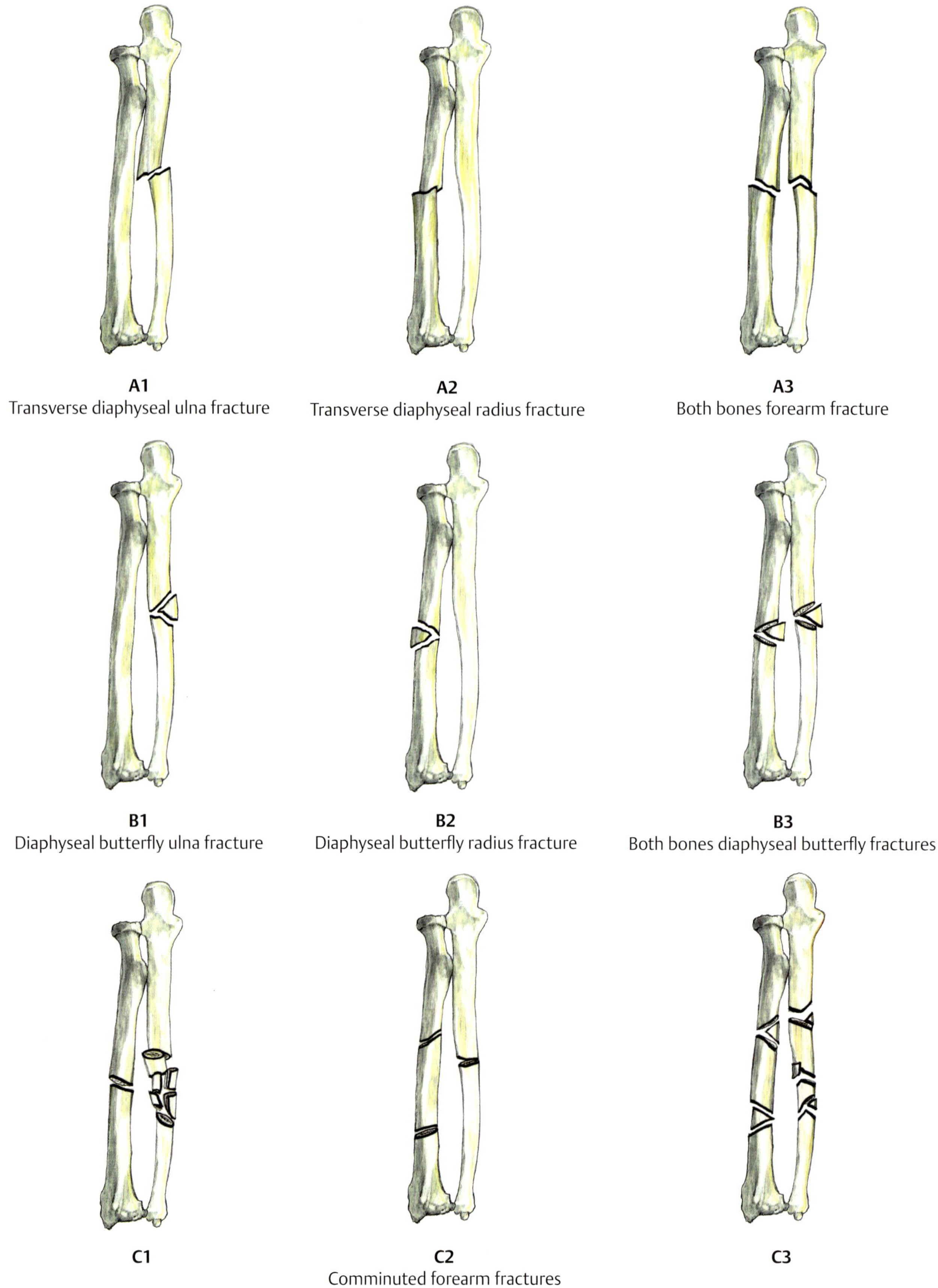

Fig. 62.6 AO/ASIF fracture classification: radius and ulna diaphysis.

Distal Radius

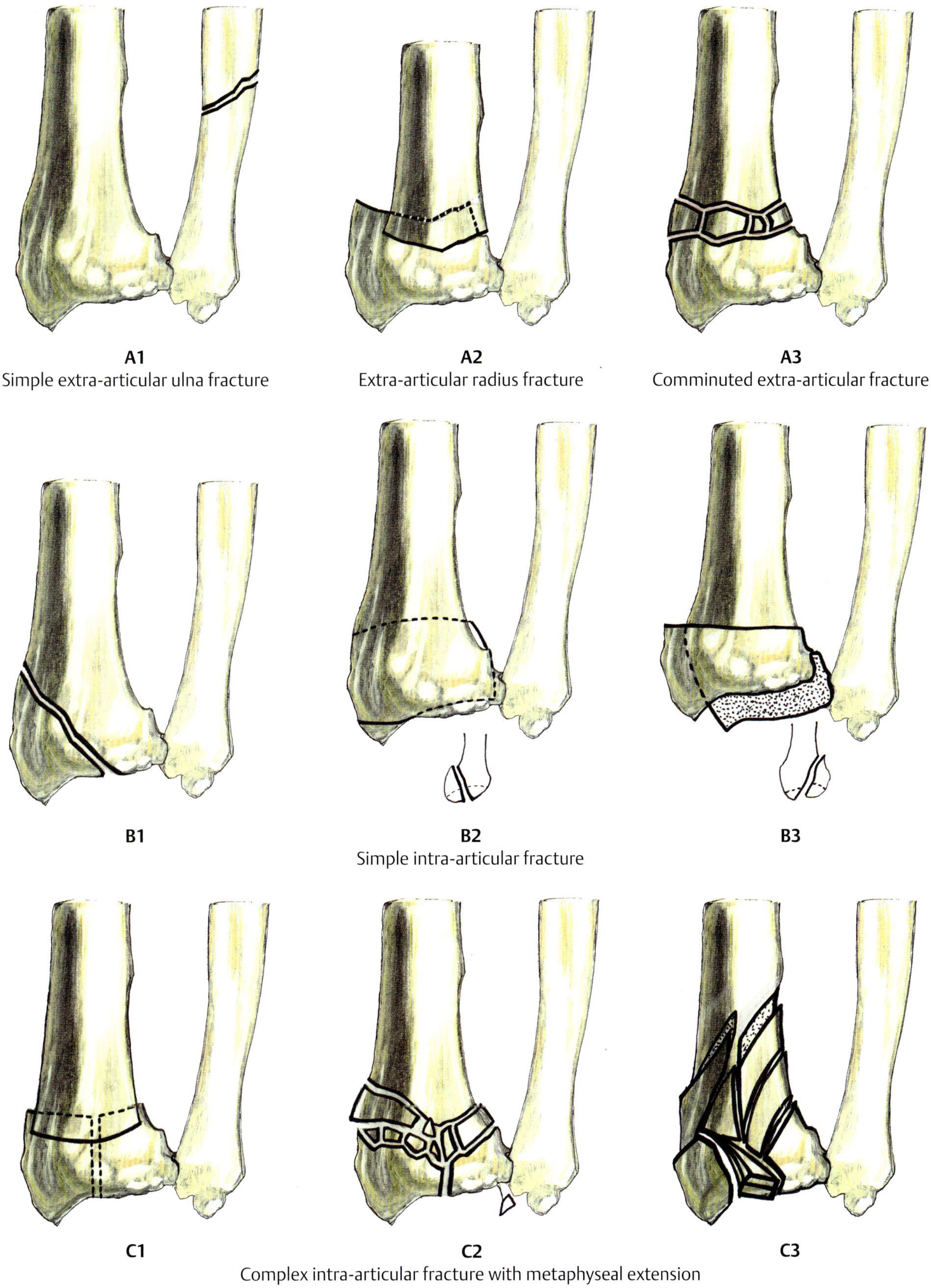

Fig. 62.7 AO/ASIF fracture classification: distal radius.

Carpal Bones

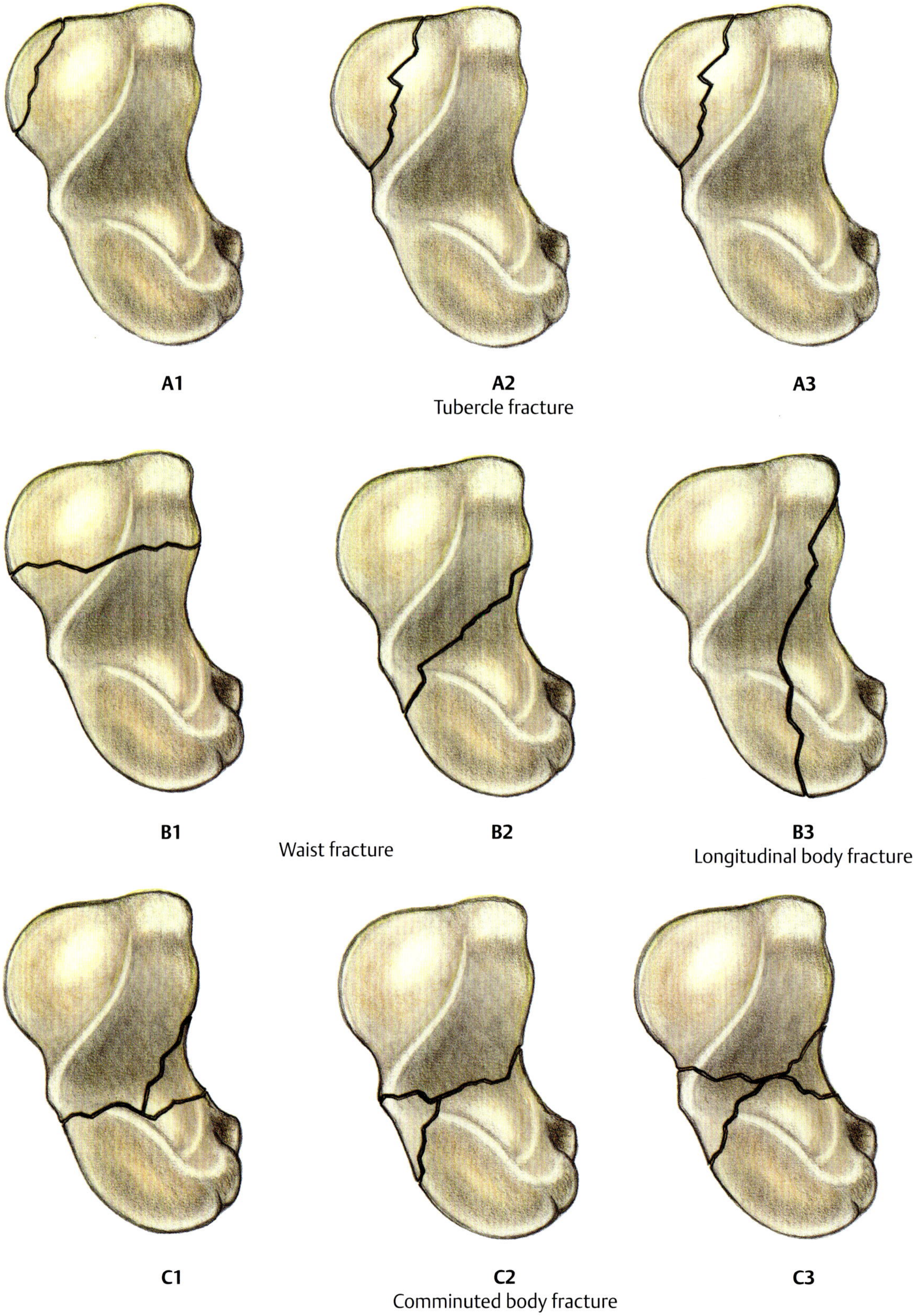

Fig. 62.8 AO/ASIF fracture classification: carpal bones.

Metacarpals and Phalanges

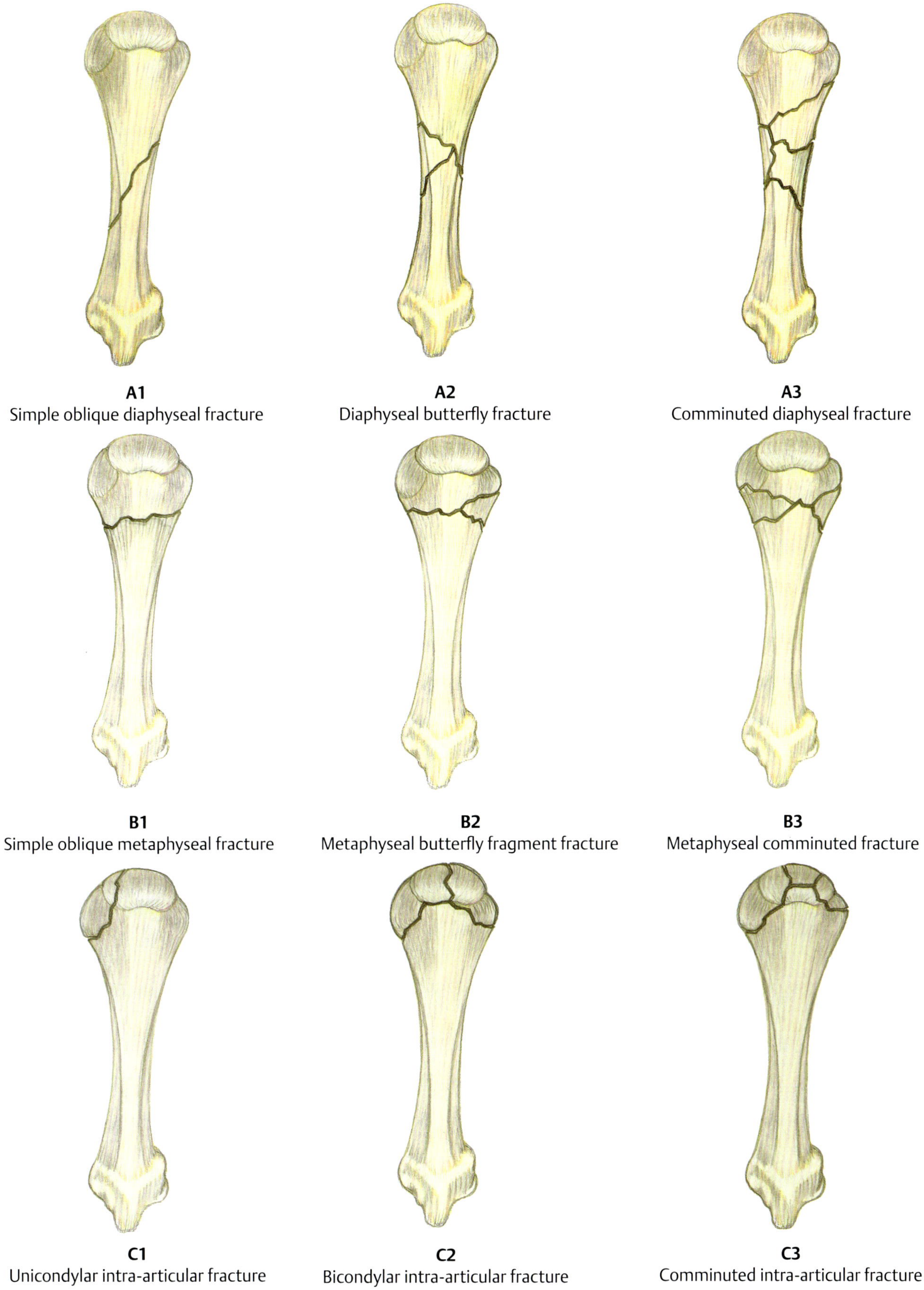

Fig. 62.9 AO/ASIF fracture classification: metacarpals and phalanges.

Chapter 63

Salter-Harris Classification of Pediatric Growth Plate Fractures

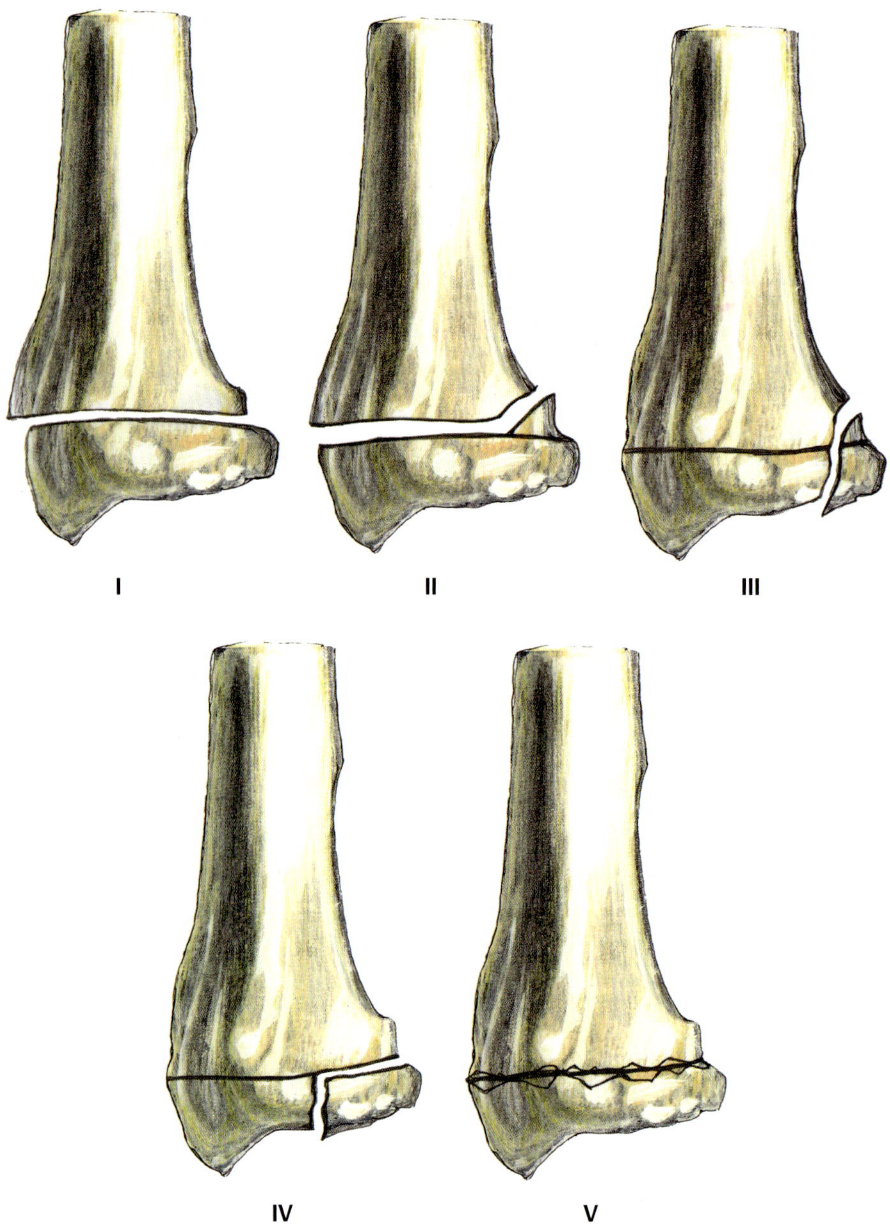

Fig. 63.1 Salter-Harris classification. (Data from Salter RB, Harris WR. Injuries involving the epiphyseal plate. Bone Joint J 1963; 45(3):623–641.)

Type I: Injury traverses horizontally across the physis (i.e., separation of the epiphysis)
Type II: Injury includes separation of a triangular piece of metaphyseal bone at one boundary of the physeal fracture
Type III: Injury traverses the physis incompletely and then extends through the epiphysis into the joint (i.e., intra-articular fracture without interference with the epiphyseal plate)
Type IV: Injury involves a vertical displaced fracture that passes from the articular surface through the epiphysis, plate, and metaphysis
Type V: Injury involves crushing of the physis without a bony fracture

Chapter 64

Classification of Nerve Injuries

In 1951, Sunderland expanded Seddon's classification to five degrees of peripheral nerve injury.

First-degree (Class I)

Seddon's neurapraxia and first-degree are the same.

Second-degree (Class II)

Seddon's axonotmesis and second-degree are the same.

Third-degree (Class III)

Third-degree is included within Seddon's Neurotmesis. Sunderland's third-degree is a nerve fiber interruption. In third-degree injury, there is a lesion of the endoneurium, but the epineurium and perineurium remain intact. Recovery from a third-degree injury is possible, but surgical intervention may be required.

Fourth-degree (Class III)

Fourth-degree is included within Seddon's Neurotmesis. In fourth-degree injury, only the epineurium remain intact. In this case, surgical repair is required.

Fifth-degree (Class III)

Fifth-degree is included within Seddon's Neurotmesis. Fifth-degree lesion is a complete transection of the nerve. Recovery is not possible without an appropriate surgical treatment

---

Data from Sunderland S. A classification of peripheral nerve injuries producing loss of function. Brain 1951;74(4):491–516.

Table 64.1 Mackinnon classification of nerve injuries

	Histopathologic changes					Tinel sign	
Degree of injury	**Myelin**	**Axon**	**Endoneurium**	**Perineurium**	**Epineurium**	**Present**	**Progresses distally**
I Neurapraxia	±	–	–	–	–	–	
II Axonotmesis	+	+	–	–	–	+	+
III	+	+	+	–	–	+	+
IV	+	+	+	+	–	+	–
V Neurotmesis	+	+	+	+	+	+	–
VI Various fibers and fascicles demonstrate various pathologic changes						+	±

Source: Data from Mackinnon SE. New directions in peripheral nerve surgery. Ann Plast Surg 1989;22(3): 257–273.

Chapter 65

Zones of Flexor Tendon Injuries

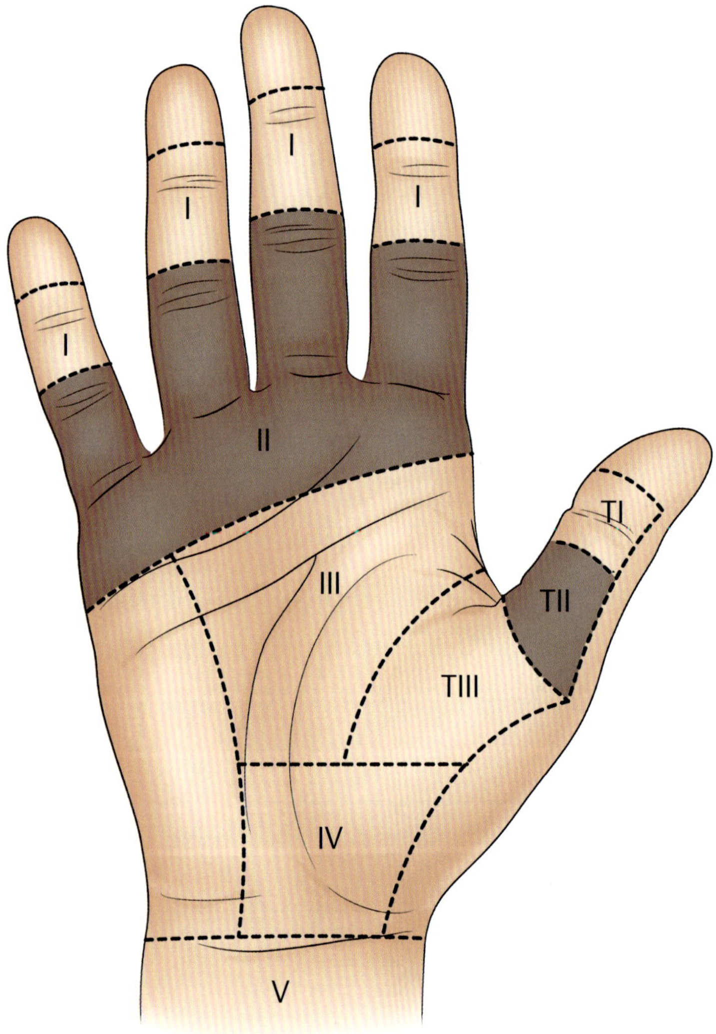

I Distal to the insertion of the FDS

II Proximal edge of the pulley system to the insertion of the FDS

III Distal end of the carpal tunnel at the A1 pulley

IV Length of the carpal tunnel

V Musculotendinous junction to the carpal tunnel

TI Distal to the IP joint

TII Distal to the MP joint

TIII Distal edge of the carpal tunnel to the proximal edge of the A1 pulley

Fig. 65.1 Zones of flexor tendon injuries. (Data from Kleinert HE, Schepel S, Gill T. Flexor tendon injuries. Surg Clin North Am 1981; 61:267–286.)

Chapter 66

Zones of Extensor Tendon Injuries

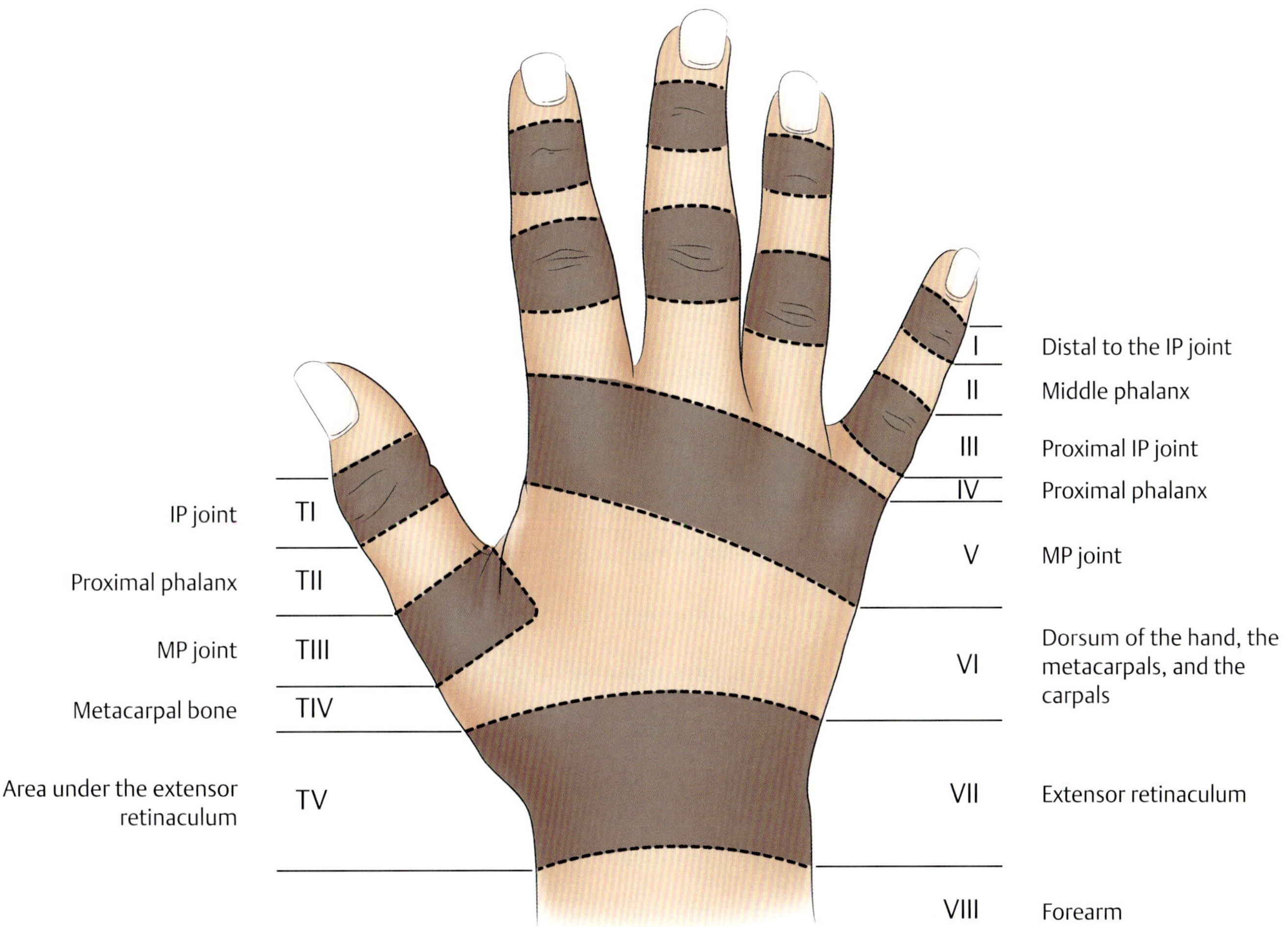

Fig. 66.1 Zones of extensor tendon injuries. (Data from Kleinert HE, Schepel S, Gill T. Flexor tendon injuries. Surg Clin North Am 1981; 61:267–286.)

Chapter 67

Carpal Instability

Box 67.1 Viegas' classification of carpal instability

I. Ulnar-sided perilunate instability
   A. Stage I: Partial to complete lunotriquetral tear (no VISI)
   B. Stage II: Complete tear of lunotriquetral ligaments, interosseous and volar (dynamic VISI)
   C. Stage III: As in Stage II plus disruption of the dorsal radiotriquetral ligament (static VISI)

II. Radial-sided perilunate instability
   A. Stage I: Partial to complete scapholunate tear (no DISI)
   B. Stage II: Complete scapholunate interosseous ligament tear plus tear of attenuation of the volar ligaments (dynamic DISI)
   C. Stage III: Complete disruption of the ligaments of Stage II plus dorsal radiotriquetral ligament disruption (static DISI)
   D. Stage IV: Complete disruption of all ligaments noted in Stage III (static DISI)

III. Dissociative
   Ligament lesion that is usually between the bones of the proximal carpal row but occasionally between the bones of the distal carpal row, the metacarpals, or even the radius and ulna

Data from Viegas SF, Patterson RM, Peterson PD, et al. Ulnar-sided perilunate instability: an anatomic and biomechanic study. J Hand Surg Am 1990;15: 268-278.

Chapter 68

Mayo Classification of Carpal Instabilities

Table 68.1 Mayo classification of carpal instabilities

	Type, site, and name	Radiographic pattern
I. CID	1.1 Proximal row CID	
	a. Unstable scaphoid fracture	DISI
	b. Scapholunate dissociation	DISI
	c. Lunotriquetral dissociation	VISI
	1.2 Distal carpal row CID	
	a. AR disruption	RT, PT
	b. AU disruption	UT, PT
	c. Combined AR and AU disruption	
	1.3 Combined proximal and distal CID	
II. CIND	2.1 Radiocarpal CIND	
	a. Volar ligament rupture	DISI, UT of entire proximal row, UT with increased SL space
	b. Dorsal ligament rupture	VISI, DT
	c. After radius malunion, Madelung deformity, scaphoid malunion, lunate malunion	
	2.2 Midcarpal CIND	
	a. Ulnar MCI from volar ligament damage	VISI
	b. Radial MCI from volar ligament damage	VISI
	c. Combined UMCI and RMCI, volar ligament damage	VISI
	d. MCI from dorsal ligament damage	DISI
	2.3 Radiocarpal–midcarpal CIND	
	a. Clip	VISI and DISI, alternating
	b. Disruption of radial and central ligaments	UT with or without VISI or DISI
III. CIC	a. Perilunate with radiocarpal instability	DISI and UT
	b. Perilunate with axial instability	AxUI and UT
	c. Radiocarpal with axial instability	AxRI and UT
	d. Scapholunate dissociation with UT	DISI and UT
IV. "Adaptive carpus"	a. Malposition of carpus with distal radius malunion	DISI or DT
	b. Malposition of carpus with scaphoid nonunion	DISI
	c. Malposition of carpus with lunate malunion	DISI or VISI
	d. Malposition of carpus with Madelung deformity	UT, DISI, PT

Source: From Carlsen BT, Shin AY. Wrist instability. Scand J Surg 2008;97(4):324–332. doi:10.1177/145749690809700409.

Chapter 69

Posttraumatic Arthritis

Stage I

Arthritis that is localized to the lateral (radial) side of the scaphoid and the radial styloid region of the distal radius

Stage II

Arthritis that extends to the entire radioscaphoid joint, with progressive radioscaphoid changes (II A) or arthritis from the radioscaphoid joint that secondarily involves the STT joint (II B)

Stage III

Arthritis that extends in a periscaphoid distribution and that involves the radioscaphoid and lunocapitate joints

Bibliography

Part I: General Principles

Adani R, Castagnetti C, Landi A. Degloving injuries of the hand and fingers. Clin Orthop Relat Res 1995;(314):19–25

Biemer E. Experience in replantation surgery in the upper extremity. Ann Acad Med Singapore 1979;8(4):393–397

Brown H. Closed crush injuries of the hand and forearm. Orthop Clin North Am 1970;1(2):253–259

Büchler U. Traumatic soft-tissue defects of the extremities. Implications and treatment guidelines. Arch Orthop Trauma Surg 1990;109(6):321–329

Chen SH, Wei FC, Noordhoff SM. Free vascularized joint transfers in acute complex hand injuries: case reports. J Trauma 1992;33(6):924–930

Chow SP, So YC, Pun WK, Luk KD, Leong JC. Thenar crush injuries. J Bone Joint Surg Br 1988;70(1):135–139

Cooney WP, Linscheid RL, Dobyns JH, eds. The Wrist—Diagnosis and Operative Treatment. St Louis, MO: CV Mosby; 1988

Garcia-Elias M, Abanco J, Salvador E, Sanchez R. Crush injury of the carpus. J Bone Joint Surg Br 1984;67(2):286–289

Germann G, Harth A, Wind G, Demir E. [Standardisation and validation of the German version 2.0 of the Disability of Arm, Shoulder, Hand (DASH) questionnaire]. Unfallchirurg 2003;106(1):13–19

Germann G, Karle B, Brüner S, Menke H. [Treatment strategy in complex hand injuries]. Unfallchirurg 2000;103(5):342–347

Green DP. Operative Hand Surgery. 4th ed. New York, NY: Churchill Livingstone; 1988

Heaps RJ, Levin LS. Hand fractures. In: Garrett WE, Speer KP, Kirkendall DT, eds. Principles and Practice of Orthopaedic Sports Medicine. Philadelphia, PA: Lippincott Williams & Wilkins; 2004

Heitmann C, Patzakis MJ, Tetsworth K, Levin LS. Musculoskeletal sepsis: principles of treatment. AAOS Instructional Course Lecture 52. 2003;733–743

Lerman OZ, Haddock N, Elliott RM, Foroohar A, Levin LS. Microsurgery of the upper extremity. J Hand Surg Am 2011;36(6):1092–1103

Levin LS, Erdmann DE. Primary and secondary microvascular reconstruction of the upper extremity. Hand Clin 2001;17(3):447–455

Lister G. The Hand: Diagnosis and Indications. 3rd ed. Edinburgh, UK: Churchill Livingstone; 1993

Megerle K, Sauerbier M, Germann G. The evolution of the pedicled radial forearm flap. Hand 2010;5(1):37–42. doi:10.1007/s11552-009-9231-6

Sherman R. The butterfly effect. Plast Reconstr Surg 2009;124(4):1357–1358. doi: 10.1097/PRS.0b013e3181b715c8

Sherman R. To reconstruct or not to reconstruct? N Engl J Med 2002;347(24):1906–1907

Sherman R, Rahban S, Pollak AN. Timing of wound coverage in extremity war injuries. J Am Acad Orthop Surg 2006;14(10):S57–S61

Simpson SG. Farm machinery injuries. J Trauma 1984; 24:150–152

Weiland AJ, Villarreal-Rios A, Kleinert HE, Kutz J, Atasoy E, Lister G. Replantation of digits and hands: analysis of surgical techniques and functional results in 71 patients with 86 replantations. J Hand Surg 1977;2(1):1–12

Part II: Techniques of Structure Repair

Beng HL, Tsai TS. The six strand technique for flexor tendon repair. In: Taras JS, Schneider LH, eds. Atlas of the Hand Clinics. Boston, MA: WB Saunders; 1996

Bickert B, Heitmann CH, Germann G. Fibulo-scapho-lunate arthrodesis as a motion-preserving procedure after tumour resection of the distal radius. J Hand Surg Br 2002;27(6):573–576

Bickert B, Sauerbier M, Germann G. Scapholunate ligament repair using the Mitek bone anchor. J Hand Surg Br 2000;25(2):188–192

Bruner JM. The zig-zag volar digital incision for flexor-tendon surgery. Plast Reconstr Surg 1976;40(6):571–574

Bunnell S. Repair of tendons in fingers and description of two new instruments. Surg Gyn Obstet 1918;26:103–110

Chen SH, Wei FC, Chen HC, Chuang CC, Noordhoff S. Miniature plates and screws in acute complex hand injury. J Trauma 1994;37(2):237–242

Erdmann D, Garcia RM, Blueschke G, Brigman BE, Levin LS. Vascularized fibula-based physis transfer for pediatric proximal humerus reconstruction. Plast Reconst Surg 2013;132(2):281e–287e

Fernandez DL, Jupiter JB. Fractures of the Distal Radius: A Practical Approach to Management. New York, NY: Springer-Verlag; 1996

Heim U. [Indications and technique of AO osteosynthesis in the treatment of the fractures of the hand]. Acta Orthop Belg 1973;39(6):957–972

Heitmann C, Erdmann D, Levin LS. Treatment of segmental defects of the humerus with an osteoseptocutaneous fibular transplant. J Bone Joint Surg Am 2002;84(12):2216–2223

Herbert TJ, Fischer WE, Leicester AW. The Herbert bone screw: a ten year perspective. J Hand Surg Br 1992; 17(4):415–419

Kessler I. The "grasping" technique for tendon repair. Hand 1973;5(3):253–255

Kirchmayr L. Zur Technik der Sehnennaht. Zbl Chir 1917; 44:906–907

Küntscher M, Tränkle M, Sauerbier M, Germann G, Bickert B. [Management of proximal scaphoid bone pseudoarthroses and fractures with the mini-Herbert screw via a dorsal approach]. Unfallchirurg 2001;104(9):813–819

Küntscher MV, Schäfer DJ, Germann G, Siebert HR. [Metacarpal fractures: treatment indications and options. Results of a multicenter study]. Chirurg 2003;74(11):1018–1025

O'Brien BM. Replantation and reconstructive microvascular surgery. Part II. Ann R Coll Surg Engl 1976;58(3):171–182

Ohlbauer M, Sauerbier M, Heitmann C, Germann G. [Improved outcome of nerve injuries in the upper extremity]. Nervenarzt 2006;77(8):922–930

Pulvertaft RG. Reconstruction of the mutilated hand. Erik Moberg Lecture 1977. Scand J Plast Reconstr Surg 1977;11(3):219–224

Saffer P. Carpal Injuries: Anatomy, Radiology, Current Treatment. New York, NY: Springer-Verlag; 1991

Sauerbier M, Tränkle M, Linsner G, Bickert B, Germann G. Midcarpal arthrodesis with complete scaphoid excision and interposition bone graft in the treatment of advanced carpal collapse (SNAC/SLAC wrist): operative technique and outcome assessment. J Hand Surg Br 2000;25(4):341–345

Scheufler O, Andresen R, Radmer S, Erdmann D, Exner K, Germann G. Hook of hamate fractures: critical evaluation of different therapeutic procedures. Plast Reconstr Surg 2005;115(2):488–497

Strickland JW. Results of flexor tendon surgery in zone II. Hand Clin 1985;1(1):167–179

Tintle SM, Levin LS. The reconstructive microsurgery ladder in orthopaedics. Injury 2013;44(3):376–385

Verdan C. Tendon Surgery of the Hand. Edinburgh, UK: Churchill Livingstone; 1979

Yajima H, Inada Y, Shono M, Tamai S. Radial forearm flap with vascularized tendons for hand reconstruction. Plast Reconstr Surg 1967;98(2):328–333

Part III: Treatment Algorithms

Atasoy E, O'Neill WL. Local flap coverage about the hand. In: Levin LS, Germann G, eds. Atlas of the Hand Clinics. Vol 3. Philadelphia, PA: WB Saunders; 1998

Baccarani A, Follmar KE, De Santis G, et al. Free vascularized tissue transfer to preserve upper extremity amputation levels. Plast Reconstr Surg 2007;120(4):971–981

Chen CL, Chiu HY, Lee JW, Yang JT. Arterialized tendocutaneous venous flap for dorsal finger reconstruction. Microsurgery 1994;15(12):886–890

Germann G, Levin S. Intrinsic flaps in the hand: new concepts in skin coverage. Tech Hand Up Extrem Surg 1997;1(1):48–61

Germann G, Rudolf KD, Levin LS, Hrabowski M. Fingertip and thumb tip wounds: changing algorithms for sensation, aesthetics, and function. J Hand Surgery Am 2017;42(4):274–284

Heitmann C, Levin LS. Alternatives to thumb replantation. Plast and Reconstr Surg 2001;110(6): 1492–1503

Levin LS. Vascularized bone grafting. In: Volgas DA, Harder Y. AO Manual of Soft-Tissue Management in Orthopaedic Trauma. AO Foundation

Levin LS, Boyer MI, Bozentka DJ, et al. Skin and soft tissue. In: Hammert WC, Boyer MI, Bozentka DJ, Calfee RP, eds. ASSH Manual of Hand Surgery. Philadelphia, PA: Lippincott Williams & Wilkins; 2010

Megerle K, Keutgen X, Müller M, Germann G, Sauerbier M. Treatment of scaphoid non-unions of the proximal third with conventional bone grafting and mini-Herbert screws: an analysis of clinical and radiological results. J Hand Surg Eur 2008;33(2):179–185. doi:10.1177/1753193408087030

Millesi H. Brachial plexus injuries. Nerve grafting. Clin Orthop Relat Res 1988;(237):36–42

Morrison WA, O'Brien BM, MacLeod AM. Thumb reconstruction with a free neurovascular wrap-around flap from the big toe. J Hand Surg Am 1980;5(6):575–577

Müller M, Germann G, Sauerbier M. Minimal invasive screw fixation and early mobilization of acute scaphoid fractures in the middle third: operative technique and early functional outcome. Tech Hand Up Extrem Surg 2008;12(2):107–113.

Ong YS, Levin LS. Hand infections. Plast Reconstr Surg 2009;124(4):225e–233e

Pestana IA, Coan B, Erdmann D, Marcus J, Levin L, Zenn MR. Early experience with fluorescent angiography in free-tissue transfer reconstruction. 2009;123(4):1239–1244

Rockwell WB, Lister GD. Soft tissue reconstruction. Coverage of hand injuries. Orthop Clin North Am 1993;24(3):411–424

Sauerbier M, Bickert B, Tränkle M, Kluge S, Pelzer M, Germann G. [Surgical treatment possibilities of advanced carpal collapse (SNAC/SLAC wrist)]. Unfallchirurg 2000;103(7):564–571

Shibu MM, Tarabe MA, Graham K, Dickson MG, Mahaffey PJ. Fingertip reconstruction with a dorsal island homodigital flap. Br J Plast Surg 1997;50(2):121–124

Stice RC, Wood MB. Neurovascular island skin flaps in the hand: functional and sensibility evaluations. Microsurgery 1987:8(3):162–167

Tsai TM, Matiko JD, Breidenbach W, Kutz JE. Venous flaps in digital revascularization and replantation. J Reconstr Microsurg 1987;3(2):113–119

Tubiana R, Duparc J. Restoration of sensibility in the hand by neurovascular skin island transfer. J Bone Joint Surg Br 1961;43(3):474–480

Zalavras CG, Patzakis MJ, Holtom PD, Sherman R. Management of open fractures. Infect Dis Clin North Am 2005;19(4):915–929.

Part IV: Clinical Examples

Altintas AA, Altintas MA, Gazyakan E, Gohla T, Germann G, Sauerbier M. Long-term results and the disabilities of the arm, shoulder, and hand score analysis after modified Brooks and D'Aubigne tendon transfer for radial nerve palsy. J Hand Surg Am 2009;34(3):474–478. doi:10.1016/j.jhsa.2008.11.012

Barisoni D, Bortolani A, Sanna A, Lorenzini M, Governa M. Free flap cover of acute burns and post-burn deformity. Eur J Plast Surg 1996;19(5):257–261

Baumeister S, Germann G, Dragu A, Tränkle M, Sauerbier M. [Functional results after proximal row carpectomy (PRC) in patients with SNAC-/SLAC-wrist stage II]. Handchir Mikrochir Plast Chir 2005;37(2):106–112. doi:10.1055/s-2004-830435

Baumeister S, Köller M, Dragu A, Germann G, Sauerbier M. Principles of microvascular reconstruction in burn and electrical burn injuries. Burns 2005;31(1):92–98

Dacho A, Grundel J, Harth A, Germann G, Sauerbier M. [Functional outcome after midcarpal arthrodesis in the treatment of advanced carpal collapse (SNAC-/SLAC-wrist)]. Handchir Mikrochir Plast Chir 2005;37(2):119–125

Germann G, Funk H, Bickert B. The fate of the dorsal metacarpal arterial system following thermal injury to the dorsal hand: a Doppler sonographic study. J Hand Surg Am 2000; 25(5):962–968

Giessler GA, Leopold A, Germann G, Heitmann C. [Blast injuries of the hands. Patterns of trauma and plastic surgical treatment]. Unfallchirurg 2006;109(11):956–963

Gregory H, Pelzer M, Gazyakan E, Sauerbier M, Germann G, Heitmann C. [Experiences with the distally based dorsal metacarpal artery (DMCA) flap and its variants in 41 cases]. Handchir Mikrochir Plast Chir 2006;38(2):75–81

Isaacs J, Levin LS. Pedicled and free tissue transfer for the treatment of recalcitrant neuralgia. Am Soc Surg Hand 2008;509–520

Kremer T, Sauerbier M, Trankle M, Dragu A, Germann G, Baumeister S. Functional results after proximal row carpectomy to salvage a wrist. Scand J Plast Reconstr Surg Hand Surg 2008;42(6):308–312. doi:10.1080/02844310802393990

Levin LS. Cutaneous tumors of the hand: Hand Surgery Update. Am Acad Orthop Surg 1999;359-368

Levin LS, Allen DM. Digital replantation including postoperative care. Tech Hand Up Extrem Surg 2002;6(4):171–177

Levin LS, Heitmann C. Applications of the vascularized fibula for the upper extremity reconstruction. Tech Hand Up Extrem Surg 2003;7(1):12–17

Levin LS, Rozell JC, Pulos N. Distal radius fractures in the elderly. J Am Acad Orthop Surg 2017;25(3):179–187

Megerle K, Bertel D, Germann G, Lehnhardt M, Hellmich S. Long-term results of dorsal intercarpal ligament capsulodesis for the treatment of chronic scapholunate instability. J Bone Joint Surg Br 2012;94(12):1660–1665. doi:10.1302/0301-620X.94B12.30007

Ray EC, Sherman R, Stevanovic M. Immediate reconstruction of a nonreplantable thumb amputation by great toe transfer. Plast Reconstr Surg 2009;123(1):259–267. doi:10.1097/PRS.0b013e3181934715

Sauerbier M, Kluge S, Bickert B, Germann G. Subjective and objective outcomes after total wrist arthrodesis in patients with radiocarpal arthrosis or Kienböck's disease. Chir Main 2000;19(4):223–231

Vetter M, Germann G, Bickert B, Sauerbier M. Current strategies for sarcoma reconstruction at the forearm and hand. J Reconstr Microsurg 2010;26(7):455–60. doi:10.1055/s-0030-1254229

Walsh M, Levin LS. Composite free tissue transfer/toe to hand. In: Rayan GM, Chung KC. Flap Reconstruction of the Upper Extremity: A Master Skills Publication. 2009, American Society for Surgery of the Hand

Zenn MR, Levin LS. Multiple digit replantation. In: Weinzweig N, Weinzweig J. The Mutilated Hand. Elsevier; 2005

Part V: Atlas of Flaps—Pearls and Pitfalls

Abdul-Hassan HS, von Drasek Ascher G, Acland RD. Surgical anatomy and blood supply of the fascial layers of the temporal region. Plast Reconstr Surg 1986;77(1):17–28

Atasoy E. Reversed cross-finger subcutaneous flap. J Hand Surg Am 1982;7(5):481–483

Atasoy E, Loakimidis E, Kasdan ML, Kutz JE, Kleinert HE. Reconstruction of the amputated finger tip with a triangular volar flap. A new surgical procedure. J Bone Joint Surg Am 1970;52(5):921–926

Baumeister S, Menke H, Wittemann M, Germann G. Functional outcome after the Moberg advancement flap in the thumb. J Hand Surg Am 2002;27(1):105–114

Braun RM, Rechnic M, Neill-Cage DJ, Schorr RT. The retrograde radial fascial forearm flap: surgical rationale, technique, and clinical application. J Hand Surg Am 1995;20(6):915–922

Cronin TD. The cross finger flap: a new method of repair. Am Surg 1951;17(5):419–425

Daniel RK, Taylor GI. Distant transfer of an island flap by microvascular anastomoses. A clinical technique. Plast Reconstr Surg 1973;52(2):111–117

Dos Santos LF. The vascular anatomy and dissection of the free scapula flap. Plast Reconst Surg 1984;73(4):599–604

Earley MJ, Milner RH. Dorsal metacarpal flaps. Br J Plast Surg 1987;40:333–341

Fischer JP, Elliott RM, Kozin SH, Levin LS. Free function muscle transfers for upper extremity reconstruction: a review of indications, techniques, and outcomes. J Hand Surg Am 2013;38(12):2485–2490. doi:10.1016/j.jhsa.2013.03.041

Flügel A, Kehrer A, Heitmann C, Germann G, Sauerbier M. Coverage of soft-tissue defects of the hand with free fascial flaps. Microsurgery 2005;25(1):47–53

Foucher G, Braun JB. A new island flap transfer from the dorsum of the index to the thumb. Plast Reconstr Surg 1979;63(3):344–349

Gang RK. The Chinese forearm flap in reconstruction of the hand. J Hand Surg Br 1990;15(1): 84–88

Geissendörffer H. [Thoughts on fingertip plasty—first description of a lateral V-Y flap]. Zbl Chir 1943;70:1107–1108

Germann G, Biedermann N, Levin LS. Intrinsic flaps in the hand. Clin Plast Surg 2011;38(4): 729–738. doi:10.1016/j.cps.2011.07.007

Germann G, Bruener S. Free flap coverage of palmar hand wounds. Tech Hand Up Extrem Surg 2000;4(4):272–281

Germann G, Rütschle S, Kania N, Raff T. The reverse pedicle heterodigital cross-finger island flap. J Hand Surg Br 1997;22(1):25–29

Germann G, Sauerbier M, Steinau HU, Wood MB. Reverse segmental pedicled ulna transfer as a salvage procedure in wrist fusion. J Hand Surg Br 2001;26(6):589–592

Germann G, Steinau HU. Functional soft-tissue coverage in skeletonizing injuries of the upper extremity using the ipsilateral latissimus dorsi myocutaneous flap. Plast Reconstr Surg 1995;96(5):1130–1135

Giessler GA, Bickert B, Sauerbier M, Germann G. [Free microvascular fibula graft for skeletal reconstruction after tumor resections in the forearm—experience with five cases]. Handchir Mikrochir Plast Chir 2004;36(5):301–307

Giessler GA, Schmidt AB, Germann G, Pelzer M. The role of fabricated chimeric free flaps in reconstruction of devastating hand and forearm injuries. J Reconstr Microsurg 2011; 27(9):567–573. doi:10.1055/s-0031-1287672

Heitmann C, Higgins LD, Levin LS. Treatment of deep infections of the shoulder with pedicled myocutaneous flaps. J Shoulder Elbow Surg 2004;13(1):13–17

Hrabowski M, Kloeters O, Germann G. Reverse homodigital dorsoradial flap for thumb soft tissue reconstruction: surgical technique. J Hand Surg Am 2010;35(4):659–662. doi:10.1016/j.jhsa.2010.01.013

Katsaros I, Schusterman M, Beppu M, Banis JC, Acland RC. The lateral upper arm flap: anatomy and clinical applications. Ann Plast Surg 1984;12(6):489–500

Kazmers NH, Thibaudeau S, Steinberger Z, Levin LS. Upper and lower extremity reconstructive applications utilizing free flaps from the medial genicular arterial system: a systematic review. Microsurgery 2016. doi:10.1002/micr.30138

Kremer T, Bickert B, Germann G, Heitmann C, Sauerbier M. Outcome assessment after reconstruction of complex defects of the forearm and hand with osteocutaneous free flaps. Plast Reconstr Surg 2006;118(2):443–454; discussion 455–456

Küntscher MV, Erdmann D, Strametz S, Sauerbier M, Germann G, Levin LS. [The use of fillet flaps in upper extremity and shoulder reconstruction]. Chirurg 2002;73(10):1019–1024

Kutler W. A new method for finger tip amputation. J Am Med Assoc 1947;133(1):29

Levin LS, Erdmann D, Germann G. The use of fillet flaps in upper extremity reconstruction. J Hand Surg Am 2002;2(1):39–44

Manktelow RT, McKee NH. Free muscle transplantation to provide active finger flexion. J Hand Surg Am 1978;3(5):416–426

Maruyama Y. The reverse dorsal metacarpal flap. Br J Plast Surg 1990;43(1):24–27

McGregor IA, Jackson IT. The groin flap. Br J Plast Surg 1972;25(1):3–16

Moberg E. Aspects of sensation in reconstructive surgery of the upper extremity. J Bone Joint Surg Am 1964;46:817–825

Nassif TM, Vidal L, Bovet JL, Baudet J. The parascapular flap: a new cutaneous microsurgical free flap. Plast Reconst Surg 1982;69(4):591–600

Pelzer M, Reichenberger M, Germann G. Osteo-periosteal-cutaneous flaps of the medial femoral condyle: a valuable modification for selected clinical situations. J Reconstr Microsurg 2010;26(5):291–294. doi:10.1055/s-0030-1248239

Pelzer M, Sauerbier M, Germann G, Tränkle M. Free "kite" flap: a new flap for reconstruction of small hand defects. J Reconstr Microsurg 2004;20(5):367–372

Quaba AA, Davison PM. The distally-based dorsal hand flap. Br J Plast Surg 1990;43(1):28–29

Rousell AR, Davies DM, Eisenberg N, Taylor GI. The anatomy of the subscapular- thoracodorsal arterial system: study of 100 cadaver dissections. Br J Plast Surg 1987;37(4):574–576

Sauerbier M, Germann G, Giessler GA, Sedigh Salakdeh M, Döll M. The free lateral arm flap—a reliable option for reconstruction of the forearm and hand. Hand 2012;7(2):163–171. doi:10.1007/s11552-012-9395-3

Taylor GI. The current status of free vascularized bone grafts. Clin Plast Surg 1983;10(1):185–209

Tränkle M, Sauerbier M, Heitmann C, Germann G. Restoration of thumb sensibility with the innervated first dorsal metacarpal artery island flap. J Hand Surg Am 2003;28(5):758–766.

Tranquilli-Leali LE. Ricostruzione dell'apice delle falangi ungueali mediante autoplastica volare peduncolata per scorrimento. Infort Trauma Lavoro 1935;1:186–193

Venkataswami R, Subramanian N. Oblique triangular flap: a new method of repair for oblique amputation of the fingertip and thumb. Plast Reconstr Surg 1980;66(2):296–300

Walsh M, Levin LS. Gracilis free flap. In: Rayan GM, Chung KC. Flap Reconstruction of the Upper Extremity: A Master Skills Publication. 2009, American Society for Surgery of the Hand

Wang HT, Erdmann D, Fletcher JW, Levin LS. Anterolateral thigh flap technique in hand and upper extremity reconstruction. Tech Hand Up Extrem Surg 2004;8(4):257–261

Zancolli EA, Angrigiani C. Posterior interosseous island forearm flap. J Hand Surg Br 1988;13(2):130–135

Part VI: Rehabilitation Protocols

AO Foundation. Locking Plate Principles. In AO Surgery Reference. www.aosurgery.org

Carlsen BT, Shin AY. Wrist instability. Scand J Surg 2008; 97(4):324–332. doi:10.1177/145749690809700409

Giessler GA, Przybilski M, Germann G, Sauerbier M, Megerle K. Early free active versus dynamic extension splinting after extensor indicis proprius tendon transfer to restore thumb extension: a prospective randomized study. J Hand Surg Am 2008;33(6):864–868. doi:10.1016/j.jhsa.2008.01.028

Levin LS. Early versus delayed closure of open fractures. Injury 2007;38(8):896–899

Mackinnon SE. New directions in peripheral nerve surgery. Ann Plast Surg 1989;22(3):257–273

Megerle K, Przybilski M, Sauerbier M, Germann G, Giessler GA. [Early active motion after transfer of the extensor indicis tendon—a randomised prospective trial]. Handchir Mikrochir Plast Chir 2008;40(3):156–159. doi:10.1055/s-2007-965140

Salter RB, Harris WR. Injuries involving the epiphyseal plate. J Bone Joint Surg Am April 1963 45-A(3): 587

Skirven TM, Osterman AL, Fedorczyk J, Amadio PC. Rehabilitation of the Hand and Upper Extremity, 6th ed. St Louis, MO: Mosby–Year Book; 2001

Smith PJ. Lister's The Hand: Diagnosis and Indications. 4th ed. Edinburgh, UK: Churchill Livingstone; 2001

Sunderland S. A classification of peripheral nerve injuries producing loss of function. Brain 1951;74(4):491–516

Viegas SF, Patterson RM, Peterson PD, et al. Ulnar-sided perilunate instability: an anatomic and biomechanic study. J Hand Surg Am 1990;15(2):268–278

Part VII: Classification and Zones of Injury

Brüner S, Wittemann M, Jester A, Blumenthal K, Germann G. Dynamic splinting after extensor tendon repair in zones V to VII. J Hand Surg Br 2003;28(3):224–227

Germann G, Wagner H, Blome-Eberwein S, Karle B, Wittemann M. Early dynamic motion versus postoperative immobilization in patients with extensor indicis proprius transfer to restore thumb extension: a prospective randomized study. J Hand Surg Am 2001;26(6):1111–1115

Küntscher M, Blazek J, Brüner S, Wittemann M, Germann G. [Functional bracing after operative treatment of metacarpal fractures]. Unfallchirurg 2002;105(12):1109–1114

Index

K

L

M

N

O

P